How to Pay for Your Degree in Nursing 2011-2013

Seventh Edition

Gail Ann Schlachter
R. David Weber

A List of: Scholarships, Fellowships, Grants, Awards, Forgivable Loans, and Other Sources of "Free Money" Set Aside to Support Study, Training, Research, and Creative Activities for Nursing Students. Plus, a Set of Five Indexes: Sponsor, Residency, Tenability, Specialty, and Deadline.

Formerly: *RSP Funding for Nursing Students and Nurses*

Reference Service Press
El Dorado Hills, California

©2011 Gail Ann Schlachter

ISBN 10: 1588412075
ISBN 13: 9781588412072

10 9 8 7 6 5 4 3 2 1

The first five editions of this directory were issued under the title *RSP Funding for Nursing Students and Nurses*.

Reference Service Press (RSP) began in 1977 with a single financial aid publication *(The Directory of Financial Aids for Women)* and now specializes in the development of financial aid resources in multiple formats, including books, large print books, disks, CD-ROMs, print-on-demand reports, eBooks, and online sources. Long recognized as a leader in the field, RSP has been called by the *Simba Report on Directory Publishing* "a true success in the world of independent directory publishers." And, both Kaplan Educational Centers and Military.com have hailed RSP as "the leading authority on scholarships."

Reference Service Press
El Dorado Hills Business Park
5000 Windplay Drive, Suite 4
El Dorado Hills, CA 95762
   (916) 939-9620
   Fax: (916) 939-9626
   E-mail: info@rspfunding.com
Visit our web site: www.rspfunding.com

Manufactured in the United States of America

Price: $30.00, plus $7 shipping.

ACADEMIC INSTITUTIONS, LIBRARIES, ORGANIZATIONS AND OTHER QUANTITY BUYERS:
Discounts on this book are available for bulk purchases. Write or call for information on our discount programs.

Contents

Introduction

WHY THIS DIRECTORY IS NEEDED

Nearly 500,000 new nurses will be needed by the year 2020, according to the latest projections from the Bureau of Labor Statistics. Hundreds of financial aid programs, representing billions of dollars, are available to help students prepare for these jobs. But, how can beginning or continuing nursing students find out about the full range of these funding opportunities?

Traditional financial aid directories don't offer much assistance. For example, the landmark *Scholarships, Fellowships, and Loans* (published by Gale Cengage) and the eclectic *Scholarship Book* (published by Prentice-Hall) just begin to scratch the surface. And the other subject-specific listings, like *Free Money for Nursing Education* (published by Medical Resource) and *Scholarships and Loans for Nursing Education* (published by the National League for Nursing), or the various Internet sites tend to be outdated or selective and lacking in detail. As a result, many nursing students (along with the counselors and librarians trying to serve them) have been unaware of the more than 800 major scholarships, fellowships, awards, grants, forgivable loans, and other sources of "free money" available specifically to them.

Now, with this new edition of *How to Pay for Your Degree in Nursing* (previously published as *RSP Funding for Nursing Students and Nurses),* that has all changed. Here, in one place, you can find out about the wide array of funding programs set aside specifically to support study, research, creative projects, and other degree-related activities by nursing students at any level, from associate degree and diploma through the doctorate. All areas of nursing are covered, ranging from general practice to administration, anesthesiology, critical care, emergency, holistic health, long-term care, midwifery, nephrology, occupational health, oncology, operating room, orthopedic, pediatric, psychiatric, rehabilitative, school health, and many others.

There's no other listing, in print or online, that's as current or comprehensive as this. That's why *American Reference Books Annual* called it "an excellent source of funding information" and "a must-have," UNC's *Research Support Newsletter* described it as a "very useful resource," *Nursing Education Perspectives* named it as an "Essential Nursing Reference," and the Foundation Center's Learning Lab selected it as one of the "most important resources" available.

WHAT'S INCLUDED?

How to Pay for Your Degree in Nursing, 2011-2013 is unique. Not only does it provides the most comprehensive coverage of nursing-related funding opportunities (more than 800 entries), but it also offers the most informative program descriptions (on the average, twice the detail found in any other source).

In addition, only funding set aside for nursing students is included. If a program doesn't support study, training, research, or creative activities specifically for this group, it's not covered here.

Third, only the biggest and best portable funding programs are covered in this book. To be listed here, a program has to offer nursing students at least $500 per year. But, most go way beyond that! And, keep in mind that this is "free" money; not one dollar awarded to you will have to be repaid! Plus, you can take the money awarded by these scholarships to any number of schools. Unlike other financial aid directories, which often list large numbers of scholarships worth only a few hundred dollars or available only to students enrolled at one specific school, all of the entries in this book are substantial and "portable" (although some portability may be restricted by other program parameters).

Fourth, many of the programs listed here have never been covered in the other financial aid directories. So, even if you have checked elsewhere, you will want to look at *How to Pay for Your Degree in Nursing* for additional leads.

Fifth, unlike other funding directories, which tend to follow a straight alphabetical arrangement, this one divides entries by educational level (undergraduates and graduate students), to help you target your search for appropriate programs. The same convenience is offered in the indexes, where sponsoring organization, geographic focus, subject, and deadline date entries specifically identify opportunities for either undergraduate or graduate students.

Further, we have tried to anticipate all the ways you might wish to search for funding; we organized the volume so you can identify programs not only by recipient group, but by program title, nursing specialty, sponsor, residency requirements, where the money can be spent, and even deadline date. Plus, we've included all the information you'll need to decide if a program is right for you: purpose, eligibility requirements, financial data, duration, special features, limitations, number awarded, and application date. You even get fax numbers, toll-free numbers, e-mail addresses, and web sites (when available) along with complete contact information, to make your requests for applications proceed smoothly.

Finally, we've included all types of "free money" in our listing:

- *Scholarships.* Programs that support studies and related activities at the undergraduate level in the United States. This is "free" money. No repayment is necessary, provided all program requirements are met.

- *Fellowships.* Programs that support studies and related activities at the graduate level in the United States. This, too, is "free" money; usually no return of service or repayment is required.

- *Grants.* Programs that provide funding to support innovative efforts, travel, projects, creative activities, or research at any level (from associate degree through doctoral) in the United States. Usually no return of service or repayment is required.

- *Awards.* Competitions, prizes, and honoraria granted in recognition of personal accomplishments, research results, creative writing, or other achievements. Prizes received solely as the result of entering contests are excluded.

- *Forgivable loans.* Also known as scholarship/loans, fellowship/loans, and loans-for-service, this is funding that converts to "free money," as long as the recipient meets specified service requirements.

WHAT'S EXCLUDED?

The focus of *How to Pay for Your Degree in Nursing* is on portable programs aimed specifically at high school seniors, high school graduates, current college students, returning college students, and beginning or continuing graduate students interested in working on a degree in nursing at any school in the United States. While the directory is intended to be the most current and comprehensive source of information on available funding, there are some programs we've specifically excluded from the listing:

- *Programs not focused on the nursing field:* Only funding opportunities set aside specifically for nursing students are described here. If you are looking for money to support study, training, research, or creative activities in other areas, check out the list of Reference Service Press's award-winning directories on the inside of the front cover. You can also look for general or other financial aid resources at your library, in a bookstore, or online.

- *Programs that do not accept applications from U.S. citizens or residents:* If a program is open only to foreign nationals or excludes Americans from applying, it is not covered.

SAMPLE ENTRY

(1) **[371]**

(2) **TYLENOL SCHOLARSHIPS**

(3) McNeil Consumer and Specialty Pharmaceuticals
c/o International Scholarship and Tuition Services
200 Crutchfield Avenue
Nashville, TN 37210
(615) 320-3149   Fax: (615) 320-3151
E-mail: contactus@applyists.com
Web: www.tylenol.com

(4) **Summary** To provide financial assistance for college or graduate school to students intending to prepare for a career in nursing or another health-related field.

(5) **Eligibility** This program is open to students who have completed at least 1 year of an undergraduate or graduate course of study at an accredited 2-year or 4-year college, university, or vocational/technical school. Applicants must be working on a degree in health education, medicine, nursing, pharmacy, or public health. Along with their application, they must submit 1) a 500-word essay on the experiences or persons that have contributed to their plans to prepare for a career in a health-related field, and 2) a 100-word summary of their professional plans. Selection is based on the essays, academic record, community involvement, and college GPA.

(6) **Financial data** Stipends are $10,000 or $5,000.

(7) **Duration** 1 year.

(8) **Additional information** This program is sponsored by McNeil Consumer and Specialty Pharmaceuticals, maker of Tylenol products, and administered by International Scholarship and Tuition Services (formerly Scholarship Program Administrators, Inc.).

(9) **Number awarded** 40 each year: 10 at $10,000 and 30 at $5,000.

(10) **Deadline** May of each year.

DEFINITION

(1) **Entry number:** Consecutive number assigned to the references and used to index the entry.

(2) **Program title:** Title of scholarship, fellowship, forgivable loan, grant, or award.

(3) **Sponsoring organization:** Name, address, and telephone number, toll-free number, fax number, e-mail address, and web site location (when information was available) for organization sponsoring the program.

(4) **Summary:** Identifies the major program requirements; read the rest of the entry for additional detail.

(5) **Eligibility:** Qualifications required of applicants, plus information on application procedure and selection process.

(6) **Financial data:** Financial details of the program, including fixed sum, average amount, or range of funds offered, expenses for which funds may and may not be applied, and cash-related benefits supplied (e.g., room and board).

(7) **Duration:** Time period for which support is provided; renewal prospects.

(8) **Additional information:** Any benefits, features, restrictions, or limitations (generally nonmonetary) associated with the program.

(9) **Number of awards:** Total number of recipients each year or other specified period.

(10) **Deadline:** The month by which applications must be submitted.

- *Funding not aimed at incoming, currently-enrolled, or returning nursing students:* If a program is not specifically for undergraduate or graduate nursing students (e.g., a contest open to adults of any age, a research grant for nursing faculty), it is excluded.

- *School-based programs:* The directory identifies "portable" programs—ones that can be used at any number of schools. Financial aid programs administered by individual schools solely for the benefit of their own students or staff are not covered. Write directly to the schools you are considering to get information on their offerings.

- *Money for study or research outside the United States:* Since there are comprehensive and up-to-date directories that describe all available funding for study and research abroad (see *Financial Aid for Research and Creative Activities Abroad* and *Financial Aid for Study and Training Abroad,* both published by Reference Service Press), only programs that support study or research in the United States are covered here.

- *Very restrictive programs:* In general, programs are excluded if they are open only to a limited geographic area (less than a state) or offer very limited financial support (under $500 per year). For descriptions of these additional programs, contact Reference Service Press and ask about licensing their complete funding database for nursing.

- *Programs that did not respond to our research inquiries:* Programs are included in *How to Pay for Your Degree in Nursing* only if the sponsors posted current information on the Internet or responded to our research requests for up-to-date information (see below for details).

WHAT'S UPDATED?

The preparation of each new edition of *How to Pay for Your Degree in Nursing* involves extensive updating and revision. To make sure that the information included here is both reliable and current, the editors at Reference Service Press 1) review and update all relevant programs currently in our funding database and 2) search exhaustively for new program leads in a variety of sources, including directories, news reports, newsletters, annual reports, and sites on the Internet. We only include program descriptions that are written directly from information supplied by the sponsoring organization in print or on the Internet (no information is ever taken from secondary sources), When that information could not be found, we sent up to four collection letters (followed by up to three telephone inquiries, if necessary) to those sponsors. Despite our best efforts, however, some sponsoring organizations still failed to respond and, as a result, their programs are not included in this edition of the directory.

The 2011-2013 edition of *How to Pay for Your Degree in Nursing* completely revises and updates the previous (sixth) edition. Programs that have ceased operations have been dropped. Similarly, programs that have broadened their scope and no longer focus on the nursing field have also been removed from the listing, as have programs with residency requirements narrower than state-wide or awards under $500. Profiles of continuing programs have been rewritten to reflect current requirements; nearly 80 percent of the continuing programs reported substantive changes in their locations, deadlines, or benefits since 2008. In addition, more than 360 new entries have been added. The result is a listing of more than 800 scholarships, fellowships, forgivable loans, grants, awards, and other funding opportunities available specifically to nursing students.

HOW THE DIRECTORY IS ORGANIZED

The directory is divided into two sections: 1) a detailed list of funding opportunities open to undergraduate and graduate nursing students; and 2) a set of indexes to help you pinpoint appropriate funding programs.

Funding for Nursing Students. The first section of the directory describes 835 scholarships, fellowships, grants, awards, forgivable loans, and other "free money" available to nursing students at any level and in any specialty. The programs listed are sponsored by 500 federal and state government agencies, professional organizations, foundations, educational associations, social and religious groups, corporations, and military/veterans organizations.

To help you focus your search, the entries in this section are grouped into two main categories:

- **Undergraduates.** Described here are 400 scholarships, grants, awards, forgivable loans, and other funding opportunities that support undergraduate study, training, research, or creative activities in nursing. These programs are open to high school seniors, high school graduates, currently-enrolled college students, and students returning to college after an absence. Money is available to support these students in any type of postsecondary institution, ranging from technical schools and community colleges to major universities.

- **Graduate Students.** Described here are 435 fellowships, grants, awards, forgivable loans, and other funding opportunities that support post-baccalaureate study, training, research, and creative activities in the field of nursing. Funding is available for all graduate-level degrees: master's, doctoral, and professional.

Entries in each of the subsections appear alphabetically by program title. Each program entry has been prepared to give you a concise but clear picture of the available funding. Information (when available) is provided on organization address and telephone numbers (including fax and toll-free), e-mail address, web site, purpose, eligibility, money awarded, duration, special features, limitations, number of awards, and application deadline. The sample entry on page 7 illustrates and explains the program entry structure.

The information provided for each of the programs covered in this section was supplied by sponsoring organizations in response to requests we sent through the end of 2010. While *How to Pay for Your Degree in Nursing* is intended to cover as comprehensively as possible the available funding, some sponsoring organizations did not respond to our research inquiries and, consequently, are not included in this edition of the directory.

Indexes. To help you find the aid you need, we have constructed five indexes; these will let you access the listings by sponsoring organization, residency, tenability, nursing specialty, and deadline date. These indexes use a word-by-word alphabetical arrangement. Note: numbers in the index refer to entry numbers, not to page numbers in the book.

Sponsoring Organization Index. This index makes it easy to identify agencies that offer funding to nursing students for study, training, research, creative, or other activities. Sponsoring organizations are listed alphabetically, word by word. In addition, we've used a code to help you identify the focus of the funding programs sponsored by these organizations: U = Undergraduates; G = Graduate Students.

Residency Index. Some programs listed in this book are restricted to residents of a particular state or region. Others are open to students wherever they live. This index helps you identify programs available only to residents in your area as well as programs that have no residency restrictions.

Tenability Index. Some programs in this book can be used only in specific cities, counties, states, or regions. Others may be used anywhere in the United States (or even abroad). Use this index to find out what programs are available to support your activities in a particular geographic area.

Specialty Index. Refer to this index when you want to identify funding in a specific area of nursing. More than two dozen specialties are indexed here, in addition to general practice: administration, anesthesiology, critical care, emergency, holistic health, long-term care, lung and respiratory, midwifery, nephrology, neuroscience, occupational health, oncology, operating room, ophthalmic, orthopedic, otorhinolaryngology and head-neck, pediatric, psychiatric, radiological, rehabilitative, school health, and others.

Calendar Index. Since most financial aid programs have specific deadline dates, some may have closed by the time you begin to look for funding. You can use the Calendar Index to identify which programs are still open. This index is arranged by student group (undergraduates and graduate students) and divided by month during which the deadline falls. Filing dates can and quite often do vary from year to year; consequently, the dates in this index should be viewed as only approximations after mid-2013.

HOW TO USE THE DIRECTORY

Here are some tips to help you get the most out of the financial aid listings in *How to Pay for Your Degree in Nursing*.

To Locate Funding by Educational Level. If you want to get an overall picture of the kind of funding that is available to support either undergraduates or graduate nursing students, turn to the appropriate category in the first section of the guide and browse through the listings there. Originally, we also intended to subdivide these two chapters by purpose (study and training versus research and creative activities). Once the compilation was complete, however, it became clear that many of the programs provided funding for both functions. Thus, further subdivision (beyond educational level) would have been unnecessarily repetitious.

To Find Information on a Particular Financial Aid Program. If you know the name and degree focus of a particular financial aid program, you can go directly to the appropriate category in the first section of the directory, where you'll find program profiles listed alphabetically by title.

To Browse Quickly Through the Listings. Look at the listings in the educational section that relates to you (undergraduates or graduate students) and read the "Summary" field in each entry. In seconds, you'll know if this is an opportunity that might apply to you. If it is, read the rest of the information in the entry to make sure you meet all of the program requirements before writing or going online for an application form. Remember: don't apply if you don't qualify!

To Locate Financial Aid Programs Sponsored by a Particular Organization. The Sponsoring Organization Index makes it easy to determine which groups are providing funding to undergraduate and graduate nursing students (approximately 500 are listed here), as well as to identify specific financial aid programs offered by a particular sponsor. Each entry number in the index is coded to indicate educational level (undergraduates and graduate students), to help you target appropriate entries.

To Locate Financial Aid Based on Residency or Where You Want to Study/Conduct Your Research. Use the Residency Index to identify funding that has been set aside for nursing students in your area. If you are looking for funding to support activities in a particular city, county, state, or region, turn to the Tenability Index. Both of these indexes are subdivided by educational level (undergraduates and graduate students), to help you identify the funding that's right for you. When using these indexes, always check the listings under the term "United States," since the programs indexed there have no geographic restrictions and can be used in any area.

To Locate Financial Aid for Study or Research in a Specific Nursing Specialty. Turn to the Specialty Index first if you are interested in identifying available funding in a specific area of nursing (more than two dozen different specialties are indexed there). As part of your search, be sure to check the listings in the index under the "General" heading; that term identifies programs supporting activities in any area of nursing (although they may be restricted in other ways). Each index entry indicates whether the funding is available to undergraduates or to graduate students.

To Locate Financial Aid by Deadline Date. If you are working with specific time constraints and want to weed out financial aid programs whose filing dates you won't be able to meet, turn first to the Calendar Index and check the program references listed under the appropriate group (undergraduates and graduate students) and month. Note: not all sponsoring organizations supplied deadline information; those programs are listed under the "Deadline not specified" entry in the index. To identify every relevant financial aid program, regardless of filing dates, read through all the entries in the chapter that matches your degree level (undergraduates or graduate students)

PLANS TO UPDATE THE DIRECTORY

This volume, covering 2011-2013, is the seventh edition of *How to Pay for Your Degree in Nursing* (which, for the first five editions, was issued under the title *RSP Funding for Nursing Students and*

Nurses). The next biennial edition of *How to Pay for Your Degree in Nursing* will cover the years 2013-2015 and will be released in mid-2013.

OTHER RELATED PUBLICATIONS

In addition to *How to Pay for Your Degree in Nursing,* Reference Service Press publishes several other titles that would be of interest to nursing students, including *The College Student's Guide to Merit and Other No-Need Funding, Money for Graduate Students in the Health Sciences,* and *Directory of Financial Aids for Women.* For more information on these and other related publications, you can 1) write to Reference Service Press' marketing department at 5000 Windplay Drive, Suite 4, El Dorado Hills, CA 95762; 2) call us at (916) 939-9620; 3) fax us at (916) 939-9626; 4) send us an e-mail message: info@rspfunding.com; or 5) visit our web site: www.rspfunding.com.

ACKNOWLEDGEMENTS

A debt of gratitude is owed all the organizations that contributed information to this edition of *How to Pay for Your Degree in Nursing.* Their generous cooperation has helped to make the seventh edition of this publication a current and comprehensive survey of funding available to undergraduate and graduate nursing students.

ABOUT THE AUTHORS

Dr. Gail Schlachter has worked for more than three decades as a library educator, a library manager, and an administrator of library-related publishing companies. Among the reference books to her credit are the biennially-issued *Directory of Financial Aids for Women* and two award-winning bibliographic guides: *Minorities and Women: A Guide to Reference Literature in the Social Sciences* (which was chosen as an "Outstanding Reference Book of the Year" by *Choice)* and *Reference Sources in Library and Information Services* (which won the first Knowledge Industry Publications "Award for Library Literature"). She is the former editor of *Reference and User Services Quarterly,* was the reference book review editor for *RQ* for 10 years, was recently elected to her fifth term on the American Library Association's governing council, and is a past president of the American Library Association's Reference and User Services Association. In recognition of her outstanding contributions to reference service, Dr. Schlachter has been named the University of Wisconsin School of Library and Information Studies "Alumna of the Year" and has been awarded both the Isadore Gilbert Mudge Citation and the Louis Shores/Oryx Press Award.

Dr. R. David Weber taught history and economics at Los Angeles Harbor College (in Wilmington, California) for many years and continues to teach history as an emeritus professor. During his years of full-time teaching there, and at East Los Angeles College, he directed the Honors Program and was frequently chosen the Teacher of the Year." He has written several critically-acclaimed reference works, including *Dissertations in Urban History* and the three-volume *Energy Information Guide.* With Gail Schlachter, he is the author of Reference Service Press' award-winning *College Student's Guide to Merit and Other No-Need Funding,* which was selected by *Choice* as one of the "Outstanding Academic Titles of the Year," *Financial Aid for the Disabled and Their Families* (named one of the "Best Reference Books of the Year" by *Library Journal),* and a number of other financial aid publications, including *Financial Aid for African Americans,* which was named the "Editor's Choice" by *Reference Books Bulletin.*

Funding for Nursing Students

Undergraduates ●

Graduate Students ●

Undergraduates

Listed alphabetically by program title are 400 scholarships, grants, awards, and other funding opportunities that support undergraduate study, training, research, and creative activities in the nursing field in the United States. Check here if you are looking for funding for undergraduates in any area of nursing, including general practice, administration, anesthesiology, critical care, emergency, holistic health, long-term care, lung and respiratory, midwifery, nephrology, neuroscience, occupational health, oncology, operating room, ophthalmic, orthopedic, otorhinolaryngology and head-neck, pediatric, psychiatric, radiological, rehabilitative, school health, etc. All of this is free money. Not one dollar will ever need to be repaid (provided all program requirements are met)!

[1]
100 GREAT IOWA NURSES SCHOLARSHIPS

Iowa Nurses Association
Attn: Iowa Nurses Foundation
1501 42nd Street, Suite 471
West Des Moines, IA 50266
(515) 225-0495   Fax: (515) 225-2201
E-mail: info@iowanurses.org
Web: www.iowanurses.org/Default.aspx?tabid=2049

Summary To provide financial assistance to students who are working on an undergraduate or graduate nursing degree at a school in Iowa.

Eligibility This program is open to pre-licensure nursing students working on an A.D.N., practicing R.N.s working on a bachelor's degree, and graduate students working on a master's degree in nursing or doctoral degree in nursing or a related field. Pre-licensure and R.N. to B.S.N. students must have completed at least 50% of the requirements for a degree; master's and doctoral students must have completed at least 12 semester hours of graduate work. Applicants must have a career plan to work in Iowa. Along with their application, they must submit brief essays on their career goals, the areas of nursing practice where they believe they have something special to offer, their interest in that area, how their interest and goals will enhance the delivery of quality health care in Iowa, and how this assistance would impact their ability to meet their educational goals. Financial need is not considered in the selection process.

Financial Data The stipend is $500 for undergraduates or $1,500 for graduate students.

Duration 1 year.

Number awarded 4 each year: 2 to students working on an A.D.N. or R.N. to B.S.N. degree and 2 to graduate students.

Deadline February of each year.

[2]
AAOHN FOUNDATION ACADEMIC SCHOLARSHIP

American Association of Occupational Health Nurses, Inc.
Attn: AAOHN Foundation
7794 Grow Drive
Pensacola, FL 32514
(850) 474-6963   Toll Free: (800) 241-8014
Fax: (850) 484-8762   E-mail: aaohn@aaohn.org
Web: www.aaohn.org/scholarships/academic-study.html

Summary To provide financial assistance to registered nurses who are working on a bachelor's or graduate degree to prepare for a career in occupational and environmental health.

Eligibility This program is open to registered nurses who are enrolled in a baccalaureate or graduate degree program. Applicants must demonstrate an interest in, and commitment to, occupational and environmental health. Along with their application, they must submit a 500-word narrative on their professional goals as they relate to the academic activity and the field of occupational and environmental health. Selection is based on that essay (50%), impact of education on applicant's career (20%), and 2 letters of recommendation (30%).

Financial Data The stipend is $3,000.

Duration 1 year; may be renewed up to 2 additional years.

Number awarded 1 each year.

Deadline January of each year.

[3]
AFTERCOLLEGE/AACN NURSING SCHOLARSHIP FUND

American Association of Colleges of Nursing
One Dupont Circle, N.W., Suite 530
Washington, DC 20036
(202) 463-6930   Fax: (202) 785-8320
E-mail: scholarship@aacn.nche.edu
Web: www.aacn.nche.edu/Education/financialaid.htm

Summary To provide financial assistance to students at institutions that are members of the American Association of Colleges of Nursing (AACN).

Eligibility This program is open to students working on a baccalaureate, master's, or doctoral degree at an AACN member school. Special consideration is given to applicants who are 1) enrolled in a master's or doctoral program to prepare for a nursing faculty career; 2) completing an R.N. to baccalaureate (B.S.N.) or master's (M.S.N) program; or 3) enrolled in an accelerated baccalaureate or master's degree nursing program. Applicants must have a GPA of 3.25 or higher. Along with their application, they must submit an essay of 200 to 250 words on their goals and aspirations as related to their education, career, and future plans. They must also register and submit their resume to AfterCollege.com.

Financial Data The stipend is $2,500.

Duration 1 year.

Additional data This program, established in 2006, is sponsored by AfterCollege, an employment web site for nursing and allied health care students.

Number awarded 8 each year: 2 for each application deadline.

Deadline January, April, July, or October of each year.

[4]
AGNES NAUGHTON RN-BSN FUND SCHOLARSHIP

Florida Nurses Association
Attn: Florida Nurses Foundation
1235 East Concord Street
P.O. Box 536985
Orlando, FL 32853-6985
(407) 896-3261   Fax: (407) 896-9042
E-mail: foundation@floridanurse.org
Web: www.floridanurse.org/foundationGrants/index.asp

Summary To provide financial assistance to Florida residents who are interested in working on a bachelor's degree in nursing at a school in the state.

Eligibility Applicants must be registered nurses who have been Florida residents for at least 1 year and have completed at least 1 semester at an accredited nursing program in the state. They must be working on a baccalaureate degree and have a GPA of 2.5 or higher. Along with their application, they must submit 1-page essays on 1) why it is necessary for them to receive this scholarship; and 2) their goals and their assessment of their potential for making a contribution to nursing and society.

Financial Data A stipend is awarded (amount not specified).

Duration 1 semester or year.

Number awarded Varies each year.

Deadline May of each year.

[5]
AIR FORCE ROTC NURSING SCHOLARSHIPS

U.S. Air Force
Attn: Headquarters AFROTC/RRUC
551 East Maxwell Boulevard
Maxwell AFB, AL 36112-5917
(334) 953-2091   Toll Free: (866) 4-AFROTC
Fax: (334) 953-6167   E-mail: afrotc1@maxwell.af.mil
Web: afrotc.com/admissions/professional-programs/nursing

Summary To provide financial assistance to college students who are interested in a career as a nurse, are interested in joining Air Force ROTC, and are willing to serve as Air Force officers following completion of their bachelor's degree.

Eligibility This program is open to U.S. citizens who are freshmen or sophomores in college and interested in a career as a nurse. Applicants must have a cumulative GPA of 2.5 or higher at the end of their freshman year and meet all other academic and physical requirements for participation in AFROTC. They must be interested in working on a nursing degree from an accredited program. At the time of Air Force commissioning, they may be no more than 31 years of age. They must be able to pass the Air Force Officer Qualifying Test (AFOQT) and the Air Force ROTC Physical Fitness Test.

Financial Data Awards are type 1 AFROTC scholarships that provide for full payment of tuition and fees plus an annual book allowance of $900. All recipients are also awarded a tax-free subsistence allowance for 10 months of each year that is $350 per month during their sophomore year, $450 during their junior year, and $500 during their senior year.

Duration 2 or 3 years, provided the recipient maintains a GPA of 2.5 or higher.

Additional data Recipients must also complete 4 years of aerospace studies courses at 1 of the 144 colleges and universities that have an Air Force ROTC unit on campus or 1 of the 984 colleges that have cross-enrollment agreements with those institutions. They must also attend a 4-week summer training camp at an Air Force base, usually between their sophomore and junior years. Following completion of their bachelor's degree, scholarship recipients earn a commission as a second lieutenant in the Air Force and serve at least 4 years.

Deadline June of each year.

[6]
AIRMAN EDUCATION AND COMMISSIONING PROGRAM

U.S. Air Force
Attn: Headquarters AFROTC/RRUE
Enlisted Commissioning Section
551 East Maxwell Boulevard
Maxwell AFB, AL 36112-6106
(334) 953-2091   Toll Free: (866) 4-AFROTC
Fax: (334) 953-6167   E-mail: enlisted@afrotc.com
Web: www.afoats.af.mil/AFROTC/EnlistedComm/AECP.asp

Summary To allow selected enlisted Air Force personnel to earn a bachelor's degree in nursing and other approved majors by providing financial assistance for full-time college study while remaining on active duty.

Eligibility Eligible to participate in this program are enlisted members of the Air Force who have been accepted at a university or college (or approved crosstown institution) that is associated with AFROTC and that offers an approved major. The majors currently supported are computer science, all ABET-accredited engineering fields (not engineering technology), foreign area studies (limited to Middle East, Africa, Asia, and Russia/Eurasia), foreign languages (limited to Arabic, Azeri, Chinese, French, Georgian, Hebrew, Hindi, Indonesian, Japanese, Kazakh, Korean, Pashto, Persian Farsi, Portuguese, Russian, Swahili, Turkish, Urdu, and Vietnamese), mathematics, meteorology, nursing, and physics. Applicants must have completed at least 1 year of time-in-service and 1 year of time-on-station. They must have scores on the Air Force Officer Qualifying Test of at least 15 on the verbal and 10 on the quantitative and be able to pass the Air Force ROTC Physical Fitness Test. Normally they should have completed at least 30 semester hours of college study with a GPA of 2.75 or higher. They must be younger than 31 years of age (39 for nursing students) or otherwise able to be commissioned before they become 35 years of age (42 for nursing students).

Financial Data While participating in this program, cadets remain on active duty in the Air Force and receive their regular salary and benefits. They also receive payment of tuition and fees up to $15,000 per year and an annual textbook allowance of $600.

Duration 1 to 3 years, until completion of a bachelor's degree.

Additional data While attending college, participants in this program attend ROTC classes at their college or university. Upon completing their degree, they are commissioned to serve in the Air Force in their area of specialization with an active-duty service commitment of at least 4 years. Further information is available from base education service officers or an Air Force ROTC unit. This program does not provide for undergraduate flying training.

Number awarded Approximately 60 each year.

Deadline February of each year.

[7]
ALABAMA NURSES FOUNDATION SCHOLARSHIPS

Alabama State Nurses Association
Attn: Alabama Nurses Foundation
360 North Hull Street
Montgomery, AL 36104-3658
(334) 262-8321   Fax: (334) 262-8578
E-mail: alabamasna@mindspring.com
Web: www.alabamanurses.org

Summary To provide financial assistance to residents of Alabama enrolled in an undergraduate or graduate program in nursing at a school in any state.

Eligibility This program is open to residents of Alabama who are enrolled in an accredited associate, baccalaureate (either initial or R.N. to B.S.N.), master's, or doctoral program in nursing. Applicants may be attending school in any state, but they should be planning to remain employed in Alabama for at least 2 years after graduation. Along with their application, they must submit a 100-word statement on their career goals. Financial need is not considered in the selection process. Priority is given to graduate students interested in teaching at a school of nursing.

Financial Data The stipend is $1,000 for undergraduates or $2,500 for graduate students.

Duration 1 year.

Number awarded 1 or more each year.

Deadline June of each year.

[8]
ALBERT E. AND FLORENCE W. NEWTON NURSING SCHOLARSHIP

Rhode Island Foundation
Attn: Funds Administrator
One Union Station
Providence, RI 02903
(401) 427-4017   Fax: (401) 331-8085
E-mail: lmonahan@rifoundation.org
Web: www.rifoundation.org

Summary To provide financial assistance to students, especially residents of Rhode Island, working on a degree in nursing.

Eligibility This program is open to 1) students enrolled in a baccalaureate nursing program; 2) students in a diploma nursing program; 3) students in a 2-year associate degree nursing program; and 4) active practicing R.N.s working on a bachelor's degree in nursing. Applicants must be studying at a nursing school on a full- or part-time basis and able to demonstrate financial need. They may be enrolled at a school in any state, but preference is given to residents of Rhode Island. Along with their application, they must submit an essay, up to 300 words, on their career goals, particularly as they relate to practicing in or advancing the field of nursing in Rhode Island.

Financial Data The stipend ranges from $500 to $2,000.

Duration 1 year; may be renewed.

Number awarded Varies each year. Recently, 8 of these scholarships were awarded: 3 new awards and 5 renewals.
Deadline April of each year.

[9]
ALCAVIS INTERNATIONAL CAREER MOBILITY SCHOLARSHIP

American Nephrology Nurses' Association
Attn: ANNA National Office
200 East Holly Avenue
P.O. Box 56
Pitman, NJ 08071-0056
(856) 256-2320   Toll Free: (888) 600-2662
Fax: (856) 589-7463   E-mail: annascholarships@ajj.com
Web: www.annanurse.org

Summary To provide financial assistance to members of the American Nephrology Nurses' Association (ANNA) who are interested in working on a baccalaureate or advanced degree in nursing.
Eligibility Applicants must be current association members, have been members for at least 2 years, be actively involved in nephrology nursing-related health care services, and be accepted or enrolled in a baccalaureate or higher degree program in nursing. Along with their application, they must submit a 250-word essay on their career and educational goals that includes the expected time frame for completing their degree, the application of the award to meet expected expenses, and the impact of the completion of the degree program on their nephrology nursing practice.
Financial Data The stipend is $2,500.
Duration 1 year.
Additional data Funds for this scholarship, first awarded in 2006, are supplied by Alcavis International, Inc.
Number awarded 1 each year.
Deadline October of each year.

[10]
ALICE/JEANNE WAGNER ENDOWMENT SCHOLARSHIP

Epsilon Sigma Alpha International
Attn: ESA Foundation
P.O. Box 270517
Fort Collins, CO 80527
(970) 223-2824   Fax: (970) 223-4456
E-mail: esainfo@esaintl.com
Web: www.esaintl.com/esaf

Summary To provide financial assistance to students interested in working on a nursing degree in college.
Eligibility This program is open to nursing students who are 1) graduating high school seniors with a GPA of 3.0 or higher or with minimum scores of 22 on the ACT or 1030 on the combined critical reading and mathematics SAT; 2) enrolled in college with a GPA of 3.0 or higher; 3) enrolled at a technical school or returning to school after an absence for retraining of job skills or obtaining a degree; or 4) engaged in online study through an accredited college, university, or vocational school. Selection is based on character (10%), leadership (20%), service (10%), financial need (30%), and scholastic ability (30%).
Financial Data The stipend is $500.
Duration 1 year; may be renewed.
Additional data Epsilon Sigma Alpha (ESA) is a women's service organization, but scholarships are available to both men and women. This scholarship was first awarded in 1987. Completed applications must be submitted to the ESA state counselor, who then verifies the information before forwarding them to the scholarship director. A $5 processing fee is required.
Number awarded 3 each year.
Deadline January of each year.

[11]
ALICE WISE MEMORIAL FUND SCHOLARSHIP

PeriAnesthesia Nurses Association of California
P.O. Box 10841
Westminster, CA 92685-0841
Toll Free: (866) 321-3582   E-mail: treasurer@panac.org
Web: www.panac.org/scholarships.html

Summary To provide financial assistance to members of the American Society of PeriAnesthesia Nurses (ASPAN) and the PeriAnesthesia Nurses Association of California (PANAC) who are interested in working on a nursing degree.
Eligibility This program is open to students working on a B.S.N. or M.S.N. degree who have been ASPAN/PANAC members for at least the past 2 consecutive years. Applicants must have compiled at least 10 points from the PANAC activity list (for the complete list of acceptable activities, contact PANAC). Selection is based on merit as indicated by involvement with PANAC on the district and state level.
Financial Data The stipend is $500.
Duration 1 year; members may not receive more than 1 scholarship or other grant in any 2-year period.
Number awarded 1 or more each year.
Deadline December of each year.

[12]
ALLIED HEALTH TO BSN SCHOLARSHIP

Society of Otorhinolaryngology and Head-Neck Nurses, Inc.
Attn: Ear, Nose and Throat Nursing Foundation
202 Julia Street
New Smyrna Beach, FL 32168
(386) 428-1695   Fax: (386) 423-7566
E-mail: info@sohnnurse.com
Web: www.sohnnurse.com/awards.html

Summary To provide financial assistance to members of the Society of Otorhinolaryngology and Head-Neck Nurses (SOHN) who are allied health providers interested in working on a bachelor's degree in nursing.
Eligibility This program is open to allied health providers who are members of SOHN practicing in otorhinolaryngology. They must be interested in working on a B.S. degree in nursing. Applicants must submit a copy of their current registration in a B.S.N. program, a copy of their latest transcript (must have at least a 3.0 GPA), a statement of current financial assistance received and required, 3 letters of recommendation, and a narrative of 500 to 750 words describing their goals in nursing and the society.
Financial Data Stipends range from $1,000 to $1,500.
Duration 1 year.
Number awarded 1 or more each year.
Deadline June of each year.

[13]
AMEDD ENLISTED COMMISSIONING PROGRAM (AECP)

U.S. Army
Attn: Recruiting Command, RCHS-SVD-AECP
1307 Third Avenue
Fort Knox, KY 40121-2726
(502) 626-0381   Toll Free: (800) 223-3735, ext. 60381
Fax: (502) 626-0952   E-mail: aecp@usarec.army.mil
Web: www.usarec.army.mil/AECP

Summary To provide financial assistance to enlisted Army personnel who are interested in completing a bachelor's degree in nursing and becoming a commissioned officer.
Eligibility This program is open to enlisted Army personnel in the active component, Reserves, or National Guard who have at least 3 but no more than 10 years of active federal service. Applicants must be interested in enrolling full time at an accredited school of nursing to work on a bachelor's degree and becoming a

licensed registered nurse. They must be U.S. citizens, have a GPA of 2.5 or higher overall and in mathematics and science courses, be between 21 and 42 years of age, be eligible to become a commissioned officer in the active component following licensure, and agree to fulfill a 3-year additional service obligation.

Financial Data The stipend is $9,000 per year for tuition and $1,000 for books. Participants are not allowed to attend a school whose tuition exceeds $9,000. They continue to draw their regular pay and allowances while attending nursing school.

Duration Participants must be able to complete all degree requirements in 24 consecutive months or less.

Number awarded Up to 100 each year.

Deadline January of each year.

[14]
AMERICAN ASSEMBLY FOR MEN IN NURSING ESSAY CONTEST

American Assembly for Men in Nursing
Education Committee
6700 Oporto-Madrid Boulevard
P.O. Box 130220
Birmingham, AL 35213
(205) 956-0146   Fax: (205) 956-0149
E-mail: aamn@aamn.org
Web: www.aamn.org/awards.html

Summary To recognize and reward nursing students who prepare outstanding creative works dealing with men's health or men's place in the nursing profession.

Eligibility This program is open to undergraduate and graduate nursing students who submit creative work in fiction, fine arts, photography, essay, or research. Applicants may be either male or female, but the submission must relate to how nursing can become more involved in men's health initiatives in order to improve the health and well-being of men and their families. They must be members of either the American Assembly for Men in Nursing or the National Student Nurses' Association.

Financial Data The award is $500. Funds may be spent at the student's discretion.

Duration The award is presented annually.

Number awarded 1 each year.

Deadline April of each year.

[15]
AMERICAN ASSOCIATION OF CRITICAL-CARE NURSES PROFESSIONAL ADVANCEMENT SCHOLARSHIPS

American Association of Critical-Care Nurses
Attn: Scholarships
101 Columbia
Aliso Viejo, CA 92656-4109
(949) 362-2000, ext. 507
Toll Free: (800) 809-CARE, ext. 507
Fax: (949) 362-2020   E-mail: scholarships@aacn.org
Web: www.aacn.org

Summary To provide financial assistance to members of the American Association of Critical-Care Nurses (AACN) who are interested in participating in professional development activities.

Eligibility This program is open to members of the association who are interested in participating in a career enrichment program. Applicants must show a direct link between the content of the learning activity they are proposing and what they need to learn in order to overcome the gaps in their knowledge and skills. Eligible programs demonstrate a relationship to nursing practice and include those that focus on communication, collaboration, mediation, leadership and governance, organizational effectiveness, informatics, political processes, safety, and quality. Students working on an academic degree may apply for funding of specific courses, but not an entire degree program over more than a year's time. They should focus on the content of a specific course and show how that content fills an individual learning gap. All applicants must submit 300-word essays that 1) describe the gaps in their knowledge and skills; 2) describe their learning plan, their goals for addressing the gaps in their knowledge and skills, and how the learning activity they are proposing will help them achieve their professional goals; and 3) list professional activities related to the proposed learning activity. Selection is based on the applicant's ability to 1) assess and articulate gaps in their own knowledge and skills; 2) set professional learning goals on the basis of identified gaps; and 3) identify and evaluate learning opportunities that will move them toward achieving their goals.

Financial Data A maximum of $3,000 per person per year is available.

Duration 1 year; recipients may reapply.

Number awarded Varies each year.

Deadline Applications may be submitted at any time, but they must be received at least 4 to 6 months prior to the beginning of the proposed activity.

[16]
AMERICAN NURSES ASSOCIATION OF MAINE SCHOLARSHIPS

American Nurses Association of Maine
Attn: Scholarship Review Committee
647 US Route 1, Suite 14
BMP 280
York, ME 03909
(207) 877-4022   E-mail: anamaine.scholarships@gmail.com
Web: www.anamaine.org

Summary To provide financial assistance to nursing students at colleges and universities in Maine.

Eligibility This program is open to undergraduates currently enrolled in a nursing program in Maine. Applicants must be a member of their school's student nurse association and have completed at least 1 semester of a clinical course. Along with their application, they must submit a 1-page statement explaining how the scholarship would help with the completion of their nursing degree.

Financial Data The stipend ranges from $250 to $500.

Duration 1 year.

Number awarded 1 or more each year.

Deadline March of each year.

[17]
ANAC STUDENT DIVERSITY MENTORSHIP SCHOLARSHIP

Association of Nurses in AIDS Care
Attn: Awards Committee
3538 Ridgewood Road
Akron, OH 44333-3122
(330) 670-0101   Toll Free: (800) 260-6780
Fax: (330) 670-0109   E-mail: anac@anacnet.org
Web: www.anacnet.org/i4a/pages/index.cfm?pageid=3321

Summary To provide financial assistance to student nurses from minority groups who are interested in HIV/AIDS nursing and in attending the national conference of the Association of Nurses in AIDS Care (ANAC).

Eligibility This program is open to student nurses from a diverse racial or ethnic background, defined to include African Americans, Hispanics/Latinos, Asians/Pacific Islanders, and American Indians/Alaskan Natives. Candidates must have a genuine interest in HIV/AIDS nursing, be interested in attending the ANAC national conference, and desire to develop a mentorship relationship with a member of the ANAC Diversity Specialty Committee. They must be currently enrolled in an accredited nursing program at any level (e.g., L.P.N., A.D.N., diploma,

B.S.N., or graduate nursing). Nominees may be recommended by themselves, nursing faculty members, or ANAC members, but their nomination must be supported by an ANAC member. Along with their nomination form, they must submit a 500-word personal statement describing their interest or experience in HIV/AIDS care and why they want to attend the ANAC conference.

Financial Data   Recipients are awarded a $1,000 scholarship (paid directly to the school), up to $599 in reimbursement of travel expenses to attend the ANAC annual conference, free conference registration, an award plaque, a free ticket to the awards ceremony at the conference, and a 1-year ANAC membership.

Duration   1 year.

Additional data   The mentor will be assigned at the conference and will maintain contact during the period of study.

Number awarded   1 each year.

Deadline   June of each year.

[18]
ANNA/ABBOTT-PAMELA BALZER CAREER MOBILITY SCHOLARSHIP

American Nephrology Nurses' Association
Attn: ANNA National Office
200 East Holly Avenue
P.O. Box 56
Pitman, NJ 08071-0056
(856) 256-2320   Toll Free: (888) 600-2662
Fax: (856) 589-7463   E-mail: annascholarships@ajj.com
Web: www.annanurse.org

Summary   To provide financial assistance to members of the American Nephrology Nurses' Association (ANNA) who are interested in working on a baccalaureate or advanced degree in nursing.

Eligibility   Applicants must be current association members, have been members for at least 2 years, be actively involved in nephrology nursing-related health care services, and be accepted or enrolled in a baccalaureate or higher degree program in nursing. Along with their application, they must submit a 250-word essay on their career and educational goals that includes the expected time frame for completing their degree, the application of the award to meet expected expenses, and the impact of the completion of the degree program on their nephrology nursing practice.

Financial Data   The stipend is $2,500.

Duration   1 year.

Additional data   Funds for this program, established in 2002, are supplied by Abbott Renal Care Group.

Number awarded   1 each year.

Deadline   October of each year.

[19]
ANNA MAY ROLANDO SCHOLARSHIP AWARD

ExceptionalNurse.com
Attn: Scholarship Committee
13019 Coastal Circle
Palm Beach Gardens, FL 33410
(561) 627-9872   Fax: (561) 776-9254
TDD: (561) 776-9442   E-mail: ExceptionalNurse@aol.com
Web: www.ExceptionalNurse.com/scholarship.php

Summary   To provide financial assistance to nursing students who have a disability.

Eligibility   This program is open to students with a documented disability who have applied to, or have already been admitted to, a college or university nursing program on a full-time basis. Preference is given to graduate students who have demonstrated a commitment to working with people with disabilities. Applicants must submit an essay on how they plan to contribute to the nursing profession and how their disability will influence their practice as a nurse. Selection is based on the essay, transcripts of high

school and/or college courses completed, activities and honors received, 3 letters of recommendation, and financial need.

Financial Data   The stipend is $500.

Duration   1 year; nonrenewable.

Number awarded   1 each year.

Deadline   May of each year.

[20]
ANNIE LOU OVERTON SCHOLARSHIP

Georgia Nurses Foundation, Inc.
Attn: Scholarship Committee
3032 Briarcliff Road, N.E.
Atlanta, GA 30329-2655
(404) 325-5536   Toll Free: (800) 324-0462
Fax: (404) 325-0407   E-mail: gnf@georgianurses.org
Web: www.georgianurses.org/scholarship_appl.htm

Summary   To provide financial assistance to Georgia residents who are working on an R.N. to B.S.N. nursing degree.

Eligibility   This program is open to residents of Georgia who are currently enrolled (full or part time) in an NLN-accredited program in nursing. Applicants must be working on an R.N. to B.S.N. degree. They must have a GPA of 2.5 or higher and be able to document financial need. Priority is given to applicants who meet the following criteria: enrolled in a Georgia school, plan to practice professional nursing in Georgia following graduation, and belong to a professional organization (e.g., Georgia Association of Nursing Students, Georgia Nurses Association, Georgia Association for Nursing Education).

Financial Data   The stipend is at least $500. Funds may be sent directly to the recipient.

Duration   1 year.

Additional data   This program is sponsored by the Georgia Nurses Association.

Number awarded   1 each year.

Deadline   June of each year.

[21]
AORN DEGREE COMPLETION RESEARCH GRANT PROGRAM

Association of periOperative Registered Nurses
Attn: Research and Nursing Resources Department
2170 South Parker Road, Suite 400
Denver, CO 80231-5711
(303) 755-6300, ext. 244 Toll Free: (800) 755-2676, ext. 244
Fax: (303) 750-2927   E-mail: rchard@aorn.org
Web: www.aorn.org

Summary   To provide funding for research to student members of the Association of periOperative Registered Nurses (AORN).

Eligibility   This program is open to student members of the association who are enrolled in an accredited baccalaureate, master's, or doctoral program. Applicants must be interested in conducting a research project that is related to perioperative nursing practice and consistent with AORN's research priorities, which emphasize patient outcomes and workforce issues. Except for generic baccalaureate nursing students, applicants must be a registered nurse with a current and valid license.

Financial Data   The maximum grant is $15,000.

Duration   These are 1-time grants.

Number awarded   Varies each year.

Deadline   March or October of each year.

[22]
AORN FOUNDATION BACCALAUREATE DEGREE IN NURSING SCHOLARSHIP

Association of periOperative Registered Nurses
Attn: AORN Foundation
2170 South Parker Road, Suite 400
Denver, CO 80231-5711
(303) 755-6300, ext. 230   Toll Free: (800) 755-2676, ext. 230
Fax: (303) 755-4219   E-mail: foundation@aorn.org
Web: www.aorn.org/AORNFoundation/Scholarships

Summary   To provide financial assistance to students who wish to work on a baccalaureate degree in a field of interest to the Association of periOperative Registered Nurses (AORN).

Eligibility   This program is open to registered nurses who are committed to perioperative nursing and are currently enrolled in an accredited baccalaureate degree program. Along with their application, they must submit 4 essays: 1) their role as a perioperative nurse and why they chose that field; 2) their professional goals and what AORN does to support those goals; 3) how they will apply their degree to perioperative nursing; and 4) how they believe AORN promotes the specialty of perioperative nursing. Financial need is not considered in the selection process. Membership in AORN is not required, but applicants are encouraged to become members.

Financial Data   A stipend is awarded (amount not specified); funds are intended to be used for payment of tuition, related fees, and books.

Duration   1 year.

Additional data   This program was established in 1991.

Number awarded   Varies each year; recently, 15 of these scholarships were awarded.

Deadline   June of each year.

[23]
AORN FOUNDATION NURSING STUDENT SCHOLARSHIPS

Association of periOperative Registered Nurses
Attn: AORN Foundation
2170 South Parker Road, Suite 400
Denver, CO 80231-5711
(303) 755-6300, ext. 230   Toll Free: (800) 755-2676, ext. 230
Fax: (303) 755-4219   E-mail: foundation@aorn.org
Web: www.aorn.org/AORNFoundation/Scholarships

Summary   To provide financial assistance to students interested in preparing for a career in nursing, especially perioperative nursing.

Eligibility   This program is open to students currently enrolled in an accredited nursing program leading to initial licensure as an R.N. The program may be for a diploma or an A.D.N., B.S.N., master's entry, or accelerated second B.S.N. degree. Applicants must submit 3 essays: 1) why they have chosen to prepare for a career in nursing and their career goals; 2) their academic and/or clinical experience or exposure to the operating room/surgical field; and 3) how they believe the Association of periOperative Registered Nurses (AORN) promotes the specialty of perioperative nursing. Financial need is not considered in the selection process. Membership in AORN is not required, but applicants are encouraged to become members.

Financial Data   A stipend is awarded (amount not specified); funds are intended to be used for payment of tuition, related fees, and books.

Duration   1 year.

Additional data   This program was established in 2001.

Number awarded   Varies each year; recently, 12 of these scholarships were awarded.

Deadline   June of each year.

[24]
ARIZONA LEGION AUXILIARY PAST PRESIDENTS' PARLEY NURSES SCHOLARSHIP

American Legion Auxiliary
Department of Arizona
4701 North 19th Avenue, Suite 100
Phoenix, AZ 85015-3727
(602) 241-1080   Fax: (602) 604-9640
E-mail: amlegauxaz@mcleodusa.net
Web: www.azlegion.org/scholar2.txt

Summary   To provide financial assistance to Arizona residents interested in working on a degree in nursing at a school in the state.

Eligibility   This program is open to student nurses who are enrolled in at least the second year at an accredited institution in Arizona, have a GPA of 2.0 or higher, are U.S. citizens, and have been residents of Arizona for at least 1 year. Immediate family members of veterans receive first preference. Along with their application, they must submit a 500-word narrative on their family background; civic, social, school, and church activities; why they feel qualified for this scholarship, and why they are preparing for a nursing career.

Financial Data   The stipend is $600, payable to the school.

Deadline   May of each year.

[25]
ARIZONA LEGION AUXILIARY PAST PRESIDENTS' PARLEY SCHOLARSHIP ASSISTANCE IN HEALTH CARE OCCUPATIONS

American Legion Auxiliary
Department of Arizona
4701 North 19th Avenue, Suite 100
Phoenix, AZ 85015-3727
(602) 241-1080   Fax: (602) 604-9640
E-mail: amlegauxaz@mcleodusa.net
Web: www.azlegion.org/scholar1.txt

Summary   To provide financial assistance to Arizona residents interested in studying a health care field in college.

Eligibility   This program is open to students enrolled or accepted for enrollment in an accredited tax-supported institution in Arizona that offers a certificate or degree in health care occupations (e.g., nurses assistant, dental assistant, licensed practical nurse, lab technician, physical therapist, or inhalation therapist). They must be U.S. citizens and residents of Arizona for at least 1 year. Immediate family members of veterans receive first preference. Along with their application, they must submit a 500-word narrative on their family, school, and church activities and their reasons for choosing a career in health care occupations. Selection is based on character (25%), financial need (30%), scholarship (25%), and initiative (20%).

Financial Data   The stipend is $500, payable to the school.

Deadline   May of each year.

[26]
ARIZONA NURSES FOUNDATION ACADEMIC SCHOLARSHIP PROGRAM

Arizona Nurses Association
Attn: Arizona Nurses Foundation
1850 East Southern Avenue, Suite 1
Tempe, AZ 85282-5832
(480) 831-0404   Fax: (480) 839-4780
E-mail: info@aznurse.org
Web: www.aznurse.org/foundation/index.html

Summary   To provide financial assistance to undergraduate and graduate students from any state enrolled in or accepted to nursing programs in Arizona.

Eligibility   This program is open to undergraduate and graduate students from any state enrolled in, or accepted for enrollment in, an academic nursing education program in Arizona. Selection is based on potential for leadership in nursing, commitment to professional nursing in Arizona, and financial need. For graduate students, priority is given to applicants planning to teach nursing.

Financial Data Stipends are $500 per semester for associate degree students, $1,000 per semester for R.N. to B.S.N. students, $1,000 per semester for direct entry B.S.N. students, $1,000 per semester for master's degree students, and $2,500 per semester for doctoral students.

Duration 1 semester; recipients may reapply.

Number awarded 18 each semester: 4 for associate degree students, 4 for R.N. to B.S.N. students, 4 for direct entry B.S.N. students, 4 for master's degree students, and 2 for doctoral students.

Deadline February or October of each year.

[27]
ARKANSAS AMERICAN LEGION AUXILIARY NURSES SCHOLARSHIP

American Legion Auxiliary
Department of Arkansas
Attn: Department Secretary
1415 West Seventh Street
Little Rock, AR 72201-2903
(501) 374-5836   Fax: (501) 372-0855
E-mail: arkaux@juno.com
Web: arklegion.homestead.com/ArkAux.html

Summary To provide financial assistance to veterans' children in Arkansas who wish to study nursing at a school in any state.

Eligibility This program is open to the children of veterans in Arkansas who served during eligibility dates for membership in the American Legion. Both the student and the parent must be residents of Arkansas. Their total family income must be less than $55,000. The student must be a high school senior planning to attend a school of nursing in any state. Along with their application, they must submit an essay of 800 to 1,000 words on what their country's flag means to them. Selection is based on character (15%), Americanism (15%), leadership (15%), financial need (15%), and scholarship (40%).

Financial Data The stipend is $500; funds are paid in 2 equal installments.

Duration 1 year.

Number awarded 1 each year.

Deadline February of each year.

[28]
ARMY FUNDED NURSE EDUCATION PROGRAM (FNEP)

U.S. Army
Attn: Recruiting Command, RCHS-SVD-FNEP
1307 Third Avenue
Fort Knox, KY 40121-2726
(502) 626-0364   Toll Free: (800) 223-3735, ext. 60364
Fax: (502) 626-0952   E-mail: fnep@usarec.army.mil
Web: www.usarec.army.mil/AECP

Summary To provide financial assistance to Army officers who are interested in completing a bachelor's or master's degree in nursing and continuing to serve in the Army Nurse Corps.

Eligibility This program is open to active component Army officers who are currently in grade O-3 and have completed at least 38 months but no more than 7 years of active federal service. Applicants must be interested in enrolling full time at an accredited school of nursing to work on a bachelor's or entry-level master's degree. They must agree to serve an additional 2 years for each year of support received for a bachelor's degree or an additional 3 years for the first year of support for a master's degree plus 1 year for each additional 6 months of support. U.S. citizenship is required.

Financial Data The stipend is $12,000 per year, including $11,000 for tuition and fees and $1,000 for books. Participants are not allowed to pay tuition in excess of $11,000 per year from other sources. If the university's tuition is more than $11,000, it must either waive the additional amount or direct the participant to another school. Army officers continue to draw their regular pay and allowances while attending nursing school.

Duration Participants must be able to complete all degree requirements in 24 consecutive months or less. They must remain enrolled full time and maintain a GPA of 2.5 or higher.

Number awarded Up to 25 each year.

Deadline February of each year.

[29]
ARMY NURSE CORPS ASSOCIATION SCHOLARSHIPS

Army Nurse Corps Association
Attn: Education Committee
P.O. Box 39235
San Antonio, TX 78218-1235
(210) 650-3534   Fax: (210) 650-3494
E-mail: education@e-anca.org
Web: e-anca.org/ANCAEduc.htm

Summary To provide financial assistance to students who have a connection to the Army and are interested in working on an undergraduate or graduate degree in nursing.

Eligibility This program is open to students attending colleges or universities that have accredited programs offering associate, bachelor's, master's, or doctoral degrees in nursing. Applicants must be 1) nursing students who plan to enter the active Army, Army National Guard, or Army Reserve and are not participating in a program funded by the active Army, Army National Guard, or Army Reserve; 2) nursing students who have previously served in the active Army, Army National Guard, or Army Reserve; 3) Army Nurse Corps officers enrolled in an undergraduate or graduate nursing program not funded by the active Army, Army National Guard, or Army Reserve; 4) enlisted soldiers in the active Army, Army National Guard, or Army Reserve who are working on a baccalaureate degree in nursing not funded by the active Army, Army National Guard, or Army Reserve; or 5) nursing students whose parent(s) or spouse are serving or have served in the active Army, Army National Guard, or Army Reserve. Along with their application, they must submit a personal statement on their professional career objectives, reasons for applying for this scholarship, financial need, special considerations, personal and academic interests, and why they are preparing for a nursing career.

Financial Data The stipend is $3,000. Funds are sent directly to the recipient's school.

Duration 1 year.

Additional data Although the sponsoring organization is made up of current, retired, and honorably discharged officers of the Army Nurse Corps, it does not have an official affiliation with the Army. Therefore, students who receive these scholarships do not incur any military service obligation.

Number awarded 1 or more each year.

Deadline March of each year.

[30]
ARMY ROTC NURSE PROGRAM

U.S. Army
ROTC Cadet Command
Attn: ATCC-OP-I-S
55 Patch Road, Building 56
Fort Monroe, VA 23651-1052
(757) 788-4552   Toll Free: (800) USA-ROTC
Fax: (757) 788-4643   E-mail: atccps@usacc.army.mil
Web: www.goarmy.com/rotc/nurse_program.jsp

Summary   To provide financial assistance to high school seniors or graduates who are interested in enrolling in Army ROTC and majoring in nursing in college.

Eligibility   Applicants for the Army Reserve Officers' Training Corps (ROTC) Nurse program must 1) be U.S. citizens; 2) be at least 17 years of age by October of the year in which they are seeking a scholarship; 3) be no more than 27 years of age when they graduate from college after 4 years; 4) score at least 1050 on the combined mathematics and critical reading SAT or 21 on the ACT; 5) have a high school GPA of 3.0 or higher; and 6) meet medical and other regulatory requirements. This program is open to ROTC scholarship applicants who wish to enroll in a nursing program at 1 of approximately 100 designated partner colleges and universities and become Army nurses after graduation.

Financial Data   This scholarship provides financial assistance toward college tuition and educational fees up to an annual amount of $17,000. In addition, a flat rate of $1,000 is provided for the purchase of textbooks, classroom supplies, and equipment. Recipients are also awarded a stipend for up to 10 months of each year that is $300 per month during their freshman year, $350 per month during their sophomore year, $450 per month during their junior year, and $500 per month during their senior year.

Duration   4 years, until completion of a baccalaureate degree. A limited number of 2-year and 3-year scholarships are also available to students who are already attending an accredited B.S.N. program on a campus affiliated with ROTC.

Additional data   This program was established in 1996 to ensure that ROTC cadets seeking nursing careers would be admitted to the upper-level division of a baccalaureate program. The 56 partnership nursing schools affiliated with Army ROTC have agreed to guarantee upper-level admission to students who maintain an established GPA during their first 2 years. During the summer, recipients have the opportunity to participate in the Nurse Summer Training Program, a paid 3- to 4-week clinical elective at an Army hospital in the United States, Germany, or Korea. Following completion of their baccalaureate degree, participants become commissioned officers in the Army Nurse Corps. Scholarship winners must serve in the military for 8 years. That service obligation may be fulfilled 1) by serving on active duty for 4 years followed by service in the Army National Guard (ARNG), the United States Army Reserve (USAR), or the Inactive Ready Reserve (IRR) for the remainder of the 8 years; or 2) by serving 8 years in an ARNG or USAR troop program unit that includes a 3- to 6-month active-duty period for initial training.

Number awarded   A limited number each year.

Deadline   November of each year.

[31]
ARMY SPECIALIZED TRAINING ASSISTANCE PROGRAM (STRAP)

U.S. Army
Human Resources Command, Health Services Division
Attn: AHRC-OPH-AN
200 Stovall Street, Room 9N47
Alexandria, VA 22332-0417
(703) 325-2330   Toll Free: (800) USA-ARMY
Fax: (703) 325-2358
Web: www.goarmy.com/amedd/postgrad.jsp

Summary   To provide funding for service to members of the United States Army Reserve (USAR) or Army National Guard (ARNG) who are engaged in additional training in designated health care fields (including nursing) that are considered critical for war time medical needs.

Eligibility   This program is open to members of the USAR or ARNG who are currently 1) medical residents (in orthopedic surgery, family practice, emergency medicine, general surgery, obstetrics/gynecology, or internal medicine); 2) dental residents (in oral surgery, prosthodontics, or comprehensive dentistry); 3) nursing students working on a master's degree in critical care or nurse anesthesia; or 4) associate degree or diploma nurses working on a bachelor's degree. Applicants must agree to a service obligation of 1 year for every 6 months of support received.

Financial Data   This program pays a stipend of $1,992 per month.

Additional data   During their obligated period of service, participants must attend Extended Combat Training (ECT) at least 12 days each year and complete the Officer Basic Leadership Course (OBLC) within the first year.

Number awarded   Varies each year.

Deadline   Applications may be submitted at any time.

[32]
ARNA/DOROTHY BUDNEK MEMORIAL SCHOLARSHIP

Association for Radiologic & Imaging Nursing
7794 Grow Drive
Pensacola, FL 32514
(850) 474-7292   Toll Free: (866) 486-2762
Fax: (850) 484-8762   E-mail: arin@dancyamc.com
Web: www.arinursing.org/awards-amp-scholarships.html

Summary   To provide financial assistance to members of the Association for Radiologic & Imaging Nursing (ARIN) who are interested in working on a higher degree in a health-related field.

Eligibility   This program is open to association members (must have been members for at least 3 years) who have a current nursing license and have returned to school to advance their nursing education. Applicants must have a GPA of 2.5 or higher at their current educational institution. Along with their application, they must submit a statement of purpose on how these funds would be utilized to further or enhance their educational goal, 2 letters of recommendation, a transcript, a statement of financial support throughout their postsecondary education, and a copy of their current nursing license.

Financial Data   The stipend is $600.

Duration   1 year.

Additional data   The ARIN was formerly named the American Radiological Nurses Association.

Number awarded   1 or more each year.

Deadline   October of each year.

[33]
ARTHUR L. DAVIS PUBLISHING AGENCY SCHOLARSHIP OF MASSACHUSETTS

Massachusetts Association of Registered Nurses
P.O. Box 285
Milton, MA 02186
(617) 990-2856   Toll Free: (866) MARN-ANA
E-mail: info@marnonline.org
Web: www.marnonline.org

Summary   To provide financial assistance to members of the Massachusetts Association of Registered Nurses (MARN) who are working on an additional degree and their children and significant others who are entering a nursing program.

Eligibility   This program is open to 1) registered nurses who have been members of MARN for at least 1 year and are enrolled in a baccalaureate, master's, or doctoral degree program in nursing, and 2) children and significant others of MARN members who have been accepted into a nursing education program. Applicants must be enrolled or planning to enroll at an accredited school of nursing in any state. They must be nominated by themselves or by a colleague. Along with their application, they must submit a 2-page essay describing their career goals and how this scholarship would assist them in achieving their goals. Financial need is not considered in the selection process.

Financial Data   The stipend is $1,000. Funds are paid jointly to the student and to the college or university and may be used for tuition and fees only.

Duration 1 year; nonrenewable.
Additional data This program is supported by the Arthur L. Davis Publishing Agency.
Number awarded 1 each year.
Deadline March of each year.

[34]
ARTHUR L. DAVIS PUBLISHING AGENCY SCHOLARSHIP OF NEW JERSEY

New Jersey State Nurses Association
Attn: Institute for Nursing
1479 Pennington Road
Trenton, NJ 08618-2661
(609) 883-5335   Toll Free: (888) UR-NJSNA
Fax: (609) 883-5343   E-mail: institute@njsna.org
Web: www.njsna.org/displaycommon.cfm?an=5
Summary To provide financial assistance to residents of New Jersey who are preparing for a career as a nurse at a school in the state.
Eligibility This program is open to residents of New Jersey who are enrolled in an associate, baccalaureate, or diploma nursing program in the state. Applicants who are R.N.s working on a higher degree in nursing are also eligible if they are members of the New Jersey State Nurses Association. Both high school graduates and adults are eligible. Selection is based on financial need, GPA, and leadership potential.
Financial Data The stipend is $1,000.
Duration 1 year.
Additional data This program is supported by the Arthur L. Davis Publishing Agency.
Number awarded 1 each year.
Deadline January of each year.

[35]
ARTHUR L. DAVIS SCHOLARSHIP AWARDS

Alabama State Nurses Association
Attn: Alabama Nurse Foundation
360 North Hull Street
Montgomery, AL 36104-3658
(334) 262-8321   Fax: (334) 262-8578
E-mail: alabamasna@mindspring.com
Web: www.alabamanurses.org
Summary To provide financial assistance to nursing students in Alabama who are working on an R.N. to B.S.N. degree or L.P.N. certificate.
Eligibility This program is open to students entering the final year of an R.N. to B.S.N. degree or L.P.N. certificate program who have a GPA of 3.0 or higher. The R.N. applicant must be a member of the Alabama Association of Nursing Students.
Financial Data The stipend is $500.
Duration 1 year.
Additional data This program is supported by the Arthur L. Davis Publishing Agency.
Number awarded 2 each year: 1 to a B.S.N. student and 1 to an L.P.N. student.
Deadline September of each year.

[36]
ARTHUR M. MILLER FUND SCHOLARSHIPS

Arthur M. Miller Fund
c/o Bank of America, N.A.
P.O. Box 1122
Wichita, KS 67201
(316) 261-4609
Summary To provide financial assistance to students working on a nursing or medical degree in Kansas.

Eligibility This program is open to students working on a nursing or medical degree in any area except osteopathy, podiatry, chiropractic, or optometry. They must be enrolled full time at a school in Kansas. Applicants working on a degree for a registered nurse must have been accepted into the professional phase of the program. Selection is based on financial need, general character, and career choice.
Financial Data The stipend is $2,000. Funds are to be used for tuition only and cannot be spent on textbooks, living expenses, or other fees.
Duration 1 year.
Number awarded Several each year.
Deadline March of each year.

[37]
ASPAN DEGREE SCHOLARSHIPS

American Society of PeriAnesthesia Nurses
Attn: Scholarship Program
90 Frontage Road
Cherry Hill, NJ 08034-1424
(856) 616-9600   Toll Free: (877) 737-9696, ext. 13
Fax: (856) 616-9601   E-mail: aspan@aspan.org
Web: www.aspan.org
Summary To provide financial assistance for additional education to members of the American Society of PeriAnesthesia Nurses (ASPAN).
Eligibility This program is open to registered nurses who have been members of the society for at least 2 years and have been employed for at least 2 years in any phase of the perianesthesia setting (preanesthesia, postanesthesia, ambulatory surgery, management, research, or education). Applicants must be interested in working on a bachelor of science in nursing, a master of science in nursing, or a doctorate in nursing. Along with their application, they must submit a statement of financial need; 2 letters of recommendation; and a narrative statement describing their level of activity or involvement in a phase of perianesthesia nursing, ASPAN and/or a component, or their community. Their statement should explain how they see their perianesthesia practice changing and benefiting as a result of their degree and how receiving this scholarship will help them obtain their professional goals and contribute to the perianesthesia community.
Financial Data The stipend is $1,000 per year; funds are sent directly to the recipient's university.
Duration 1 year; recipients may not reapply for additional funding until 3 years have elapsed.
Number awarded At least 2 each year.
Deadline June of each year.

[38]
ASSE AMERICA RESPONDS MEMORIAL SCHOLARSHIP

American Society of Safety Engineers
Attn: ASSE Foundation
1800 East Oakton Street
Des Plaines, IL 60018
(847) 768-3435   Fax: (847) 768-3434
E-mail: agabanski@asse.org
Web: www.asse.org/foundation/scholarships/scholarships.php
Summary To provide financial assistance to upper-division student members of the American Society of Safety Engineers (ASSE).
Eligibility This program is open to ASSE student members who are majoring in occupational safety, health, and environment or a closely-related field (e.g., industrial or environmental engineering, environmental science, industrial hygiene, occupational health nursing). Applicants must be full-time students who have completed at least 60 semester hours with a GPA of 3.0 or higher. Along with their application, they must submit 2 essays of 300

words or less: 1) why they are seeking a degree in occupational safety and health or a closely-related field, a brief description of their current activities, and how those relate to their career goals and objectives; and 2) why they should be awarded this scholarship (including career goals and financial need). U.S. citizenship is required.

Financial Data The stipend is $1,000 per year.

Duration 1 year; recipients may reapply.

Additional data This program was established to honor the ASSE members who died in the September 11, 2001 World Trade Center attacks.

Number awarded 1 each year.

Deadline November of each year.

[39]
ASSE UPS DIVERSITY SCHOLARSHIPS

American Society of Safety Engineers
Attn: ASSE Foundation
1800 East Oakton Street
Des Plaines, IL 60018
(847) 768-3435   Fax: (847) 768-3434
E-mail: agabanski@asse.org
Web: www.asse.org/foundation/scholarships/scholarships.php

Summary To provide financial assistance to minority upper-division student members of the American Society of Safety Engineers (ASSE).

Eligibility This program is open to ASSE student members who are U.S. citizens and members of minority ethnic or racial groups. Applicants must be majoring in occupational safety, health, and environment or a closely-related field (e.g., industrial or environmental engineering, environmental science, industrial hygiene, occupational health nursing). They must be full-time students who have completed at least 60 semester hours with a GPA of 3.0 or higher. Along with their application, they must submit 2 essays of 300 words or less: 1) why they are seeking a degree in occupational safety and health or a closely-related field, a brief description of their current activities, and how those relate to their career goals and objectives; and 2) why they should be awarded this scholarship (including career goals and financial need).

Financial Data The stipend is $5,250 per year.

Duration 1 year; recipients may reapply.

Additional data Funding for this program is provided by the UPS Foundation.

Number awarded 2 each year.

Deadline November of each year.

[40]
ASSOCIATION OF BRETHREN CARING MINISTRIES NURSING SCHOLARSHIPS

Church of the Brethren
Attn: Caring Ministries
1451 Dundee Avenue
Elgin, IL 60120-1694
(847) 742-5100, ext. 300   Toll Free: (800) 323-8039
Fax: (847) 742-6103
Web: www.brethren.org

Summary To provide financial assistance to members of the Church of the Brethren working on an undergraduate or graduate degree in nursing.

Eligibility This program is open to students who are members of the Church of the Brethren or employed in a Church of the Brethren agency. Applicants must be enrolled in a L.P.N., R.N., or graduate program in nursing. Along with their application, they must submit 1) a statement describing their reasons for wanting to enter nursing or continue their nursing education, including something of their aspirations for service in the profession; and 2) a description of how the scholarship will assist them in reaching their educational and career goals.

Financial Data The stipend is $2,000 for R.N. and graduate nurse candidates or $1,000 for L.P.N. candidates.

Duration 1 year. Recipients are eligible for only 1 scholarship per degree.

Number awarded Varies each year.

Deadline March of each year.

[41]
ASSOCIATION OF JEWISH REGISTERED NURSES SCHOLARSHIP

Association of Jewish Registered Nurses
c/o Nona Dorman, Scholarship Chairperson
31 Woodland Street, 6L
Hartford, CT 06105
(860) 724-2323

Summary To provide financial assistance to Jewish residents of Connecticut who are interested in studying at a school of nursing.

Eligibility This program is open to Jewish residents of Connecticut who are enrolled or planning to enroll in an accredited college program in nursing. Selection is based on academic record and community service.

Financial Data The stipend is $500.

Duration 1 year.

Number awarded 1 each year.

Deadline April of each year.

[42]
ASSOCIATION OF REHABILITATION NURSES BSN SCHOLARSHIP

Association of Rehabilitation Nurses
Attn: Scholarship Program
4700 West Lake Avenue
Glenview, IL 60025-1485
(847) 375-4710   Toll Free: (800) 229-7530
Fax: (888) 458-0456   E-mail: info@rehabnurse.org
Web: www.rehabnurse.org/awards/allscholar.html

Summary To provide financial assistance to members of the Association of Rehabilitation Nurses (ARN) who are working on a bachelor's degree in nursing.

Eligibility This program is open to ARN members who are currently practicing rehabilitation nursing and have at least 2 years of experience in the field. Applicants must be enrolled in a B.S.N. degree program and have successfully completed at least 1 course. Along with their application, they must submit a 1- to 3-page summary of their professional and educational goals that includes 1) involvement in ARN at the national and local levels; 2) continuing education participation in the past 3 to 5 years; 3) professional publications or presentations; 4) community involvement, particularly relating to advocating for individuals with disabilities; and 5) efforts they have made to improve their rehabilitation nursing practice and the delivery of care in their work setting. Financial need is not considered in the selection process.

Financial Data The stipend is $1,000.

Duration 1 year.

Number awarded 1 or more each year.

Deadline May of each year.

[43]
ASSOCIATION OF UNITED NURSES SCHOLARSHIPS

Scholarship Administrative Services, Inc.
Attn: AUN Program
457 Ives Terrace
Sunnyvale, CA 94087

Summary To provide financial assistance to undergraduate and graduate students working on a degree in nursing.

Eligibility This program is open to full-time students working on or planning to work on an undergraduate or graduate degree in nursing. Applicants must have a GPA of 3.0 or higher and be able to demonstrate a record of involvement in extracurricular and work activities related to nursing. Along with their application, they must submit a 1,000-word essay on their educational and career goals, why they believe nursing is essential to America, and why they have decided to prepare for a career in nursing. Financial need is not considered in the selection process.

Financial Data The stipend is $5,000 per year.

Duration 1 year; may be renewed 1 additional year if the recipient maintains full-time enrollment and a GPA of 3.0 or higher.

Additional data This program is sponsored by the Association of United Nurses (AUN) and administered by Scholarship Administrative Services, Inc. AUN was established in 2005 to encourage more American students to consider a career as a nurse. Requests for applications should be accompanied by a self-addressed stamped envelope, the student's e-mail address, and the source where they found the scholarship information.

Number awarded Up to 20 each year.

Deadline April of each year.

[44]
BANNER HEALTH SYSTEM NORTH COLORADO MEDICAL CENTER NIGHTINGALE SCHOLARSHIP

Colorado Nurses Foundation
7400 East Arapahoe Road, Suite 211
Centennial, CO 80112
(303) 694-4728   Fax: (303) 694-4869
E-mail: mail@cnfound.org
Web: www.cnfound.org/scholarships.html

Summary To provide financial assistance to undergraduate and graduate nursing students in Colorado who are willing to work at a designated facility following graduation.

Eligibility This program is open to Colorado residents who are enrolled in an approved nursing program in the state. Applicants may be 1) second-year students in an associate degree program; 2) junior or senior level B.S.N. undergraduate students; 3) R.N.s enrolled in a baccalaureate or higher degree program in a school of nursing; 4) R.N.s with a master's degree in nursing, currently practicing in Colorado and enrolled in a doctoral program; or 5) students in the second or third year of a Doctorate Nursing Practice (D.N.P.) program. They must be willing to work for a Banner Health Facility following graduation. Undergraduates must have a GPA of 3.25 or higher and graduate students must have a GPA of 3.5 or higher. Selection is based on professional philosophy and goals, dedication to the improvement of patient care in Colorado, demonstrated commitment to nursing, critical thinking skills, potential for leadership, involvement in community and professional organizations, recommendations, GPA, and financial need.

Financial Data The stipend is $1,000.

Duration 1 year.

Number awarded 1 each year.

Deadline October of each year.

[45]
BARBARA PALO FOSTER MEMORIAL SCHOLARSHIP

Ulman Cancer Fund for Young Adults
Attn: Scholarship Program Coordinator
10440 Little Patuxent Parkway, Suite 1G
Columbia, MD 21044
(410) 964-0202, ext. 106   Toll Free: (888) 393-FUND
E-mail: scholarship@ulmanfund.org
Web: www.ulmanfund.org/Services/tabid/53/Default.aspx

Summary To provide financial assistance to undergraduate and graduate nursing students who have a parent with cancer.

Eligibility This program is open to nursing students who have or have lost a parent to cancer. Applicants must be younger than 35 years of age and enrolled in, or planning to enroll in, an undergraduate or graduate program in nursing. They must demonstrate an interest in furthering patient education, focusing on persons from medically underserved communities and/or women's health issues. Along with their application, they must submit an essay of at least 1,000 words on the ways in which their experiences as a member of a marginalized group within the cancer community (i.e., young adults affected by cancer) have taught them lessons that inspire them to be of service to other socially, politically, and or economically marginalized people in the healthcare system. Selection is based on demonstrated dedication to community service, commitment to educational and professional goals, use of their cancer experience to impact the lives of other young adults affected by cancer, medical hardship, and financial need.

Financial Data The stipend is $2,500. Funds are paid directly to the educational institution.

Duration 1 year; nonrenewable.

Additional data Recipients must agree to complete 50 hours of community service.

Number awarded 1 each year.

Deadline April of each year.

[46]
BASIC MIDWIFERY STUDENT SCHOLARSHIPS

American College of Nurse-Midwives
Attn: ACNM Foundation, Inc.
8403 Colesville Road, Suite 1550
Silver Spring, MD 20910-6374
(240) 485-1850   Fax: (240) 485-1818
Web: www.midwife.org/foundation_award.cfm

Summary To provide financial assistance for midwifery education to student members of the American College of Nurse-Midwives (ACNM).

Eligibility This program is open to ACNM members who are currently enrolled in an accredited basic midwife education program and have successfully completed 1 academic or clinical semester/quarter or clinical module. Applicants must submit a 150-word essay on their midwifery career plans and a 100-word essay on their intended future participation in the local, regional, and/or national activities of the ACNM. Selection is based on leadership potential, financial need, academic history, and potential for future professional contribution to the organization.

Financial Data The stipend is $3,000.

Duration 1 year.

Additional data This program includes the following named scholarships: the A.C.N.M. Foundation Memorial Scholarship, the TUMS Calcium for Life Scholarship (presented by GlaxoSmithKline), the Edith B. Wonnell CNM Scholarship, and the Margaret Edmundson Scholarship.

Number awarded Varies each year; recently, 4 of these scholarships were awarded.

Deadline March of each year.

[47]
BCSP MICHAEL ORN SCHOLARSHIP

American Society of Safety Engineers
Attn: ASSE Foundation
1800 East Oakton Street
Des Plaines, IL 60018
(847) 768-3435   Fax: (847) 768-3434
E-mail: agabanski@asse.org
Web: www.asse.org/foundation/scholarships/scholarships.php

Summary To provide financial assistance to upper-division and graduate student members of the American Society of Safety Engineers (ASSE).

Eligibility   This program is open to ASSE student members who are working on an undergraduate or graduate degree in occupational safety, health, and environment or a closely-related field (e.g., industrial or environmental engineering, environmental science, industrial hygiene, occupational health nursing). Undergraduates must be full-time students who have completed at least 60 semester hours with a GPA of 3.0 or higher. Graduate students must also be enrolled full time, have completed at least 9 semester hours with a GPA of 3.5 or higher, and have earned a GPA of 3.0 or higher as an undergraduate. Along with their application, they must submit 2 essays of 300 words or less: 1) why they are seeking a degree in occupational safety and health or a closely-related field, a brief description of their current activities, and how those relate to their career goals and objectives; and 2) why they should be awarded this scholarship (including career goals and financial need). U.S. citizenship is not required.

Financial Data   The stipend is $1,000 per year.

Duration   1 year; recipients may reapply.

Additional data   This program is supported by the Board of Certified Safety Professionals (BCSP).

Number awarded   1 each year.

Deadline   November of each year.

[48]
BERNICE PICKENS PARSONS FUND SCHOLARSHIPS

Greater Kanawha Valley Foundation
Attn: Scholarship Coordinator
1600 Huntington Square
900 Lee Street, East
P.O. Box 3041
Charleston, WV 25331-3041
(304) 346-3620   Toll Free: (800) 467-5909
Fax: (304) 346-3640   E-mail: shoover@tgkvf.org
Web: www.tgkvf.org/scholar.htm

Summary   To provide financial assistance to residents of West Virginia who are interested in studying designated fields (including nursing) at a school in any state.

Eligibility   This program is open to residents of West Virginia who are working or planning to work full time on a degree or certificate in the fields of library science, nursing, or paraprofessional legal work at a college or university in any state. Applicants must have an ACT score of 20 or higher, be able to demonstrate good moral character and financial need, and have a GPA of 2.5 or higher. Preference is given to residents of Jackson County.

Financial Data   Stipends average $1,000 per year.

Duration   1 year; may be renewed.

Number awarded   Varies each year; recently, 4 of these scholarships were awarded.

Deadline   January of each year.

[49]
BERTHA P. SINGER SCHOLARSHIP

Oregon Student Assistance Commission
Attn: Grants and Scholarships Division
1500 Valley River Drive, Suite 100
Eugene, OR 97401-2146
(541) 687-7395   Toll Free: (800) 452-8807, ext. 7395
Fax: (541) 687-7414   TDD: (800) 735-2900
E-mail: awardinfo@osac.state.or.us
Web: www.osac.state.or.us/osac_programs.html

Summary   To provide financial assistance to residents of Oregon who are interested in studying nursing at a school in the state.

Eligibility   This program is open to residents of Oregon who are studying nursing at a college in the state and have a cumulative GPA of 3.0 or higher. Applicants must provide documentation of enrollment in the third year of a 4-year nursing degree program or the second year of a 2-year associate degree nursing program.

Financial Data   Stipend amounts vary; recently, they were at least $1,087.

Duration   1 year.

Number awarded   Varies each year; recently, 23 of these scholarships were awarded.

Deadline   February of each year.

[50]
BOARD OF CERTIFICATION FOR EMERGENCY NURSING UNDERGRADUATE SCHOLARSHIPS

Emergency Nurses Association
Attn: ENA Foundation
915 Lee Street
Des Plaines, IL 60016-6569
(847) 460-4100   Toll Free: (800) 900-9659, ext. 4100
Fax: (847) 460-4004   E-mail: foundation@ena.org
Web: www.ena.org

Summary   To provide financial assistance for baccalaureate study to nurses who are members of the Emergency Nurses Association (ENA) and are certified by the Board of Certification for Emergency Nursing (BCEN).

Eligibility   This program is open to nurses (R.N., L.P.N., L.V.N.) who have a current BCEN credential (CEN, CFRN, CTRN, or CPEN) and are working on a bachelor's degree. Applicants must have been members of ENA for at least 12 months and have a GPA of 3.0 or higher. They must submit a 1-page statement on their professional and educational goals and how this scholarship will help them attain those goals. Selection is based on content and clarity of the goal statement (45%), professional association involvement (35%), presentation of the application (10%), and letters of reference (10%).

Financial Data   The stipend is $2,000.

Duration   1 year; nonrenewable.

Additional data   Support for this program is provided by BCEN.

Number awarded   1 each year.

Deadline   May of each year.

[51]
BRAINTRACK NURSING SCHOLARSHIP

BrainTrack
c/o FutureMeld, LLC
221 Boston Post Road East
Marlborough, MA 01772
(978) 451-0471   E-mail: info@braintrack.com
Web: www.braintrack.com/about-braintrack-scholarships.htm

Summary   To provide financial assistance to students and nurses working on an undergraduate or graduate degree in nursing.

Eligibility   This program is open to students preparing for a career in nursing as an L.P.N. or R.N. and to nurses advancing their education by working on an associate, bachelor's, master's, or doctoral degree. Applicants must have completed at least 1 semester of study as a full- or part-time student in an on-campus and/or online program. They must be a U.S. citizen, have permanent resident status, or have an appropriate student visa. Along with their application, they must submit essays between 200 and 800 words each on 1) what led them to choose nursing as a career path; 2) what they have enjoyed most and least during their nursing degree program so far; 3) what they wish they had known about selecting and entering their nursing school that would be helpful to others going into nursing. Selection is based entirely on the creativity, focus, overall thoughtfulness, accuracy, and practical value of their essays.

Financial Data   Stipends are $1,000 or $500.

Duration   1 year.

Number awarded   4 each year: 2 at $1,000 and 2 at $500.

Deadline   October or February of each year.

[52]
BREAKTHROUGH TO NURSING SCHOLARSHIPS

National Student Nurses' Association
Attn: Foundation
45 Main Street, Suite 606
Brooklyn, NY 11201
(718) 210-0705   Fax: (718) 797-1186
E-mail: nsna@nsna.org
Web: www.nsna.org

Summary To provide financial assistance to minority undergraduate and graduate students who wish to prepare for careers in nursing.

Eligibility This program is open to students currently enrolled in state-approved schools of nursing or pre-nursing associate degree, baccalaureate, diploma, generic master's, generic doctoral, R.N. to B.S.N., R.N. to M.S.N., or L.P.N./L.V.N. to R.N. programs. Graduating high school seniors are not eligible. Support for graduate education is provided only for a first degree in nursing. Applicants must be members of a racial or ethnic minority underrepresented among registered nurses (American Indian or Alaska Native, Hispanic or Latino, Native Hawaiian or other Pacific Islander, Black or African American, or Asian). They must be committed to providing quality health care services to underserved populations. Along with their application, they must submit a 200-word description of their professional and educational goals and how this scholarship will help them achieve those goals. Selection is based on academic achievement, financial need, and involvement in student nursing organizations and community health activities. U.S. citizenship or permanent resident status is required.

Financial Data Stipends range from $1,000 to $2,500. A total of approximately $155,000 is awarded each year by the foundation for all its scholarship programs.

Duration 1 year.

Additional data Applications must be accompanied by a $10 processing fee.

Number awarded Varies each year. Recently, 5 of these scholarships were awarded: 2 sponsored by the American Association of Critical-Care Nurses and 3 sponsored by the Mayo Clinic.

Deadline January of each year.

[53]
BROTHER FRANCES SMITH SCHOLARSHIP

Connecticut Nurses' Association
Attn: Connecticut Nurses' Foundation
377 Research Parkway, Suite 2D
Meriden, CT 06450-7155
(203) 238-1207   Fax: (203) 238-3437
E-mail: info@ctnurses.org
Web: www.ctnurses.org/displaycommon.cfm?an=12

Summary To provide financial assistance to Connecticut residents interested in preparing for a career as a licensed practical nurse (L.P.N.) or working on a degree in nursing at a school in any state.

Eligibility This program is open to residents of Connecticut who are entering or enrolled at an accredited practical nurse education program in any state to earn a license as an L.P.N. or work on an associate, bachelor's, master's, or doctoral degree. Selection is based on employment experience; professional, community, and student activities; a statement of educational and practice goals; and financial need.

Financial Data The stipend depends on the qualifications of the recipient and the availability of funds.

Duration 1 year.

Number awarded 1 or more each year.

Deadline June of each year.

[54]
CALIFORNIA LEGION AUXILIARY PAST PRESIDENTS' PARLEY NURSING SCHOLARSHIPS

American Legion Auxiliary
Department of California
Veterans War Memorial Building
401 Van Ness Avenue, Room 113
San Francisco, CA 94102-4586
(415) 861-5092   Fax: (415) 861-8365
E-mail: calegionaux@calegionaux.org
Web: www.calegionaux.org/scholarships.htm

Summary To provide financial assistance to California residents who are current military personnel, veterans, or members of their families and interested in studying nursing at a school in the state.

Eligibility This program is open to California residents who are currently serving on active military duty, veterans who served during war time, or the spouse, widow(er), or child of such a veteran. Applicants must be entering or continuing students of nursing at an accredited institution of higher learning in California. Financial need is considered in the selection process.

Financial Data Stipends range up to $2,000.

Duration 1 year.

Number awarded Varies each year.

Deadline April of each year.

[55]
CAPPEX HEALTH CAREERS AND NURSING SCHOLARSHIP

Cappex.com, LLC
600 Laurel Avenue
Highland Park, IL 60035
Web: www.cappex.com

Summary To provide financial assistance for college to high school senior who complete a profile for Cappex.com and who plan to major in a health-related field in college.

Eligibility Applicants for this scholarship must first complete an online profile for Cappex.com which will enable colleges and universities to contact them for recruiting purposes. They must be U.S. citizens or permanent residents planning to attend an accredited college or university in the United States. This scholarship is designed for students who plan to major in nursing, medicine, dentistry, veterinary medicine, health and clinical science, health services administration, or health technology (medical, dental, laboratory).

Financial Data The stipend is $1,000.

Duration 1 year.

Number awarded 1 each year.

Deadline August of each year.

[56]
CAPTAIN SALLY TOMPKINS NURSING AND APPLIED HEALTH SCIENCES SCHOLARSHIP

United Daughters of the Confederacy-Virginia Division
c/o Janice Busic, Education Committee Chair
P.O. Box 356
Honaker, VA 24260
E-mail: 2vp@vaudc.org
Web: vaudc.org/gift.html

Summary To provide financial assistance for college to women who are Confederate descendants from Virginia and working on a degree in nursing.

Eligibility This program is open to women residents of Virginia interested in working on a degree in nursing. Applicants must be 1) lineal descendants of Confederates, or 2) collateral descendants and also members of the Children of the Confederacy or the United Daughters of the Confederacy. They must submit proof of the Confederate military record of at least 1 ancestor, with the company and regiment in which he served. They must also submit a personal letter pledging to make the best possible use of the scholarship; describing their health, social, family, religious, and fraternal connections within the community; and reflecting on what a Southern heritage means to them (using the term "War Between the States" in lieu of "Civil War"). They must have a GPA of 3.0 or higher and be able to demonstrate financial need.

Financial Data The amount of the stipend depends on the availability of funds. Payment is made directly to the college or university the recipient attends.

Duration 1 year; may be renewed up to 3 additional years if the recipient maintains a GPA of 3.0 or higher.

Number awarded This scholarship is offered whenever a prior recipient graduates or is no longer eligible.

Deadline April of the years in which a scholarship is available.

[57]
CAROLINE E. HOLT NURSING SCHOLARSHIP

National Society Daughters of the American Revolution
Attn: Committee Services Office, Scholarships
1776 D Street, N.W.
Washington, DC 20006-5303
(202) 628-1776
Web: www.dar.org/natsociety/edout_scholar.cfm

Summary To provide financial assistance to undergraduate nursing students.

Eligibility This program is open to undergraduate students currently enrolled in accredited schools of nursing who have completed at least 1 year. Applicants must be sponsored by a local chapter of the Daughters of the American Revolution (DAR). Selection is based on academic excellence, commitment to field of study, and financial need. U.S. citizenship is required.

Financial Data The stipend is $1,000.

Duration 1 year; nonrenewable.

Number awarded Varies each year.

Deadline February of each year.

[58]
CCHEST PATRICK J. CONROY SCHOLARSHIP

American Society of Safety Engineers
Attn: ASSE Foundation
1800 East Oakton Street
Des Plaines, IL 60018
(847) 768-3435   Fax: (847) 768-3434
E-mail: agabanski@asse.org
Web: www.asse.org/foundation/scholarships/scholarships.php

Summary To provide financial assistance to undergraduate student members of the American Society of Safety Engineers (ASSE).

Eligibility This program is open to ASSE student members who are working on an undergraduate degree in occupational safety, health, and environment or a closely-related field (e.g., industrial or environmental engineering, environmental science, industrial hygiene, occupational health nursing). Applicants must be full-time students who have completed at least 60 semester hours with a GPA of 3.0 or higher. Along with their application, they must submit 2 essays of 300 words or less: 1) why they are seeking a degree in occupational safety and health or a closely-related field, a brief description of their current activities, and how those relate to their career goals and objectives; and 2) why they should be awarded this scholarship (including career goals and financial need). U.S. citizenship is not required.

Financial Data The stipend is $1,000 per year.

Duration 1 year; recipients may reapply.

Additional data This program, established in 2008, is supported by the Council on Certification of Health, Environmental and Safety Technologists (CCHEST).

Number awarded 1 each year.

Deadline November of each year.

[59]
CENTENNIAL SCHOLARSHIP

New Jersey State Nurses Association
Attn: Institute for Nursing
1479 Pennington Road
Trenton, NJ 08618-2661
(609) 883-5335   Toll Free: (888) UR-NJSNA
Fax: (609) 883-5343   E-mail: institute@njsna.org
Web: www.njsna.org/displaycommon.cfm?an=5

Summary To provide financial assistance to New Jersey residents who are preparing for a career as a nurse at a school in the state.

Eligibility Applicants must be New Jersey residents currently enrolled in a diploma, associate, baccalaureate, or master's nursing program located in the state. Registered nurses in an R.N.-B.S.N. program are also eligible if they are members of the New Jersey State Nurses Association. Selection is based on financial need, GPA, and leadership potential.

Financial Data The stipend is $1,000.

Duration 1 year.

Number awarded 1 each year.

Deadline January of each year.

[60]
CENTRAL INDIANA ASSE SCHOLARSHIP

American Society of Safety Engineers
Attn: ASSE Foundation
1800 East Oakton Street
Des Plaines, IL 60018
(847) 768-3435   Fax: (847) 768-3434
E-mail: agabanski@asse.org
Web: www.asse.org/foundation/scholarships/scholarships.php

Summary To provide financial assistance to upper-division and graduate student members of the American Society of Safety Engineers (ASSE) from Indiana.

Eligibility This program is open to ASSE student members who are working on an undergraduate or graduate degree in occupational safety, health, and environment or a closely-related field (e.g., industrial or environmental engineering, environmental science, industrial hygiene, occupational health nursing). Priority is given to residents of Indiana attending school in the state or anywhere in the United States and to nonresidents attending school in Indiana. Undergraduates must be full-time students who have completed at least 60 semester hours with a GPA of 3.0 or higher. Graduate students must also be enrolled full time, have completed at least 9 semester hours with a GPA of 3.5 or higher, and have earned a GPA of 3.0 or higher as an undergraduate. Along with their application, they must submit 2 essays of 300 words or less: 1) why they are seeking a degree in occupational safety and health or a closely-related field, a brief description of their current activities, and how those relate to their career goals and objectives; and 2) why they should be awarded this scholarship (including career goals and financial need). U.S. citizenship is not required.

Financial Data The stipend is $1,500 per year.

Duration 1 year; recipients may reapply.

Additional data This program is supported by the Central Indiana Chapter of ASSE.

Number awarded 1 each year.

Deadline November of each year.

[61]
CHARLES KUNZ MEMORIAL UNDERGRADUATE SCHOLARSHIP

Emergency Nurses Association
Attn: ENA Foundation
915 Lee Street
Des Plaines, IL 60016-6569
(847) 460-4100   Toll Free: (800) 900-9659, ext. 4100
Fax: (847) 460-4004   E-mail: foundation@ena.org
Web: www.ena.org

Summary To provide financial assistance for baccalaureate study to nurses who are members of the Emergency Nurses Association (ENA).

Eligibility This program is open to nurses (R.N., L.P.N., L.V.N.) who are working on a bachelor's degree. Applicants must have been members of the association for at least 12 months and have a GPA of 3.0 or higher. They must submit a 1-page statement on their professional and educational goals and how this scholarship will help them attain those goals. Selection is based on content and clarity of the goal statement (45%), professional association involvement (35%), presentation of the application (10%), and letters of reference (10%).

Financial Data The stipend is $3,000.

Duration 1 year; nonrenewable.

Number awarded 1 each year.

Deadline May of each year.

[62]
CHARLOTTE LIDDELL SCHOLARSHIP

Florida Nurses Association
Attn: Florida Nurses Foundation
1235 East Concord Street
P.O. Box 536985
Orlando, FL 32853-6985
(407) 896-3261   Fax: (407) 896-9042
E-mail: foundation@floridanurse.org
Web: www.floridanurse.org/foundationGrants/index.asp

Summary To provide financial assistance to Florida residents who are interested in working on an undergraduate or graduate degree in nursing.

Eligibility Applicants must have been Florida residents for at least 1 year and have completed at least 1 semester at an accredited nursing program in the state. They may be working on an associate, baccalaureate, master's, or doctoral degree. Undergraduates must have a GPA of 2.5 or higher and graduate students 3.0 or higher. Preference is given to students focusing on psychiatric nursing and attending school in south Florida. Along with their application, they must submit 1-page essays on 1) why it is necessary for them to receive this scholarship; and 2) their goals and their assessment of their potential for making a contribution to nursing and society.

Financial Data A stipend is awarded (amount not specified).

Duration 1 semester or year.

Number awarded 1 or more each year.

Deadline May of each year.

[63]
CHESAPEAKE UROLOGY ASSOCIATES SCHOLARSHIP

Central Scholarship Bureau
1700 Reisterstown Road, Suite 220
P.O. Box 37064
Baltimore, MD 21297-3064
(410) 415-5558   Fax: (410) 415-5501
E-mail: info@centralsb.org
Web: www.centralsb.org

Summary To provide financial assistance to residents of Maryland working on a degree in a health-related field at a college in any state.

Eligibility This program is open to residents of Maryland who are enrolled full time at a college or university in any state. Applicants must be working on a degree in pre-medicine, pre-nursing, or an ancillary health field. Applicants must have a GPA of 3.0 or higher and a family income less than $91,000 per year. Selection is based on demonstrated commitment to the medical field, academic achievement, and financial need. U.S. citizenship or permanent resident status is required.

Financial Data The stipend is $5,000.

Duration 1 year.

Additional data This program was established in 2006.

Number awarded 3 each year.

Deadline May of each year.

[64]
CHIMSS SCHOLARSHIP

Healthcare Information and Management Systems Society-
  Colorado Chapter
c/o Bob Barrett, Treasurer
4375 Golden Glow View, Number 102
Colorado Springs, CO 80922
E-mail: academic@chimss.org
Web: www.chimss.org/scholarship/scholarship.html

Summary To provide financial assistance to residents of Colorado working on an undergraduate or graduate degree in health care informatics at a school in any state.

Eligibility This program is open to Colorado residents currently enrolled in an undergraduate, master's, or Ph.D. program in any state in health care informatics or a sub-specialty, such as nursing informatics or healthcare information management. Applicants must submit a 500-word essay on how they will impact the field of health care informatics and 2 letters of recommendation.

Financial Data The stipend is $2,500. The winner also receives a 1-year complimentary membership in the Colorado Healthcare Information and Management Systems Society (CHIMSS).

Duration 1 year.

Number awarded 2 each year.

Deadline April of each year.

[65]
CLAIRE MARTIN MEMORIAL SCHOLARSHIPS

New Hampshire Nurse Practitioner Association
Attn: Executive Director
P.O. Box 820
New London, NH 03257-0820
(603) 848-4341   Fax: (603) 526-7841
E-mail: lkcarpenter@tds.net
Web: www.npweb.org

Summary To provide financial assistance to residents of New Hampshire who are interested in working on an undergraduate or graduate degree in nursing at a school in any state.

Eligibility This program is open to residents of New Hampshire who are enrolled or planning to enroll at a college or university in any state to work on an undergraduate or graduate degree in nursing. Applicants must submit a 250-word essay on why they chose nursing as a career and the qualities they possess that will help them succeed. Financial need is not considered in the selection process.

Financial Data The stipend is $500.

Duration 1 year.

Number awarded 4 each year.

Deadline August of each year.

[66]
CLARK-PHELPS SCHOLARSHIP

Oregon Student Assistance Commission
Attn: Grants and Scholarships Division
1500 Valley River Drive, Suite 100
Eugene, OR 97401-2146
(541) 687-7395   Toll Free: (800) 452-8807, ext. 7395
Fax: (541) 687-7414   TDD: (800) 735-2900
E-mail: awardinfo@osac.state.or.us
Web: www.osac.state.or.us/osac_programs.html

Summary To provide financial assistance to residents of Oregon and Alaska who are interested in studying nursing, dentistry, or medicine at schools in Oregon.

Eligibility This program is open to residents of Oregon and Alaska who are currently enrolled or planning to enroll at a public college or university in Oregon. Applicants must be interested in working on a 4-year or graduate degree in nursing, a doctoral degree in dentistry, or a doctoral degree in medicine. Preference is given to applicants who are interested in studying at Oregon Health and Science University, including the nursing programs at Eastern Oregon University, Southern Oregon University, and Oregon Institute of Technology.

Financial Data A stipend is awarded (amount not specified).

Duration 1 year; recipients may reapply.

Additional data This program is administered by the Oregon Student Assistance Commission (OSAC) with funds provided by the Oregon Community Foundation, 1221 S.W. Yamhill, Suite 100, Portland, OR 97205, (503) 227-6846, Fax: (503) 274-7771.

Number awarded Varies each year.

Deadline February of each year.

[67]
CLIFFORD JORDAN SCHOLARSHIP

Florida Council of periOperative Registered Nurses
c/o Carol Morris, Scholarship Chair
223 S.E. Ninth Terrace
Cape Coral, FL 33990
(239) 458-8539   E-mail: Christmascat721@aol.com
Web: community.aorn.org:8080

Summary To provide financial assistance to nursing students and registered nurses in Florida who are working on a degree to advance their career as a perioperative nurse.

Eligibility This program is open to residents of Florida who are 1) students in the final year of an accredited nursing program, or 2) perioperative nurses. Students must have a GPA of 3.0 or higher and be planning to work in a perioperative setting after graduation. Current perioperative nurses must be interested in working on a diploma to A.D.N., diploma/A.D.N., A.D.N. to M.S.N., B.S.N. to M.S.N., degree in hospital administration or health care administration, or Ph.D. in nursing. Applicants must submit information on their educational history, professional activities, civic and school activities, work experience, personal philosophy of perioperative nursing, and reasons for applying. Financial need is not considered.

Financial Data A stipend is awarded (amount not specified).

Duration 1 year.

Number awarded 1 or more each year.

Deadline June of each year.

[68]
CNA FOUNDATION SCHOLARSHIPS

American Society of Safety Engineers
Attn: ASSE Foundation
1800 East Oakton Street
Des Plaines, IL 60018
(847) 768-3435   Fax: (847) 768-3434
E-mail: agabanski@asse.org
Web: www.asse.org/foundation/scholarships/scholarships.php

Summary To provide financial assistance to upper-division and graduate student members of the American Society of Safety Engineers (ASSE).

Eligibility This program is open to ASSE student members who are working on an undergraduate or graduate degree in occupational safety, health, and environment or a closely-related field (e.g., industrial or environmental engineering, environmental science, industrial hygiene, occupational health nursing). Undergraduates must be full-time students who have completed at least 60 semester hours with a GPA of 3.0 or higher. Graduate students must also be enrolled full time, have completed at least 9 semester hours with a GPA of 3.5 or higher, and have earned a GPA of 3.0 or higher as an undergraduate. Along with their application, they must submit 2 essays of 300 words or less: 1) why they are seeking a degree in occupational safety and health or a closely-related field, a brief description of their current activities, and how those relate to their career goals and objectives; and 2) why they should be awarded this scholarship (including career goals and financial need). U.S. citizenship is not required.

Financial Data The stipend is $4,650 per year.

Duration 1 year; recipients may reapply.

Additional data This program, established in 2006, is supported by the CNA Foundation.

Number awarded 2 each year.

Deadline November of each year.

[69]
COLLEGE NETWORK MOLN MEMBER SCHOLARSHIPS

Minnesota Organization of Leaders in Nursing
1821 University Avenue West, Suite S256
St. Paul, MN 55104
(651) 999-5344   Fax: (651) 917-1835
E-mail: office@moln.org
Web: www.moln.org/sections/scholarships.php

Summary To provide financial assistance to members of the Minnesota Organization of Leaders in Nursing (MOLN) who are interested in returning to school to earn an additional degree in nursing.

Eligibility This program is open to MOLN members (must have been voting members for at least 12 months) who are currently enrolled or have been admitted to a relevant bachelor's, master's, or doctoral degree program. Applicants must have a GPA of 3.0 or higher in their current academic work. Along with their application, they must submit a 2-page essay on their goals in returning to school to complete a degree, how attainment of this degree will facilitate their professional development as a leader in nursing, and how their educational and career goals relate to the goals of MOLN. Selection is based on the essay, a letter of recommendation, and transcripts. Financial need is not considered.

Financial Data A total of $3,000 is available to MOLN members who attend a partnership university in The College Network and an additional $1,000 is available to MOLN members who attend a college or university of their choice.

Duration 1 year.

Additional data This program is sponsored by The College Network.

Number awarded Varies each year.

Deadline June of each year.

[70]
COLON FURR MEMORIAL NURSING SCHOLARSHIP

American Legion
Department of North Carolina
4 North Blount Street
P.O. Box 26657
Raleigh, NC 27611-6657
(919) 832-7506   Fax: (919) 832-6428
E-mail: nclegion@nc.rr.com
Web: nclegion.org/colonfurr.htm

Summary To provide financial assistance to nursing students at colleges in North Carolina.

Eligibility This program is open to North Carolina residents currently enrolled in a 1-year Licensed Practical Nurse program or a 2-, 3-, or 4-year program leading to certification as a registered nurse. The school must be in North Carolina. Applicants must be endorsed by their local post of the American Legion; each post may endorse only 1 applicant per year. Financial need is not considered in the selection process.

Financial Data The stipend is $600; funds are paid directly to the college.

Duration 1 year.

Additional data This program was established in 1992.

Number awarded Varies each year; since the program was established, it has awarded more than 100 of these scholarships.

Deadline September of each year.

[71]
COLORADO LEGION AUXILIARY PAST PRESIDENT'S PARLEY NURSE'S SCHOLARSHIP

American Legion Auxiliary
Department of Colorado
7465 East First Avenue, Suite D
Denver, CO 80230
(303) 367-5388   Fax: (303) 367-5388
E-mail: ala@impactmail.net
Web: www.freewebs.com/ala-colorado

Summary To provide financial assistance to war time veterans and their descendants in Colorado who are interested in attending school in the state to prepare for a career in nursing.

Eligibility This program is open to 1) daughters, sons, spouses, granddaughters, and great-granddaughters of veterans, and 2) veterans who served in the armed forces during eligibility dates for membership in the American Legion. Applicants must be Colorado residents who have been accepted by an accredited school of nursing in the state. Along with their application, they must submit a 500-word essay on the topic, "Americanism." Selection is based on scholastic ability (25%), financial need (25%), references (13%), a 500-word essay on Americanism (25%), and dedication to chosen field (12%).

Financial Data Stipends range from $500 to $1,000.

Duration 1 year; nonrenewable.

Number awarded Varies each year, depending on the availability of funds.

Deadline April of each year.

[72]
COLORADO NURSES ASSOCIATION NIGHTINGALE SCHOLARSHIP

Colorado Nurses Foundation
7400 East Arapahoe Road, Suite 211
Centennial, CO 80112
(303) 694-4728   Fax: (303) 694-4869
E-mail: mail@cnfound.org
Web: www.cnfound.org/scholarships.html

Summary To provide financial assistance to undergraduate and graduate nursing students in Colorado who are members of the Colorado Nurses Association (CNA) or Colorado Student Nurses Association (CSNA).

Eligibility This program is open to Colorado residents who have been accepted as a student in an approved nursing program in the state. Applicants may be 1) second-year students in an associate degree program; 2) junior or senior level B.S.N. undergraduate students; 3) R.N.s enrolled in a baccalaureate or higher degree program in a school of nursing; 4) R.N.s with a master's degree in nursing, currently practicing in Colorado and enrolled in a doctoral program; or 5) students in the second or third year of a Doctorate Nursing Practice (D.N.P.) program. They must be current members of CNA or CSNA. Undergraduates must have a GPA of 3.25 or higher and graduate students must have a GPA of 3.5 or higher. Selection is based on professional philosophy and goals, dedication to the improvement of patient care in Colorado, demonstrated commitment to nursing, critical thinking skills, potential for leadership, involvement in community and professional organizations, recommendations, GPA, and financial need.

Financial Data The stipend is $1,000.

Duration 1 year.

Number awarded 1 each year.

Deadline October of each year.

[73]
COLORADO NURSES FOUNDATION SCHOLARSHIPS

Colorado Nurses Foundation
7400 East Arapahoe Road, Suite 211
Centennial, CO 80112
(303) 694-4728   Fax: (303) 694-4869
E-mail: mail@cnfound.org
Web: www.cnfound.org/scholarships.html

Summary To provide financial assistance to undergraduate and graduate nursing students in Colorado.

Eligibility This program is open to Colorado residents who have been accepted as a student in an approved nursing program in the state. Applicants may be 1) second-year students in an associate degree program; 2) junior or senior level B.S.N. undergraduate students; 3) R.N.s enrolled in a baccalaureate or higher degree program in a school of nursing; 4) R.N.s with a master's degree in nursing, currently practicing in Colorado and enrolled in a doctoral program; or 5) students in the second or third year of a Doctorate Nursing Practice (D.N.P.) program. They must be committed to practicing nursing in Colorado. Undergraduates must have a GPA of 3.25 or higher and graduate students must have a GPA of 3.5 or higher. Selection is based on professional philosophy and goals, dedication to the improvement of patient care in Colorado, demonstrated commitment to nursing, critical thinking skills, potential for leadership, involvement in community and professional organizations, recommendations, GPA, and financial need.

Financial Data The stipend is $1,000.

Duration 1 year.

Additional data The program includes the following named scholarships: the Johnson and Johnson Nightingale Scholarship, the Donor Alliance Nightingale Scholarship, the National Jewish Health Nightingale Scholarship, the Colorado Trust Nightingale Scholarship, the Colorado Nurses Association District 3 Scholarship, the Colorado Nurses Association District 16 Scholarship in Honor of Eleanor Bent, the University of Colorado Denver College of Nursing Scholarship (limited to students in the nursing program at the University of Colorado at Denver), the Denver Metro Regional Nightingale Scholarship, the Exempla Lutheran Medical Center Nightingale Scholarship, the Medical Center of Aurora Nightingale Scholarship, the Rose Medical Center Nightingale Scholarship, the St. Anthony's Hospitals Nightingale Scholarship, the Nightingale Scholarships, the Arthur L. Davis Publishing Agency Scholarship, the Colorado Organization of Nurse Leaders Scholarship in Memory of Dorothy Babcock, the LaFawn Biddle Nightingale Scholarship, and the Patty Walter Memorial Scholarship (limited to graduate students in urology or oncology at the University of Northern Colorado).

Number awarded   Varies each year; recently, 15 of these scholarships were awarded.

Deadline   October of each year.

[74]
COLUMBIA-WILLAMETTE CHAPTER PRESIDENT SCHOLARSHIP

American Society of Safety Engineers
Attn: ASSE Foundation
1800 East Oakton Street
Des Plaines, IL 60018
(847) 768-3435   Fax: (847) 768-3434
E-mail: agabanski@asse.org
Web: www.asse.org/foundation/scholarships/scholarships.php

Summary   To provide financial assistance to upper-division students, especially those from Oregon or Washington, majoring in fields related to occupational safety and health.

Eligibility   This program is open to undergraduate students who are majoring in occupational safety, health, and environment or a closely-related field (e.g., industrial or environmental engineering, environmental science, industrial hygiene, occupational health nursing). Priority is given to residents of Oregon and Washington attending school within those states, to nonresidents attending school in those states, and to residents of those states attending school anywhere in the United States. Applicants must be full-time students who have completed at least 60 semester hours with a GPA of 3.0 or higher and be ASSE student members. Along with their application, they must submit 2 essays of 300 words or less: 1) why they are seeking a degree in occupational safety and health or a closely-related field, a brief description of their current activities, and how those relate to their career goals and objectives; and 2) why they should be awarded this scholarship (including career goals and financial need). U.S. citizenship is not required.

Financial Data   The stipend is $1,000 per year.

Duration   1 year; recipients may reapply.

Additional data   This program, established in 2008, is supported by the Columbia-Willamette Chapter of the American Society of Safety Engineers (ASSE).

Number awarded   1 each year.

Deadline   November of each year.

[75]
COMMUNITY CARE ORGANIZATION COLLEGE-TO-WORK PROGRAM

Wisconsin Foundation for Independent Colleges, Inc.
Attn: College-to-Work Program
4425 North Port Washington Road, Suite 402
Glendale, WI 53212
(414) 273-5980   Fax: (414) 273-5995
E-mail: wfic@wficweb.org
Web: www.wficweb.org/4.html

Summary   To provide financial assistance and work experience to students at member institutions of the Wisconsin Foundation for Independent Colleges (WFIC) who are interested in preparing for a career in human services (including nursing).

Eligibility   This program is open to full-time sophomores, juniors, and seniors at WFIC member colleges and universities. Applicants must be majoring in nursing, occupational therapy, physical therapy, psychology, recreation therapy, social work, sociology, or other human service-related field. They must be interested in a summer internship at Community Care Organization in Milwaukee, Wisconsin. Along with their application, they must submit a cover letter that describes their career aspirations, explains why this internship would be beneficial to them in their career search and educational pursuits, what they hope to gain from this experience (both personally and professionally), and what made them want to apply for this internship.

Financial Data   The stipends are $3,000 for the scholarship and $2,000 for the internship.

Duration   1 year for the scholarship; 10 weeks during the summer for the internship.

Additional data   The WFIC member schools are Alverno College, Beloit College, Cardinal Stritch University, Carroll College, Carthage College, Concordia University of Wisconsin, Edgewood College, Lakeland College, Lawrence University, Marian College, Marquette University, Milwaukee Institute of Art & Design, Milwaukee School of Engineering, Mount Mary College, Northland College, Ripon College, St. Norbert College, Silver Lake College, Viterbo University, and Wisconsin Lutheran College. This program is sponsored by Community Care Organization, Inc.

Number awarded   1 each year.

Deadline   Deadline not specified.

[76]
CONNECTICUT CHAPTER HFMA SCHOLARSHIPS

Healthcare Financial Management Association-Connecticut
   Chapter
c/o Cassandra L. Mitchell, Scholarship Committee Chair
UConn Health Center/John Dempsey Hospital
263 Farmington Avenue
Farmington, CT 06030-5355
(860) 679-2916   Fax: (860) 679-3071
E-mail: mitchellc@uche.edu
Web: www.cthfma.org/site/epage/18079_473.htm

Summary   To recognize and reward, with scholarships, undergraduate and graduate students in fields related to health care financial management (including nursing) at colleges and universities in Connecticut who submit outstanding essays on topics in the field.

Eligibility   This competition is open to undergraduate and graduate students at colleges and universities in Connecticut, children of members of the Connecticut chapter of the Healthcare Financial Management Association (HFMA) attending a school outside of Connecticut, residents of Connecticut commuting to a college or university in a state that borders the state, and Connecticut health care industry employees who are currently attending college. Applicants must be enrolled in a business, finance, accounting, or information systems program and have an interest in health care or be enrolled in a nursing or allied health program. They must submit an essay, up to 5 pages, on a topic that changes annually but relates to financing of health care. Finalists may be interviewed.

Financial Data   The first-place winner (undergraduate or graduate) receives a $4,000 award and the second-place winner (undergraduate or graduate) receives a $1,000 award. Both winners also receive membership in the Connecticut chapter of HFMA, a 1-year subscription to *Healthcare Financial Management,* and waiver of chapter program fees for 1 year.

Duration   1 year.

Number awarded   2 each year: 1 for an undergraduate and 1 for a graduate student.

Deadline   March of each year.

[77]
CONNECTICUT LEGION AUXILIARY PAST PRESIDENTS PARLEY' EDUCATION GRANTS

American Legion Auxiliary
Department of Connecticut
287 West Street
P.O. Box 266
Rocky Hill, CT 06067-0266
(860) 721-5945   Fax: (860) 721-5828
E-mail: ctalahq@juno.com

Summary To provide financial assistance to Connecticut residents who are the children or grandchildren of women veterans and interested in attending college in any state.

Eligibility This program is open to children and grandchildren of ex-servicewomen who have been members for at least 5 years of the American Legion or American Legion Auxiliary in Connecticut. If no children or grandchildren of ex-servicewomen apply, the program is open to children or grandchildren of members of the Connecticut Department of the American Legion, American Legion Auxiliary, or Sons of the American Legion who have been members for at least 5 years. Applicants must be between 16 and 23 years of age, have a high academic standing, and be able to demonstrate financial need. They must be attending or planning to attend a college, university, technical school, or professional school in any state.

Financial Data The maximum stipend is $500.

Duration 1 year.

Number awarded At least 4 each year. At least 1 of those awards is designated for a nursing student.

Deadline February of each year.

[78]
CONNECTICUT NURSES' FOUNDATION SCHOLARSHIPS

Connecticut Nurses' Association
Attn: Connecticut Nurses' Foundation
377 Research Parkway, Suite 2D
Meriden, CT 06450-7155
(203) 238-1207   Fax: (203) 238-3437
E-mail: info@ctnurses.org
Web: www.ctnurses.org/displaycommon.cfm?an=12

Summary To provide financial assistance to Connecticut residents interested in preparing for a career as a registered nurse (R.N.) or working on a degree in nursing at a school in any state.

Eligibility This program is open to residents of Connecticut who are entering or enrolled at an accredited school of nursing in any state to earn an R.N. certificate or work on an associate, bachelor's, master's, or doctoral degree. Selection is based on employment experience; professional, community, and student activities; a statement of educational and practice goals; and financial need.

Financial Data The stipend depends on the qualifications of the recipient and the availability of funds.

Duration 1 year.

Additional data This program includes the following named scholarships: the Dominion Enterprises Scholarship, the Frank Chant Memorial Scholarship, and the Polly Barey Scholarship.

Number awarded 1 or more each year.

Deadline June of each year.

[79]
CONNIE SCHEFFER PUBLIC HEALTH NURSE ENDOWED SCHOLARSHIP

Kansas State Nurses Association
Attn: Kansas Nurses Foundation
1109 S.W. Topeka Boulevard
Topeka, KS 66612-1602
(785) 233-8638   Fax: (785) 233-5222
E-mail: ksna@ksna.net
Web: www.nursingworld.org/SNAS/KS/Knf.htm

Summary To provide financial assistance to residents of Kansas who are working on a degree in public health nursing at the undergraduate, master's, or doctoral level at a school in the state.

Eligibility This program is open to students who are working on a nursing degree on the undergraduate or graduate level at a school in Kansas. Applicants must have a GPA of 3.0 or higher. Along with their application, they must submit a personal narrative describing their anticipated role in nursing in the state of Kansas. Preference is given to full-time students. The following priority is used in awarding scholarships: 1) R.N.s working on B.S.N.s and employed in public health settings; and 2) graduate and postgraduate nursing students in public health nursing or public health (e.g., M.P.H. degree).

Financial Data The stipend is $500.

Duration 1 year.

Number awarded 1 each year.

Deadline June of each year.

[80]
C.R. BARD FOUNDATION NURSING SCHOLARSHIP

Independent College Fund of New Jersey
797 Springfield Avenue
Summit, NJ 07901-1107
(908) 277-3424   Fax: (908) 277-0851
E-mail: scholarships@njcolleges.org
Web: www.njcolleges.org/i_about_schol_students.html

Summary To provide financial assistance to students enrolled at member institutions of the Independent College Fund of New Jersey (ICFNJ) who are working on a bachelor's degree in nursing.

Eligibility This program is open to students enrolled full time at ICJNF-member institutions that offer a program in nursing (Bloomfield College, Fairleigh Dickinson University, College of Saint Elizabeth, Felician College, Georgian Court University, Monmouth University, Saint Peter's College, or Seton Hall University). Applicants must be entering at least the second semester of their sophomore year or the second semester of the second year of their nursing program. They must have a GPA of 3.0 or higher, be a U.S. citizen or eligible to work in the United States, be able to demonstrate financial need, and be planning to prepare for a career in the health industry. Along with their application, they must submit a 200-word statement on why they want to prepare for the profession of nursing or a career in the health industry, what they hope to accomplish, and their qualifications for the award. Selection is based on the quality of that statement, academic performance, extracurricular activities, demonstrated leadership, and financial need.

Financial Data The stipend is $2,500 per year.

Duration 1 year; may be renewed.

Additional data This program is sponsored by C.R. Bard, Inc.

Number awarded 8 each year.

Deadline March of each year.

[81]
CUTTING EDGE CAREERS SCHOLARSHIP

Cappex.com, LLC
600 Laurel Avenue
Highland Park, IL 60035
Web: www.cappex.com

Summary To provide financial assistance for college to high school seniors who complete a profile for Cappex.com and who plan to prepare for a career in designated fields.

Eligibility Applicants for this scholarship must first complete an online profile for Cappex.com which will enable colleges and universities to contact them for recruiting purposes. They must be U.S. citizens or permanent residents planning to attend an accredited college or university in the United States. In completing their profile, they must describe their extracurricular, leadership, and volunteer activities and why they want to prepare for a career in their field.. This scholarship is reserved for high school seniors who plan to prepare for a career in business, computer and information sciences, criminal justice, health care and nursing, design, digital media, or culinary arts.

Financial Data The stipend is $1,000.

Duration 1 year.

Number awarded 1 each year.

Deadline July of each year.

[82]
CYNTHIA HUNT-LINES SCHOLARSHIP

Minnesota Nurses Association
Attn: Minnesota Nurses Association Foundation
1625 Energy Park Drive, Suite 200
St. Paul, MN 55108
(651) 414-2822   Toll Free: (800) 536-4662, ext. 122
Fax: (651) 695-7000   E-mail: linda.owens@mnnurses.org
Web: www.mnnurses.org

Summary To provide financial assistance to members of the Minnesota Nurses Association (MNA) and the Minnesota Student Nurses Association (MSNA) who are single parents and interested in working on a baccalaureate or master's degree in nursing.

Eligibility This program is open to MNA and MSNA members who are enrolled or entering a baccalaureate or master's program in nursing in Minnesota or North Dakota. Applicants must be single parents, at least 21 years of age, with at least 1 dependent. Along with their application, they must submit: a current transcript; a short essay describing their interest in nursing, their long-range career goals, and how their continuing education will have an impact on the profession of nursing in Minnesota; a description of their financial need; and 2 letters of support.

Financial Data The stipend is $2,000 per year.

Duration 1 year; may be renewed.

Number awarded 1 each year.

Deadline May of each year.

[83]
DAKOTA CORPS SCHOLARSHIP PROGRAM

Education Assistance Corporation
115 First Avenue S.W.
Aberdeen, SD 57401
Toll Free: (800) 874-9033   E-mail: eac@eac-easci.org
Web: www.state.sd.us/dakotacorps/default.html

Summary To provide scholarship/loans to high school seniors in South Dakota who plan to attend a college or university in the state and work in the state in nursing or another critical need occupation following graduation.

Eligibility This program is open to seniors graduating from high schools in South Dakota who are U.S. citizens or nationals. Applicants must plan to attend a participating college, university, technical college, or tribal college in the state and major in a field to prepare for a career in a critical need occupation; currently, those are 1) teaching K-12 music, special education, or foreign language in a public, private, or parochial school; 2) teaching high school mathematics or science in a public, private, or parochial school; or 3) working as a licensed practical nurse, registered nurse, or other allied health care provider. They must have a GPA of 2.8 or higher and an ACT score of at least 24 (or the SAT equivalent). Applications must be submitted within 1 year after high school graduation or release from active duty of a component of the U.S. armed forces. Along with their application, they must submit a short essay explaining what has attracted them to their profession and to remaining in South Dakota for employment. Selection is based on that essay, GPA, test scores, activities, honors, and community service.

Financial Data At public colleges, universities, technical colleges, and tribal colleges, awards provide full payment of tuition and generally-applicable fees up to 16 credit hours. At private colleges and universities, awards provide the same amount as at a public 4-year college; the remaining tuition and generally-applicable fees must be covered by the participating college through an institutional scholarship or tuition waiver. This is a scholarship loan program; recipients must commit to work in a critical need occupation in South Dakota for a period of time equal to the number of years of scholarship support received plus 1 additional year. If recipients fail to complete their commitment, the scholarship converts to a low-interest loan that much be repaid.

Duration 1 year; may be renewed up to 3 additional years, provided the recipient maintains a GPA of 2.8 or higher and remains enrolled full time.

Additional data This program is supported by Great Plains Education Foundation, Avera Health, Sanford Health, Allianz Global Investors Distributors LLC, Great Western Bank, and the South Dakota Department of Labor.

Number awarded A limited number each year.

Deadline January of each year.

[84]
DAVID E. KNOX MEMORIAL NURSING SCHOLARSHIP

Alaska Community Foundation
Attn: Scholarships
400 L Street, Suite 100
Anchorage, AK 99501
(907) 334-6700   Fax: (907) 334-5780
E-mail: info@alaskacf.org
Web: www.alaskacf.org

Summary To provide grants-for-service to residents of Alaska who are interested in studying nursing at a school in any state and then practicing in a small community in Alaska.

Eligibility This program is open to residents of Alaska who are graduating high school seniors or students already enrolled full time at a college or university in any state. Applicants must be interested in working on a degree (R.N. or B.S.N.) in nursing and be willing to commit to a 1-year service obligation as a nurse in a small (less than 50,000 residents) community in Alaska. They must have a GPA of 3.0 or higher and be able to demonstrate financial need. Along with their application, they must submit a 1,000-word essay describing how their background is relevant to their interest in preparing for a nursing career, their educational goals and objectives, their plan and timeframe for meeting those goals, and their specific qualifications for this scholarship. Preference is given to applicants who wish to practice in operating rooms.

Financial Data The stipend is $2,500 per year. If recipients fail to honor their service commitment, they must repay all funds received.

Duration 1 year; recipients may reapply.

Number awarded 1 or more each year.
Deadline January of each year.

[85]
DAVID IDEN MEMORIAL SAFETY SCHOLARSHIPS

American Society of Safety Engineers
Attn: ASSE Foundation
1800 East Oakton Street
Des Plaines, IL 60018
(847) 768-3435   Fax: (847) 768-3434
E-mail: agabanski@asse.org
Web: www.asse.org/foundation/scholarships/scholarships.php

Summary To provide financial assistance to minority upper-division student members of the American Society of Safety Engineers (ASSE).

Eligibility This program is open to ASSE student members who are majoring in occupational safety, health, and environment or a closely-related field (e.g., industrial or environmental engineering, environmental science, industrial hygiene, occupational health nursing). Applicants must be full-time students who have completed at least 60 semester hours with a GPA of 3.0 or higher. Along with their application, they must submit 2 essays of 300 words or less: 1) why they are seeking a degree in occupational safety and health or a closely-related field, a brief description of their current activities, and how those relate to their career goals and objectives; and 2) why they should be awarded this scholarship (including career goals and financial need). U.S. citizenship is not required.

Financial Data The stipend is $5,250 per year.
Duration 1 year; recipients may reapply.
Additional data Funding for this program is provided by the UPS Foundation.
Number awarded 4 each year.
Deadline November of each year.

[86]
DELAWARE NURSING INCENTIVE PROGRAM

Delaware Higher Education Commission
Carvel State Office Building, Fifth Floor
820 North French Street
Wilmington, DE 19801-3509
(302) 577-5240   Toll Free: (800) 292-7935
Fax: (302) 577-6765   E-mail: dhec@doe.k12.de.us
Web: www.doe.k12.de.us

Summary To provide scholarship/loans to Delaware residents who are interested in studying nursing at a school in any state.

Eligibility This program is open to residents of Delaware who are enrolled or planning to enroll full time in an accredited program in any state leading to certification as an R.N. or L.P.N. High school seniors must rank in the upper half of their class and have a cumulative GPA of 2.5 or higher. Current undergraduate students must be enrolled full time and have a GPA of 2.5 or higher. Also eligible are 1) current state employees (they are not required to be Delaware residents and may enroll part time); and 2) registered nurses with 5 or more years of state service (they must be working on a bachelor of science in nursing degree, but they may enroll full or part time). U.S. citizenship or eligible non-citizen status is required.

Financial Data Awards up to the cost of tuition, fees, and other direct educational expenses are available. This is a scholarship/loan program; if the recipient performs required service at a state-owned hospital or clinic in Delaware, the loan is forgiven at the rate of 1 year of service for each year of assistance. Recipients who fail to perform the required service must repay the loan in full.

Duration 1 year; may be renewed for up to 3 additional years, provided the recipient maintains a GPA of 2.75 or higher.
Number awarded Up to 50 each year.
Deadline March of each year.

[87]
DERMATOLOGY NURSES' ASSOCIATION CAREER MOBILITY SCHOLARSHIPS

Dermatology Nurses' Association
Attn: Recognition Program
15000 Commerce Parkway, Suite C
Mt. Laurel, NJ 08055
Toll Free: (800) 454-4DNA   Fax: (856) 439-0525
E-mail: dna@dnanurse.org
Web: www.dnanurse.org

Summary To provide financial assistance to members of the Dermatology Nurses' Association (DNA) who are working on an undergraduate or graduate degree.

Eligibility Applicants for these scholarships must 1) have been members of the association for at least 2 years, 2) be employed in the specialty of dermatology, and 3) be working on a degree or advanced degree in nursing. Selection is based on a letter in which applicants describe their professional goals, proposed course of study, time frame for completion of study, funds necessary to meet their educational needs, and financial need.

Financial Data The stipend is $2,500.
Duration 1 year.
Number awarded 1 or more each year.
Deadline September of each year.

[88]
DERMATOLOGY NURSES' ASSOCIATION NEW NURSE EDUCATIONAL SCHOLARSHIP

Dermatology Nurses' Association
Attn: Recognition Program
15000 Commerce Parkway, Suite C
Mt. Laurel, NJ 08055
Toll Free: (800) 454-4DNA   Fax: (856) 439-0525
E-mail: dna@dnanurse.org
Web: www.dnanurse.org

Summary To provide financial assistance to members of the Dermatology Nurses' Association (DNA) who are studying to become an L.P.N., L.V.N., or R.N.

Eligibility Applicants for this scholarships must be associate members of the association, active in community service, and accepted as a student in a certified nursing program to become an L.P.N., L.V.N., or R.N. Selection is based on a letter in which applicants describe their professional goals, proposed course of study, time frame for completion of study, funds necessary to meet their educational goals, financial need, and their most important achievement as a nursing student or their inspiration to study dermatology nursing.

Financial Data The stipend is $2,000.
Duration 1 year.
Number awarded 1 each year.
Deadline September of each year.

[89]
DISTRICT 6 GENERIC SCHOLARSHIPS FOR FLORIDA

Florida Nurses Association
Attn: Florida Nurses Foundation
1235 East Concord Street
P.O. Box 536985
Orlando, FL 32853-6985
(407) 896-3261   Fax: (407) 896-9042
E-mail: foundation@floridanurse.org
Web: www.floridanurse.org/foundationGrants/index.asp

Summary To provide financial assistance to residents of Florida who are interested in working on an undergraduate or graduate degree in nursing.

Eligibility Applicants must have been residents of Florida for at least 1 year and have completed at least 1 semester at an accredited nursing program in the state. They may be working on an associate, baccalaureate, master's, or doctoral degree. Undergraduates must have a GPA of 2.5 or higher and graduate students a GPA of 3.0 or higher. Along with their application, they must submit 1-page essays on 1) why it is necessary for them to receive this scholarship; and 2) their goals and their assessment of their potential for making a contribution to nursing and society.

Financial Data A stipend is awarded (amount not specified).

Duration 1 semester or year.

Number awarded 4 each year.

Deadline May of each year.

[90]
DIVERSITY COMMITTEE SCHOLARSHIP

American Society of Safety Engineers
Attn: ASSE Foundation
1800 East Oakton Street
Des Plaines, IL 60018
(847) 768-3435   Fax: (847) 768-3434
E-mail: agabanski@asse.org
Web: www.asse.org/foundation/scholarships/scholarships.php

Summary To provide financial assistance to upper-division and graduate student members of the American Society of Safety Engineers (ASSE) who come from diverse groups.

Eligibility This program is open to ASSE student members who are majoring in occupational safety, health, and environment or a closely-related field (e.g., industrial or environmental engineering, environmental science, industrial hygiene, occupational health nursing). Undergraduates must be full-time students who have completed at least 60 semester hours with a GPA of 3.0 or higher. Graduate students must also be enrolled full time, have completed at least 9 semester hours with a GPA of 3.5 or higher, and have earned a GPA of 3.0 or higher as an undergraduate. Along with their application, they must submit 2 essays of 300 words or less: 1) why they are seeking a degree in occupational safety and health or a closely-related field, a brief description of their current activities, and how those relate to their career goals and objectives; and 2) why they should be awarded this scholarship (including career goals and financial need). A goal of this program is to support individuals regardless of race, ethnicity, gender, religion, personal beliefs, age, sexual orientation, physical challenges, geographic location, university, or specific area of study. U.S. citizenship is not required.

Financial Data The stipend is $1,000 per year.

Duration 1 year; recipients may reapply.

Number awarded 1 each year.

Deadline November of each year.

[91]
DNA 30 STUDENT SCHOLARSHIP

Colorado Society of Advanced Practice Nurses
Attn: Colorado Nurses Association, DNA 30
P.O. Box 100158
Denver, CO 80250-0158
(303) 757-7483   Toll Free: (800) 757-7310
Fax: (303) 757-8833   E-mail: CSAPN@msn.com
Web: www.enpnetwork.com

Summary To provide financial assistance to registered nurses in Colorado who are interested in working on a degree in advanced practice.

Eligibility This program is open to Colorado residents who are R.N.s preparing to become advanced practice nurses and advanced practice nurses working on an advanced degree in nursing (M.S. or higher). Applicants must submit brief statements on why they should be the recipient of this scholarship, their goals after they finish school, in the nursing activities and organizations in which they are involved, the community service activities in which they have been involved, and how they would use this

scholarship. Membership in the Colorado Society of Advanced Practice Nurses (DNA 30 of the Colorado Nurses Association) is not required, but members received preference.

Financial Data The stipend is $750.

Duration 1 year; recipients may reapply.

Number awarded 2 each year.

Deadline May of each year.

[92]
DON JONES EXCELLENCE IN SAFETY SCHOLARSHIP

American Society of Safety Engineers
Attn: ASSE Foundation
1800 East Oakton Street
Des Plaines, IL 60018
(847) 768-3435   Fax: (847) 768-3434
E-mail: agabanski@asse.org
Web: www.asse.org/foundation/scholarships/scholarships.php

Summary To provide financial assistance to upper-division students at southeastern universities who are majoring in fields related to occupational safety and health.

Eligibility This program is open to undergraduate students who are majoring in occupational safety, health, and environment or a closely-related field (e.g., industrial or environmental engineering, environmental science, industrial hygiene, occupational health nursing). Priority is given first to students at Southeastern Louisiana University in Hammond, Louisiana, second to students at other colleges and universities in Louisiana, and third to students at colleges and universities within the southeastern region of the United States. Applicants must be full- or part-time students who have completed at least 60 semester hours with a GPA of 3.0 or higher. Full-time students must be ASSE student members; part-time students must be ASSE general or professional members. Along with their application, they must submit 2 essays of 300 words or less: 1) why they are seeking a degree in occupational safety and health or a closely-related field, a brief description of their current activities, and how those relate to their career goals and objectives; and 2) why they should be awarded this scholarship (including career goals and financial need). U.S. citizenship is not required.

Financial Data The stipend is $1,000 per year.

Duration 1 year; recipients may reapply.

Additional data This program is supported by the Greater Baton Rouge Chapter of the American Society of Safety Engineers (ASSE).

Number awarded 1 each year.

Deadline November of each year.

[93]
DOROTHY E. GENERAL SCHOLARSHIP

Seattle Foundation
Attn: African American Scholarship Program
1200 Fifth Avenue, Suite 1300
Seattle, WA 98101-3151
(206) 622-2294   Fax: (206) 622-7673
E-mail: scholarships@seattlefoundation.org
Web: www.seattlefoundation.org/page32313.cfm

Summary To provide financial assistance to African Americans from any state working on an undergraduate or graduate degree in a field related to health care.

Eligibility This program is open to African American undergraduate and graduate students who are preparing for a career in a health care profession, including public health, medicine, nursing, or dentistry; pre-professional school students are also eligible. Applicants must be able to demonstrate financial need, academic competence, and leadership of African American students. They may be residents of any state attending school in any state. Along with their application, they must submit a 2-page essay describing their future aspirations, including their career goals and how their study of health care will help them achieve those goals and contribute to the African American community.

Financial Data The stipend is $1,000 per year. Payments are made directly to the recipient's educational institution.

Duration 1 year; may be renewed.

Number awarded 1 or more each year.

Deadline February of each year.

[94]
DR. SANDRA J. TUNAJEK SCHOLARSHIP FOR NURSE ANESTHESIA EDUCATION

American Association of Nurse Anesthetists
Attn: AANA Foundation
222 South Prospect Avenue
Park Ridge, IL 60068-4001
(847) 655-1170   Fax: (847) 692-6968
E-mail: foundation@aana.com
Web: www.aanafoundation.com

Summary To provide financial assistance to members of the American Association of Nurse Anesthetists (AANA) who are residents of Kentucky pursuing further education at a program in any state.

Eligibility This program is open to members of the association who are residents of Kentucky attending a nurse anesthesia program in any state. Applicants may be working on an entry-level or advanced degree. They must intend to practice in Kentucky after graduation. Along with their application, they must submit a 200-word essay describing why they have chosen nurse anesthesia as a profession and their professional goals for the future. Financial need is also considered in the selection process.

Financial Data The stipend is $1,500.

Duration 1 year.

Additional data This program, which began in 2008, is sponsored by the Kentucky Association of Nurse Anesthetists. The application processing fee is $25.

Number awarded 1 each year.

Deadline March of each year.

[95]
ECLIPSYS CLINICAL INFORMATICS SCHOLARSHIP

Healthcare Information and Management Systems Society
Attn: HIMSS Foundation
230 East Ohio Street, Suite 500
Chicago, IL 60611-3270
(312) 915-9277   Fax: (312) 664-6143
E-mail: foundation@himss.org
Web: www.himss.org/foundation/schlr_Eclipsys.asp

Summary To provide financial assistance to student members of the Healthcare Information and Management Systems Society (HIMSS) who are working on an undergraduate or graduate degree in health care information management.

Eligibility This program is open to upper-division and graduate students working full time on a degree in a health care information management systems field. Applicants must be members of HIMSS. They may be studying in any relevant field, but preference is given to students enrolled in a nursing, medical, or health informatics program. Along with their application, they must submit a personal statement that includes their career goals, past achievements, and future goals. Selection is based on that statement, academic achievement, and financial need.

Financial Data The stipend is $5,000. The award includes an all-expense paid trip to the annual conference and exhibition of HIMSS.

Duration 1 year; nonrenewable.

Additional data This scholarship, first offered in 2008, is sponsored by Eclipsys Corporation.

Number awarded 1 each year.

Deadline October of each year.

[96]
EDWARD J. AND VIRGINIA M. ROUTHIER NURSING SCHOLARSHIP

Rhode Island Foundation
Attn: Funds Administrator
One Union Station
Providence, RI 02903
(401) 427-4017   Fax: (401) 331-8085
E-mail: lmonahan@rifoundation.org
Web: www.rifoundation.org

Summary To provide financial assistance to undergraduate and graduate students enrolled in nursing programs in Rhode Island.

Eligibility This program is open to students enrolled or accepted at an accredited nursing program in Rhode Island. Applicants must be 1) registered nurses (R.N.s) enrolled in a nursing baccalaureate degree program; 2) students enrolled in a baccalaureate nursing program; or 3) R.N.s working on a graduate degree (master's or Ph.D.). They must be able to demonstrate financial need and a commitment to practice in Rhode Island. Along with their application, they must submit an essay, up to 300 words, on their career goals, particularly as they relate to practicing in or advancing the field of nursing in Rhode Island.

Financial Data The stipend ranges from $500 to $3,000 per year.

Duration 1 year; may be renewed.

Number awarded Varies each year. Recently, 11 of these scholarships were awarded: 6 new awards and 5 renewals.

Deadline April of each year.

[97]
EDWIN P. GRANBERRY, JR. SCHOLARSHIP

American Society of Safety Engineers
Attn: ASSE Foundation
1800 East Oakton Street
Des Plaines, IL 60018
(847) 768-3435   Fax: (847) 768-3434
E-mail: agabanski@asse.org
Web: www.asse.org/foundation/scholarships/scholarships.php

Summary To provide financial assistance to undergraduate student members of the American Society of Safety Engineers (ASSE), especially those at schools in designated southeastern states.

Eligibility This program is open to ASSE student members who are majoring in occupational safety, health, and environment or a closely-related field (e.g., industrial or environmental engineering, environmental science, industrial hygiene, occupational health nursing). Priority is given to students at schools in ASSE Region IV (Louisiana, Alabama, Mississippi, Georgia, Florida, Puerto Rico, and the U.S. Virgin Islands). Applicants must be full-time students who have completed at least 60 semester hours with a GPA of 3.0 or higher. Along with their application, they must submit 2 essays of 300 words or less: 1) why they are seeking a degree in occupational safety and health or a closely-related field, a brief description of their current activities, and how those relate to their career goals and objectives; and 2) why they should be awarded this scholarship (including career goals and financial need). U.S. citizenship is not required.

Financial Data The stipend is $1,000 per year.

Duration 1 year; recipients may reapply.

Number awarded 1 each year.

Deadline November of each year.

[98]
ELEANOR BINDRUM SCHOLARSHIP

Florida Nurses Association
Attn: Florida Nurses Foundation
1235 East Concord Street
P.O. Box 536985
Orlando, FL 32853-6985
(407) 896-3261   Fax: (407) 896-9042
E-mail: foundation@floridanurse.org
Web: www.floridanurse.org/foundationGrants/index.asp

Summary To provide financial assistance to Florida residents who are interested in working on an undergraduate or graduate degree in nursing.

Eligibility Applicants must have been Florida residents for at least 1 year and have completed at least 1 semester at an accredited nursing program in the state. They may be working on an associate, baccalaureate, master's, or doctoral degree. Preference is given to perioperative nurses returning to school in south Florida. Undergraduates must have a GPA of 2.5 or higher and graduate students a GPA of 3.0 or higher. Along with their application, they must submit 1-page essays on 1) why it is necessary for them to receive this scholarship; and 2) their goals and their assessment of their potential for making a contribution to nursing and society.

Financial Data A stipend is awarded (amount not specified).
Duration 1 semester or year.
Number awarded 1 or more each year.
Deadline May of each year.

[99]
ELIZABETH GARDE NATIONAL SCHOLARSHIP

Danish Sisterhood of America
Attn: Donna Hansen, Scholarship Chair
1605 South 58th Street
Lincoln, NE 68506
(402) 488-5820   E-mail: djhansen@windstream.net
Web: www.danishsisterhood.org/dssScholGrant.asp

Summary To provide financial assistance for nursing or medical education to members or relatives of members of the Danish Sisterhood of America.

Eligibility This program is open to members or the family of members of the sisterhood who have been members for at least 1 year. Applicants must be working on an undergraduate or graduate degree in the nursing or medical profession. They must have a GPA of 3.0 or higher.

Financial Data The stipend is $850.
Duration 1 year; nonrenewable.
Number awarded 1 each year.
Deadline February of each year.

[100]
EMILY S. GARRISON NURSING SCHOLARSHIP

United Methodist Church-Greater New Jersey Conference
Conference Board of Higher Education and Ministry
Attn: Scholarship Committee
1001 Wickapecko Drive
Ocean, NJ 07712-4733
(732) 359-1040   Toll Free: (877) 677-2594, ext. 1040
Fax: (732) 359-1049   E-mail: Lperez@gnjumc.org
Web: www.gnjumc.org/grants_loans_and_scholarship

Summary To provide financial assistance to members of United Methodist Churches in New Jersey who are attending college in any state to prepare for a career in nursing.

Eligibility This program is open to members of congregations affiliated with the Greater New Jersey Conference of the United Methodist Church. Applicants must be enrolled in a program in any state leading to a bachelor's degree in nursing to prepare for a nursing career. Along with their application, they must submit a

statement on why they wish to be considered for this scholarship, including information on their financial need and Christian commitment.

Financial Data A stipend is awarded (amount not specified).
Duration 1 year.
Additional data This program is sponsored by Greater New Jersey Conference United Methodist Women.
Number awarded 1 each year.
Deadline March of each year.

[101]
EPILEPSY FOUNDATION BEHAVIORAL SCIENCES STUDENT FELLOWSHIPS

Epilepsy Foundation
Attn: Research Department
8301 Professional Place
Landover, MD 20785-2237
(301) 459-3700   Toll Free: (800) EFA-1000
Fax: (301) 577-2684   TDD: (800) 332-2070
E-mail: grants@efa.org
Web: www.epilepsyfoundation.org/research/grants.cfm

Summary To provide funding to undergraduate and graduate students interested in working on a summer research training project in a behavioral science field relevant to epilepsy.

Eligibility This program is open to undergraduate and graduate students in a behavioral science program relevant to epilepsy research or clinical care, including, but not limited to, sociology, social work, psychology, anthropology, nursing, economics, vocational rehabilitation, counseling, and political science. Applicants must be interested in working on an epilepsy research project under the supervision of a qualified mentor. Because the program is designed as a training opportunity, the quality of the training plans and environment are considered in the selection process. Other selection criteria include the quality of the proposed project, the relevance of the proposed work to epilepsy, the applicant's interest in the field of epilepsy, the applicant's qualifications, and the mentor's qualifications, including his or her commitment to the student and the project. U.S. citizenship is not required, but the project must be conducted in the United States. Applications from women, members of minority groups, and people with disabilities are especially encouraged. The program is not intended for students working on a dissertation research project.

Financial Data The grant is $3,000.
Duration 3 months during the summer.
Additional data This program is supported by the American Epilepsy Society, Abbott Laboratories, Ortho-McNeil Pharmaceutical Corporation, and Pfizer Inc.
Number awarded Varies each year.
Deadline February of each year.

[102]
ERNESTINE F. SHAW ENDOWED SCHOLARSHIP

Kansas State Nurses Association
Attn: Kansas Nurses Foundation
1109 S.W. Topeka Boulevard
Topeka, KS 66612-1602
(785) 233-8638   Fax: (785) 233-5222
E-mail: ksna@ksna.net
Web: www.nursingworld.org/SNAS/KS/Knf.htm

Summary To provide financial assistance to residents of Kansas who are working on a degree in nursing at the undergraduate, master's, or doctoral level at a school in the state.

Eligibility This program is open to students who are working on a nursing degree on the undergraduate or graduate level at a school in Kansas. Preference is given to residents of Sedgwick and Sumner counties. Applicants must have a GPA of 3.0 or higher. Along with their application, they must submit a personal narrative describing their anticipated role in nursing in the state of

Kansas. Preference is given to full-time students. The following priority is used in awarding scholarships: 1) students enrolled in undergraduate R.N. nursing programs; 2) R.N.s working on B.S.N.s; and 3) graduate and postgraduate nursing students.

Financial Data The stipend is $500.

Duration 1 year.

Additional data This program was established in 2008.

Number awarded 1 each year.

Deadline June of each year.

[103]
ETHICON UNDERGRADUATE SCHOLARSHIPS

Emergency Nurses Association
Attn: ENA Foundation
915 Lee Street
Des Plaines, IL 60016-6569
(847) 460-4100   Toll Free: (800) 900-9659, ext. 4100
Fax: (847) 460-4004   E-mail: foundation@ena.org
Web: www.ena.org

Summary To provide financial assistance for baccalaureate study to nurses who are members of the Emergency Nurses Association (ENA).

Eligibility This program is open to nurses (R.N., L.P.N., L.V.N.) who are working on a bachelor's degree. Applicants must have been members of the association for at least 12 months and have a GPA of 3.0 or higher. They must submit a 1-page statement on their professional and educational goals and how this scholarship will help them attain those goals. Selection is based on content and clarity of the goal statement (45%), professional association involvement (35%), presentation of the application (10%), and letters of reference (10%).

Financial Data The stipend is $2,500.

Duration 1 year; nonrenewable.

Additional data This program is supported by Ethicon, Inc.

Number awarded 4 each year.

Deadline May of each year.

[104]
EUNICE M. SMITH SCHOLARSHIPS

North Carolina Nurses Association
Attn: North Carolina Foundation for Nursing
103 Enterprise Street
P.O. Box 12025
Raleigh, NC 27605-2025
(919) 821-4250   Toll Free: (800) 626-2153
Fax: (919) 829-5807   E-mail: rns@ncnurses.org
Web: www.ncnurses.org/ncfn.asp

Summary To provide financial assistance to registered nurses in North Carolina who are interested in pursing additional education on a part-time basis.

Eligibility This program is open to registered nurses in North Carolina who are interested in pursuing additional education at the baccalaureate, master's, or doctoral level on a part-time basis. Applicants must be North Carolina residents (for at least 12 months prior to application), must be admitted to a program in North Carolina offering a nursing degree on the baccalaureate, master's, or Ph.D. level, must be enrolled part time but for at least 6 hours per semester, and must have a cumulative GPA of 3.0 or higher. Selection is based on GPA, professional involvement, community involvement, potential for contribution to the profession, and honors and certifications. Preference is given to members of the North Carolina Nurses Association.

Financial Data The stipend is $2,500 per year for graduate students or $1,000 per year for undergraduates.

Duration 1 year.

Additional data This program was established in 1995.

Number awarded 1 or more each year.

Deadline May of each year.

[105]
EVA VIEIRA MEMORIAL SCHOLARSHIP

Luso-American Education Foundation
Attn: Administrative Director
7080 Donlon Way, Suite 202
P.O. Box 2967
Dublin, CA 94568
(925) 828-3883   Fax: (925) 828-3883
E-mail: odom@luso-american.org
Web: www.luso-american.org

Summary To provide financial assistance to high school seniors in California who are of Portuguese descent and interested in studying nursing at a school in any state.

Eligibility This program is open to seniors graduating from high schools in California who are of Portuguese descent. Applicants must be planning to enroll at a 4-year college or university in any state that has an accredited nursing program. They must have a GPA of 3.0 or higher. Along with their application, they must submit transcripts, SAT or ACT scores, and 3 letters of recommendation. Special consideration is given to 1) first generation college-bound students, and 2) students from a farming family.

Financial Data The stipend is $1,000.

Duration 1 year; may be renewed up to 3 additional years.

Number awarded 1 each year.

Deadline February of each year.

[106]
EVELYN JOHNSON ENTREKIN SCHOLARSHIP

South Carolina Nurses Foundation, Inc.
Attn: Awards Committee Chair
1821 Gadsden Street
Columbia, SC 29201
(803) 252-4781   Fax: (803) 779-3870
E-mail: brownk1@aol.com
Web: www.scnursesfoundation.org/index_files/Page316.htm

Summary To provide financial assistance to nursing students enrolled in a bachelor's degree program in South Carolina.

Eligibility This program is open to residents of South Carolina who are entering their junior or senior year of a bachelor of science in nursing program in the state. Applicants must have a GPA of 3.0 or higher and be able to demonstrate financial need. They must intend to seek employment in South Carolina after graduation.

Financial Data The stipend is $1,500.

Duration 1 year.

Number awarded 1 or 2 each year.

Deadline May of each year.

[107]
FADONA/LTC SCHOLARSHIP

Florida Association Directors of Nursing Administration/Long Term Care
200 Butler Street, Suite 305
West Palm Beach, FL 33407
(561) 659-2167   Fax: (561) 659-1291
E-mail: fadona@fadona.org
Web: www.fadona.org/scholarship.html

Summary To provide financial assistance to individuals employed in long-term care in Florida who are interested in continuing their education.

Eligibility This program is open to currently licensed R.N.s, L.P.N.s, or certified nursing assistants (C.N.A.s) employed in the long-term care industry in Florida. R.N.s must be currently accepted or enrolled in a baccalaureate or master's degree program in nursing, gerontology program, undergraduate or graduate program in health care management, or nurse practitioner program. L.P.N.s must be currently accepted or enrolled in an R.N. program or undergraduate health care management program. C.N.A.s must be currently accepted or enrolled in an R.N. or L.P.N. program. All applicants must have at least 2 years of employment in the long-term care field (a list of employers and dates of employment is required). They must be either a member of the Florida Association Directors of Nursing Administration/ Long Term Care or sponsored by a member. Financial need is not considered in the selection process.

Financial Data The stipend is at least $500. Funds are paid directly to the college, university, or accredited L.P.N. school.

Duration 1 year.

Number awarded 1 or more each year.

Deadline October of each year.

[108]
FILIPINO NURSES' ORGANIZATION OF HAWAII SCHOLARSHIP

Hawai'i Community Foundation
Attn: Scholarship Department
1164 Bishop Street, Suite 800
Honolulu, HI 96813
(808) 566-5570   Toll Free: (888) 731-3863
Fax: (808) 521-6286   E-mail: scholarships@hcf-hawaii.org
Web: www.hawaiicommunityfoundation.org

Summary To provide financial assistance to Hawaii residents of Filipino ancestry who are interested in preparing for a career as a nurse.

Eligibility This program is open to Hawaii residents of Filipino ancestry who are interested in studying in Hawaii or the mainland as full-time undergraduate or graduate students and majoring in nursing. They must be able to demonstrate academic achievement (GPA of 2.7 or higher), good moral character, and financial need. Along with their application, they must submit a short statement indicating their reasons for attending college, their planned course of study, and their career goals.

Financial Data The amounts of the awards depend on the availability of funds and the need of the recipient; recently, stipends averaged $1,000.

Duration 1 year.

Number awarded Varies each year; recently, 2 of these scholarships were awarded.

Deadline February of each year.

[109]
FLORENCE WHIPPLE SCHOLARSHIP

Idaho Nurses Association
Attn: Idaho Nurses Foundation
3525 Piedmont Road
Building 5, Suite 300
Atlanta, GA 30305
(404) 760-2803   Toll Free: (888) 721-8904
Fax: (404) 240-0998   E-mail: ed@idahonurses.org
Web: www.idahonurses.org

Summary To provide financial assistance to members of the Idaho Nurses Association (INA) and other residents of Idaho who are interested in obtaining training in nursing.

Eligibility This program is open to 1) INA members who are registered nurses and have been accepted to an accredited school of nursing to work on an advanced degree, and 2) residents of Idaho who are interesting in continuing their education at a school of nursing in or outside of Idaho. Applicants must be able to demonstrate financial need and a potential for making a definite contribution to nursing.

Financial Data The stipend varies; recently, it was $646.

Duration 1 year; may be renewed up to 2 additional years.

Additional data This program was established in 1956 as the Florence Whipple Scholarship and Loan Fund. The loan program was eventually closed.

Number awarded Varies each year; recently, 5 of these scholarships were awarded.

Deadline Deadline not specified.

[110]
FLORIDA NURSES FOUNDATION SCHOLARSHIPS

Florida Nurses Association
Attn: Florida Nurses Foundation
1235 East Concord Street
P.O. Box 536985
Orlando, FL 32853-6985
(407) 896-3261   Fax: (407) 896-9042
E-mail: foundation@floridanurse.org
Web: www.floridanurse.org/foundationGrants/index.asp

Summary To provide financial assistance to Florida residents who are interested in working on an undergraduate or graduate degree in nursing.

Eligibility Applicants must have been Florida residents for at least 1 year and have completed at least 1 semester at an accredited nursing program in the state. They may be working on an associate, baccalaureate, master's, or doctoral degree. Undergraduates must have a GPA of 2.5 or higher and graduate students a GPA of 3.0 or higher. Along with their application, they must submit 1-page essays on 1) why it is necessary for them to receive this scholarship; and 2) their goals and their assessment of their potential for making a contribution to nursing and society.

Financial Data A stipend is awarded (amount not specified).

Duration 1 semester or year.

Additional data This program includes the following named programs open to all qualified applicants: the Edna Hicks Fund Scholarships, the Mary York Scholarships, the Undine Sams and Friends Scholarships, and the Ruth Finamore Scholarships.

Number awarded Varies each year.

Deadline May of each year.

[111]
FLORIDA NURSING STUDENTS ASSOCIATION FINANCIAL NEED SCHOLARSHIPS

Florida Nursing Students Association
c/o Florida Nurses Association
P.O. Box 536985
Orlando, FL 32853-6985
(408) 896-3261   Fax: (408) 896-9042
Web: www.fnsa.net/resource/scholarships

Summary To provide financial assistance to students from any state who are enrolled at nursing schools in Florida.

Eligibility This program is open to students from any state who are currently enrolled at a school of nursing in Florida. Applicants must be able to demonstrate financial need.

Financial Data The stipend depends on the need of the recipient.

Duration 1 year.

Additional data This program is sponsored by the Florida Nurses Association Foundation.

Number awarded Several each year.

Deadline October of each year.

[112]
FOUNDATION FOR NEONATAL RESEARCH AND EDUCATION SCHOLARSHIPS

Academy of Neonatal Nursing
Attn: Foundation for Neonatal Research and Education
200 East Holly Avenue
P.O. Box 56
Pitman, NJ 08071-0056
(856) 256-2343   Fax: (856) 589-7463
E-mail: FNRE@ajj.com
Web: www.inurse.com/fnre/scholarship.htm

Summary To provide financial assistance to neonatal nurses interested in working on a degree.
Eligibility Applicants must be professionally active neonatal nurses engaged in a service, research, or educational role that contributes directly to the health care of neonates or to the neonatal nursing profession. They must be an active member of a professional association dedicated to enhancing neonatal nursing and the care of neonates. Participation in ongoing professional education in neonatal nursing must be demonstrated by at least 10 contact hours in neonatal content over the past 24 months. Qualified nurses must have been admitted to a college or school of higher education to work on 1 of the following: bachelor of science in nursing, master of science in nursing for advanced practice in neonatal nursing, doctoral degree in nursing, or master's or post-master's degree in nursing administration or business management. They must have a GPA of 3.0 or higher. Along with their application, they must submit a 250-word statement on how they plan to make a significant difference in neonatal nursing practice. Financial need is not considered in the selection process.
Financial Data The stipends are $1,500 or $1,000.
Duration 1 year.
Additional data The Foundation for Neonatal Research and Education was established in 1992 by the National Association of Neonatal Nurses (NANN), 2270 Northpoint Parkway, Santa Rosa, CA 95407, (707) 568-2168. Originally housed at the NANN office, it moved to its current location in 1998.
Number awarded Varies each year.
Deadline April of each year.

[113]
FRANCES W. HARRIS SCHOLARSHIP

New England Regional Black Nurses Association, Inc.
P.O. Box 190690
Boston, MA 02119
(617) 524-1951
Web: www.nerbna.org/org/scholarships.html

Summary To provide financial assistance to nursing students from New England who have contributed to the African American community.
Eligibility The program is open to residents of the New England states who are enrolled full time in a NLN-accredited generic diploma, associate, or bachelor's nursing program in any state. Applicants must have at least 1 full year of school remaining. Along with their application, they must submit a 3-page essay that covers their career aspirations in the nursing profession; how they have contributed to the African American or other communities of color in such areas as work, volunteering, church, or community outreach; an experience that has enhanced their personal and/or professional growth; and any financial hardships that may hinder them from completing their education.
Financial Data A stipend is awarded (amount not specified).
Duration 1 year.
Number awarded 1 or more each year.
Deadline March of each year.

[114]
FRANK LANZA MEMORIAL SCHOLARSHIPS

Phi Theta Kappa
Attn: Scholarship Programs Director
1625 Eastover Drive
P.O. Box 13729
Jackson, MS 39236-3729
(601) 984-3539   Fax: (601) 984-3546
E-mail: scholarship.programs@ptk.org
Web: www.ptk.org/scholarships/franklanza

Summary To provide financial assistance to community college students who are working on an associate degree in registered nursing, respiratory care, or emergency medical services.
Eligibility This program is open to full-time students, part-time students, and international students who have completed at least 50% of the course work for an associate degree in registered nursing, respiratory care, or emergency medical services at an accredited community college. Pre-major students, certificate students, and students who already have an associate or higher degree are not eligible. Applicants must have a GPA of 3.0 or higher and be able to demonstrate financial need.
Financial Data The stipend is $1,000.
Duration 1 year.
Additional data Funds for this program, which began in 2009, are supplied by Medical Education Technologies, Inc., L-3 Communications, the American Association of Community Colleges, and Phi Theta Kappa.
Number awarded Up to 25 each year.
Deadline October of each year.

[115]
FRIENDS OF NURSING SCHOLARSHIPS

Friends of Nursing
Attn: Scholarship Chair
P.O. Box 735
Englewood, CO 80151-0735
(303) 449-5318   E-mail: asmith2498@aol.com
Web: www.friendsofnursing.org/scholarships.htm

Summary To provide financial assistance to residents of any state who are working on an undergraduate or graduate degree in nursing at a school in Colorado.
Eligibility This program is open to registered nurses and nursing students who are residents of any state and working on a B.S.N. or higher degree at an NLN-accredited school of nursing in Colorado. Applicants must be enrolled at least as juniors and have a GPA of 3.0 or higher. Along with their application, they must submit a 3-page essay in which they identify a health care issue in Colorado that they believe will have a major impact on nursing in the future, a discussion of their professional nursing beliefs, and a description of their career goals (including how they anticipate their education or research will contribute or help them achieve those goals). Financial need is considered in the selection process.
Financial Data A stipend is awarded (amount not specified).
Duration 1 year.
Number awarded 1 or more each year.
Deadline October of each year.

[116]
GALLAGHER KOSTER HEALTH CAREERS SCHOLARSHIP PROGRAM

Gallagher Koster
Attn: Scholarship
500 Victory Road
Quincy, MA 02171
(617) 770-9889   Toll Free: (800) 457-5599
Fax: (617) 479-0860
E-mail: scholarship@gallagherkoster.com
Web: www.gallagherkoster.com/scholarship

Summary To provide financial assistance to undergraduate students working on a degree in a health-related field.
Eligibility This program is open to full-time undergraduates entering their second-to-last or final year of study in a health-related field, including (but not limited to) pre-medicine, nursing, public and community health, physical therapy, occupational therapy, pharmacy, biology, chemistry, physiology, social work, dentistry, or optometry. Applicants must have a GPA of 3.0 or higher and be able to demonstrate financial need. Along with their appli-

cation, they must submit a 1-page essay describing their personal goals, including their reasons for preparing for a career in health care. Selection is based on motivation to pursue a career in health care, academic excellence, dedication to community service, and financial need.

Financial Data The stipend is $5,000 per year.

Duration 1 year; may be renewed 1 additional year.

Additional data This program began in 2001.

Number awarded 5 each year.

Deadline May of each year.

[117]
GARDNER FOUNDATION INS EDUCATION SCHOLARSHIP

Infusion Nurses Society
Attn: Gardner Foundation
315 Norwood Park South
Norwood, MA 02062
(781) 440-9408   Toll Free: (800) 694-0298
Fax: (781) 440-9409   E-mail: ins@ins1.org
Web: www.ins1.org/i4a/pages/index.cfm?pageid=3344

Summary To provide financial assistance to members of the Infusion Nurses Society (INS) who are interested in continuing their education.

Eligibility This program is open to INS members interested in a program of continuing education, including working on a college or graduate degree or attending a professional meeting or seminar. Applicants must demonstrate how the continuing education activity will enhance their infusion career, describe their professional goals, and explain how the scholarship will be used.

Financial Data The stipend is $1,000.

Duration This is a 1-time award.

Number awarded 2 each year.

Deadline January of each year.

[118]
GAY WALLENTINE MEMORIAL NURSES SCHOLARSHIP

St. Alexius Foundation
Attn: Department of Development
900 East Broadway Avenue
P.O. Box 5510
Bismarck, ND 58506-5510
(701) 530-7065   Fax: (701) 530-8984
TDD: (701) 530-5555
Web: www.st.alexius.org

Summary To provide financial assistance to North Dakota residents interested in working on a nursing degree.

Eligibility Nursing students who are residents of North Dakota are eligible to apply.

Financial Data Typically, the stipend ranges from $500 to $1,500 each year, depending upon the interest earned by the endowment.

Duration 1 year, beginning in September.

Additional data This scholarship is named for a former director of critical care services at the St. Alexius Medical Center.

Number awarded 1 each year.

Deadline May of each year.

[119]
GENEVIEVE SARAN RICHMOND AWARD

ExceptionalNurse.com
Attn: Scholarship Committee
13019 Coastal Circle
Palm Beach Gardens, FL 33410
(561) 627-9872   Fax: (561) 776-9254
TDD: (561) 776-9442   E-mail: ExceptionalNurse@aol.com
Web: www.ExceptionalNurse.com/scholarship.php

Summary To provide financial assistance to nursing students who have a disability.

Eligibility This program is open to students with a documented disability who have applied to, or have already been admitted to, a college or university nursing program on a full-time basis. Applicants must submit an essay on how they plan to contribute to the nursing profession and how their disability will influence their practice as a nurse. Selection is based on the essay, transcripts of high school and/or college courses completed, activities and honors received, 3 letters of recommendation, and financial need.

Financial Data The stipend is $500.

Duration 1 year; nonrenewable.

Number awarded 1 each year.

Deadline May of each year.

[120]
GEORGE B. BOLAND NURSES TRAINING TRUST FUND

National Forty and Eight
Attn: Voiture Nationale
777 North Meridian Street
Indianapolis, IN 46204-1170
(317) 634-1804   Fax: (317) 632-9365
E-mail: voiturenationale@msn.com
Web: fortyandeight.org/40_8programs.htm

Summary To provide financial assistance to students working on an undergraduate degree in nursing.

Eligibility This program is open to students working full time on an associate or bachelor's degree in nursing. Applications must be submitted to the local Voiture of the Forty and Eight in the county of student's permanent residence; if the county organization has exhausted all of its nurses training funds, it will provide the student with an application for this scholarship. Students who are receiving assistance from the Eight and Forty Lung and Respiratory Disease Nursing Scholarship Program of the American Legion are not eligible. Financial need must be demonstrated.

Financial Data Grants may be used to cover tuition, required fees, room and board or similar living expenses, and other school-related expenses.

Additional data National Forty and Eight is the Honor Society of the American Legion. Students may not apply directly to the National Forty and Eight for these scholarships.

Number awarded Varies each year; recently, 2,131 students received more than $1,100,000 in these scholarships.

Deadline Deadline not specified.

[121]
GEORGE GUSTAFSON HSE MEMORIAL SCHOLARSHIP

American Society of Safety Engineers
Attn: ASSE Foundation
1800 East Oakton Street
Des Plaines, IL 60018
(847) 768-3435   Fax: (847) 768-3434
E-mail: agabanski@asse.org
Web: www.asse.org/foundation/scholarships/scholarships.php

Summary To provide financial assistance to upper-division and graduate student members of the American Society of Safety Engineers (ASSE), especially those from Texas.

Eligibility This program is open to ASSE student members who are working on an undergraduate or graduate degree in occupational safety, health, and environment or a closely-related field (e.g., industrial or environmental engineering, environmental science, industrial hygiene, occupational health nursing). Priority is given to residents of Texas or students attending a university in the state. Undergraduates must be full-time students who have completed at least 60 semester hours with a GPA of 3.0 or higher. Graduate students must also be enrolled full time, have completed at least 9 semester hours with a GPA of 3.5 or higher, and have earned a GPA of 3.0 or higher as an undergraduate. Along with their application, they must submit 2 essays of 300 words or less: 1) why they are seeking a degree in occupational safety and health or a closely-related field, a brief description of their current activities, and how those relate to their career goals and objectives; and 2) why they should be awarded this scholarship (including career goals and financial need). U.S. citizenship is not required.

Financial Data The stipend is $2,500 per year.

Duration 1 year; recipients may reapply.

Additional data This program, established in 2006, is supported by the Texas Safety Foundation.

Number awarded 1 each year.

Deadline November of each year.

[122]
GEORGIA ANN BERNARD HALL AWARD FOR EXCELLENCE

Mississippi Nurses Association
Attn: Mississippi Nurses Foundation
31 Woodgreen Place
Madison, MS 39110
(601) 898-0850   Fax: (601) 898-0190
E-mail: foundation@msnurses.org
Web: msnursesfoundation.com/scholarships

Summary To provide financial assistance to African American students enrolled at Mississippi schools of nursing.

Eligibility This program is open to African American residents of Mississippi currently enrolled as juniors or seniors at a public school of nursing in the state. Applicants must be members of the Mississippi Association of Student Nurses and working on a B.S.N. degree. Along with their application, they must submit a 3-page essay on their role model of excellence. Selection is based on that essay, school of nursing activities, community activities, and awards and honors.

Financial Data The stipend is $500.

Duration 1 year.

Number awarded 1 each year.

Deadline September of each year.

[123]
GEORGIA CHAPTER ANNUAL SCHOLARSHIP

American Society of Safety Engineers
Attn: ASSE Foundation
1800 East Oakton Street
Des Plaines, IL 60018
(847) 768-3435   Fax: (847) 768-3434
E-mail: agabanski@asse.org
Web: www.asse.org/foundation/scholarships/scholarships.php

Summary To provide financial assistance to upper-division student members of the American Society of Safety Engineers (ASSE) from Georgia.

Eligibility This program is open to ASSE student members who are majoring in occupational safety, health, and environment or a closely-related field (e.g., industrial or environmental engineering, environmental science, industrial hygiene, occupational health nursing). Applicants must be residents of Georgia, although they may attend school in any state. They must be full-

time students who have completed at least 60 semester hours with a GPA of 3.0 or higher. Along with their application, they must submit 2 essays of 300 words or less: 1) why they are seeking a degree in occupational safety and health or a closely-related field, a brief description of their current activities, and how those relate to their career goals and objectives; and 2) why they should be awarded this scholarship (including career goals and financial need). U.S. citizenship is not required.

Financial Data The stipend is $2,000 per year.

Duration 1 year; recipients may reapply.

Number awarded 1 each year.

Deadline November of each year.

[124]
GEORGIA LEGION AUXILIARY PAST PRESIDENT PARLEY NURSING SCHOLARSHIP

American Legion Auxiliary
Department of Georgia
3035 Mt. Zion Road
Stockbridge, GA 30281-4101
(678) 289-8446   E-mail: amlegaux@bellsouth.net
Web: www.galegion.org/auxiliary.htm

Summary To provide financial assistance to daughters of veterans in Georgia who are interested in attending college in any state to prepare for a career in nursing.

Eligibility This program is open to George residents who are 1) interested in nursing education and 2) the daughters of veterans. Applicants must be sponsored by a local unit of the American Legion Auxiliary. Selection is based on a statement explaining why they want to become a nurse and why they need a scholarship, a transcript of all high school or college grades, and 4 letters of recommendation (1 from a high school principal or superintendent, 1 from the sponsoring American Legion Auxiliary local unit, and 2 from other responsible people).

Financial Data The amount of the award depends on the availability of funds.

Number awarded Varies, depending upon funds available.

Deadline May of each year.

[125]
GEORGIA NURSES FOUNDATION SCHOLARSHIPS

Georgia Nurses Foundation, Inc.
Attn: Scholarship Committee
3032 Briarcliff Road, N.E.
Atlanta, GA 30329-2655
(404) 325-5536   Toll Free: (800) 324-0462
Fax: (404) 325-0407   E-mail: gnf@georgianurses.org
Web: www.georgianurses.org/scholarship_appl.htm

Summary To provide financial assistance to Georgia residents who are working on a nursing degree, at any level, at an accredited school, college, or university.

Eligibility This program is open to residents of Georgia who are currently enrolled (full or part time) in an NLN-accredited program in nursing. Applicants may be working on a degree at any level (including associate, baccalaureate, master's, or doctoral). They must have a GPA of 2.5 or higher and be able to document financial need. Priority is given to applicants who meet the following criteria: enrolled in a Georgia school, plan to practice professional nursing in Georgia following graduation, and belong to a professional organization (e.g., Georgia Association of Nursing Students, Georgia Nurses Association, Georgia Association for Nursing Education).

Financial Data The stipend is at least $500. Funds may be sent directly to the recipient.

Duration 1 year.

Number awarded Varies each year.

Deadline June of each year.

[126]
GERALDINE GEE NURSING FUND SCHOLARSHIP

Greater Kanawha Valley Foundation
Attn: Scholarship Coordinator
1600 Huntington Square
900 Lee Street, East
P.O. Box 3041
Charleston, WV 25331-3041
(304) 346-3620   Toll Free: (800) 467-5909
Fax: (304) 346-3640   E-mail: shoover@tgkvf.org
Web: www.tgkvf.org/scholar.htm

Summary To provide financial assistance to residents of West Virginia who are working on a degree in nursing at a school in any state.

Eligibility This program is open to residents of West Virginia who are have completed at least their freshman year of a nursing program at a college or university anywhere in the country. Preference is given to residents of Boone County. Applicants must have an ACT score of 20 or higher, be able to demonstrate good moral character and financial need, and have a GPA of 2.5 or higher.

Financial Data The stipend is $500 per year.

Duration 1 year; may be renewed provided the recipient maintains a GPA of 3.0 or higher.

Number awarded 1 or more each year.

Deadline January of each year.

[127]
GERALDINE K. MORRIS AWARD

Army Engineer Officers' Wives' Club
c/o Nancy Temple, Chair
P.O. Box 6332
Alexandria, VA 22306-6332
E-mail: scholarships@aeowc.com
Web: www.aeowc.com/scholarships.html

Summary To provide financial assistance to the children of officers and civilians who served in the Army Corps of Engineers and are interested in studying nursing in college.

Eligibility This program is open to children of 1) U.S. Army Corps of Engineers officers and warrant officers who are on active duty, retired, or deceased while on active duty or after retiring from active duty; or 2) civilians (GS-1 through GS-9) assigned to U.S. Army Corps of Engineers. Applicants must be high school seniors planning to enroll in a program leading to a nursing degree or certification. Selection is based on academic and extracurricular achievement during high school. U.S. citizenship is required.

Financial Data The stipend ranges from $1,000 to $2,000.

Duration 1 year.

Additional data This program was established in 2006.

Number awarded 1 each year.

Deadline February of each year.

[128]
GERRIE HELWIG SCHOLARSHIP

Florida Council of periOperative Registered Nurses
c/o Carol Morris, Scholarship Chair
223 S.E. Ninth Terrace
Cape Coral, FL 33990
(239) 458-8539   E-mail: Christmascat721@aol.com

Summary To provide financial assistance to nursing students interested in preparing for a career as a perioperative nurse.

Eligibility This program is open to students in Florida who have completed at least 2 semesters in an accredited nursing program. Applicants must have a GPA of 3.0 or higher and be planning to work in a perioperative setting after graduation. They must be planning to complete (or already have completed) an internship in perioperative nursing. Along with their application, they must sub-mit a 250-word essay on their reasons for entering a career in perioperative nursing. Selection is based on the essay, professional activities, civic and school activities, and work experience. Financial need is not considered.

Financial Data The stipend is $500.

Duration 1 year.

Number awarded 1 or more each year.

Deadline September of each year.

[129]
GLENN AND GRETA SNELL ENDOWMENT FUND SCHOLARSHIP

Kansas State Nurses Association
Attn: Kansas Nurses Foundation
1109 S.W. Topeka Boulevard
Topeka, KS 66612-1602
(785) 233-8638   Fax: (785) 233-5222
E-mail: ksna@ksna.net
Web: www.nursingworld.org/SNAS/KS/Knf.htm

Summary To provide financial assistance to residents of Kansas who are working on a degree in nursing at the undergraduate, master's, or doctoral level at a school in the state.

Eligibility This program is open to students who are working on a nursing degree on the undergraduate or graduate level at a school in Kansas. Applicants must have a GPA of 3.0 or higher. Along with their application, they must submit a personal narrative describing their anticipated role in nursing in the state of Kansas. Preference is given to full-time students. The following priority is used in awarding scholarships: 1) students enrolled in undergraduate R.N. nursing programs and employed by Hutchinson Hospital; 2) R.N.s working on B.S.N.s and employed by Hutchinson Hospital; 3) R.N.s accepted by a nursing program to prepare for a faculty position in Kansas; and 4) R.N.s with a B.S.N. and accepted by a graduate program with a major in nursing supervision or administration for a position in Kansas.

Financial Data The stipend is $1,000.

Duration 1 year.

Number awarded 1 each year.

Deadline June of each year.

[130]
GOLD COUNTRY SECTION AND REGION II SCHOLARSHIP

American Society of Safety Engineers
Attn: ASSE Foundation
1800 East Oakton Street
Des Plaines, IL 60018
(847) 768-3435   Fax: (847) 768-3434
E-mail: agabanski@asse.org
Web: www.asse.org/foundation/scholarships/scholarships.php

Summary To provide financial assistance to upper-division and graduate student members of the American Society of Safety Engineers (ASSE) from designated western states.

Eligibility This program is open to ASSE student members who are working on an undergraduate or graduate degree in occupational safety, health, and environment or a closely-related field (e.g., industrial or environmental engineering, environmental science, industrial hygiene, occupational health nursing). Priority is given to residents of ASSE Region II (Arizona, Colorado, Idaho, Montana, Nevada, New Mexico, Utah, and Wyoming). Undergraduates must be full-time students who have completed at least 60 semester hours with a GPA of 3.0 or higher. Graduate students must also be enrolled full time, have completed at least 9 semester hours with a GPA of 3.5 or higher, and have had a GPA of 3.0 or higher as an undergraduate. Along with their application, they must submit 2 essays of 300 words or less: 1) why they are seeking a degree in occupational safety and health or a closely-related field, a brief description of their current activities, and how those relate to their career goals and objectives; and 2) why they should be awarded this scholarship (including career goals and financial need). U.S. citizenship is not required.

Financial Data The stipend is $1,000 per year.

Duration 1 year; recipients may reapply.

Number awarded 1 each year.

Deadline November of each year.

[131]
GOOD SAMARITAN FOUNDATION SCHOLARSHIPS

Good Samaritan Foundation
5615 Kirby Drive, Suite 308
Houston, TX 77005
(713) 529-4646   Fax: (713) 521-1169
Web: www.gsftx.org/scholarships

Summary To provide financial assistance to student nurses enrolled in a program in nursing at an accredited university in Texas.

Eligibility This program is open to residents of Texas who have attained the clinical level of their nursing education. Applicants must be enrolled at an institution in Texas in an accredited nursing program at the L.V.N., Diploma, A.D.N., B.S.N., M.S.N., Ph.D., D.S.N., or D.N.P. level. They must be U.S. citizens or eligible to work in the United States and be planning to work as a nurse in Texas after graduation. Financial need is considered in the selection process. A personal interview is required.

Financial Data Scholarship awards may be used for clinical education expenses: tuition, fees, books, and some copying and seminars. Undergraduate awards are based on the amount of the tuition fees of that school and its nursing program. Graduate awards are paid on a reimbursement basis up to a pre-determined amount per semester.

Duration 1 year.

Additional data This program began in 1951.

Number awarded Varies each year. Since the program began, it has awarded more than 12,000 scholarships worth more than $14.6 million.

Deadline There are no formal deadlines, but applications should be received at least 8 weeks before the start of the semester.

[132]
GREATER BOSTON CHAPTER LEADERSHIP AWARD

American Society of Safety Engineers
Attn: ASSE Foundation
1800 East Oakton Street
Des Plaines, IL 60018
(847) 768-3435   Fax: (847) 768-3434
E-mail: agabanski@asse.org
Web: www.asse.org/foundation/scholarships/scholarships.php

Summary To provide financial assistance to upper-division and graduate students at colleges and universities in New England who are members or family of members of the American Society of Safety Engineers (ASSE).

Eligibility This program is open to undergraduate and graduate students who are working on a degree in occupational safety, health, and environment or a closely-related field (e.g., industrial or environmental engineering, environmental science, industrial hygiene, occupational health nursing). Applicants must be 1) a member of an ASSE chapter in New England; 2) the spouse or child of an ASSE chapter member in New England; or 3) a member of an ASSE student section in New England. Undergraduates must be full-time students who have completed at least 60 semester hours with a GPA of 3.0 or higher. Graduate students must also be enrolled full time, have completed at least 9 semester hours with a GPA of 3.5 or higher, and have earned a GPA of 3.0 or higher as an undergraduate. Along with their application,

they must submit 2 essays of 300 words or less: 1) why they are seeking a degree in occupational safety and health or a closely-related field, a brief description of their current activities, and how those relate to their career goals and objectives; and 2) why they should be awarded this scholarship (including career goals and financial need). U.S. citizenship is not required.

Financial Data Stipends are $2,000 or $1,000 per year.

Duration 1 year; recipients may reapply.

Number awarded 2 each year: 1 at $2,000 and 1 at $1,000.

Deadline November of each year.

[133]
GREATER CHICAGO CHAPTER SCHOLARSHIP

American Society of Safety Engineers
Attn: ASSE Foundation
1800 East Oakton Street
Des Plaines, IL 60018
(847) 768-3435   Fax: (847) 768-3434
E-mail: agabanski@asse.org
Web: www.asse.org/foundation/scholarships/scholarships.php

Summary To provide financial assistance to upper-division and graduate student members of the American Society of Safety Engineers (ASSE) from designated midwestern states.

Eligibility This program is open to ASSE student members who are working on an undergraduate or graduate degree in occupational safety, health, and environment or a closely-related field (e.g., industrial or environmental engineering, environmental science, industrial hygiene, occupational health nursing). Priority is given to students who reside or attend school in ASSE Region V (Illinois, Iowa, Kansas, Minnesota, Missouri, Nebraska, North Dakota, South Dakota, and Wisconsin). Undergraduates must be full-time students who have completed at least 60 semester hours with a GPA of 3.0 or higher. Graduate students must also be enrolled full time, have completed at least 9 semester hours with a GPA of 3.5 or higher, and have earned a GPA of 3.0 or higher as an undergraduate. Along with their application, they must submit 2 essays of 300 words or less: 1) why they are seeking a degree in occupational safety and health or a closely-related field, a brief description of their current activities, and how those relate to their career goals and objectives; and 2) why they should be awarded this scholarship (including career goals and financial need). U.S. citizenship is not required.

Financial Data The stipend is $1,000 per year.

Duration 1 year; recipients may reapply.

Additional data This program, established in 2008, is sponsored by the Greater Chicago Chapter of ASSE.

Number awarded 1 each year.

Deadline November of each year.

[134]
GULF COAST PAST PRESIDENT'S SCHOLARSHIP

American Society of Safety Engineers
Attn: ASSE Foundation
1800 East Oakton Street
Des Plaines, IL 60018
(847) 768-3435   Fax: (847) 768-3434
E-mail: agabanski@asse.org
Web: www.asse.org/foundation/scholarships/scholarships.php

Summary To provide financial assistance to upper-division students majoring in fields related to occupational safety and health.

Eligibility This program is open to undergraduate students who are majoring in occupational safety, health, and environment or a closely-related field (e.g., industrial or environmental engineering, environmental science, industrial hygiene, occupational health nursing). Although the program is sponsored by the Gulf Coast (Texas) chapter of the American Society of Safety Engineers (ASSE), there are no geographical restrictions on eligibility. Applicants may be full- or part-time students, but they must have completed at least 60 semester hours with a GPA of 3.0 or higher. Full-time students must be ASSE student members; part-time students must be ASSE general or professional members. Along with their application, they must submit 2 essays of 300 words or less: 1) why they are seeking a degree in occupational safety and health or a closely-related field, a brief description of their current activities, and how those relate to their career goals and objectives; and 2) why they should be awarded this scholarship (including career goals and financial need). U.S. citizenship is not required.

Financial Data The stipend is $1,000 per year.

Duration 1 year; recipients may reapply.

Number awarded 2 each year.

Deadline November of each year.

[135]
GUSTAVUS B. CAPITO FUND SCHOLARSHIPS

Greater Kanawha Valley Foundation
Attn: Scholarship Coordinator
1600 Huntington Square
900 Lee Street, East
P.O. Box 3041
Charleston, WV 25331-3041
(304) 346-3620   Toll Free: (800) 467-5909
Fax: (304) 346-3640   E-mail: shoover@tgkvf.org
Web: www.tgkvf.org/scholar.htm

Summary To provide financial assistance to residents of West Virginia who are working on a degree in nursing at a university in the state.

Eligibility This program is open to residents of West Virginia who are working or planning to work full time on a degree in nursing at a college or university in the state that has an accredited nursing program. Applicants must have an ACT score of 20 or higher, be able to demonstrate good moral character and financial need, and have a GPA of 2.5 or higher.

Financial Data Stipends average $1,000 per year.

Duration 1 year; may be renewed.

Number awarded Varies each year; recently, 6 of these scholarships were awarded.

Deadline January of each year.

[136]
HACU/AETNA NURSING SCHOLARSHIP

Hispanic Association of Colleges and Universities
Attn: National Scholarship Program
8415 Datapoint Drive, Suite 400
San Antonio, TX 78229
(210) 692-3805   Fax: (210) 692-0823
TDD: (800) 855-2880   E-mail: scholarships@hacu.net
Web: www.hacu.net

Summary To provide financial assistance to undergraduate students who are preparing for a career in nursing at institutions that belong to the Hispanic Association of Colleges and Universities (HACU).

Eligibility This program is open to full- or part-time undergraduate students who are enrolled at a 2- or 4-year HACU member institution. Applicants must be preparing for a career in nursing. They must have a GPA of 3.0 or higher and be able to demonstrate financial need. Along with their application, they must submit an essay of 200 to 250 words that describes their academic and/or career goals, where they expect to be and what they expect to be doing 10 years from now, and what skills they can bring to an employer.

Financial Data The stipend is $2,500.

Duration 1 year; nonrenewable.

Additional data This program is sponsored by Aetna, Inc. and administered by HACU.

Number awarded Varies each year.

Deadline May of each year.

[137]
HAITIAN AMERICAN NURSES ASSOCIATION SCHOLARSHIPS

Haitian American Nurses Association
Attn: Chair of the Education Committee
P.O. Box 694933
Miami, FL 33269
(305) 609-7498   E-mail: info@hana84.org
Web: www.hana84.org/scholarshipinfo.html

Summary To provide financial assistance to students who are of Haitian descent and enrolled in an accredited nursing program.

Eligibility This program is open to nursing students who are of Haitian descent and enrolled at a school in the state. Applicants must have a GPA of 3.0 or higher. Along with their application, they must submit a 1-page essay on why they selected nursing as a career. An interview is required.

Financial Data A stipend is awarded (amount not specified).

Duration 1 year; nonrenewable.

Number awarded Varies each year; recently, 3 of these scholarships were awarded.

Deadline March of each year.

[138]
HAROLD F. POLSTON SCHOLARSHIP

American Society of Safety Engineers
Attn: ASSE Foundation
1800 East Oakton Street
Des Plaines, IL 60018
(847) 768-3435   Fax: (847) 768-3434
E-mail: agabanski@asse.org
Web: www.asse.org/foundation/scholarships/scholarships.php

Summary To provide financial assistance to upper-division and graduate student members of the American Society of Safety Engineers (ASSE), especially those in specified categories.

Eligibility This program is open to ASSE student members who are working on an undergraduate or graduate degree in occupational safety, health, and environment or a closely-related field (e.g., industrial or environmental engineering, environmental science, industrial hygiene, occupational health nursing). Priority is given first to members of the Middle Tennessee Chapter of ASSE, second to students at Middle Tennessee State University in Murfreesboro, Tennessee or Murray State University in Murray, Kentucky, and third to residents of ASSE Region VII (Indiana, Kentucky, Michigan, Ohio, Tennessee, or West Virginia). Undergraduates must be full-time students who have completed at least 60 semester hours with a GPA of 3.0 or higher. Graduate students must also be enrolled full time, have completed at least 9 semester hours with a GPA of 3.5 or higher, and have earned a GPA of 3.0 or higher as an undergraduate. Along with their application, they must submit 2 essays of 300 words or less: 1) why they are seeking a degree in occupational safety and health or a closely-related field, a brief description of their current activities, and how those relate to their career goals and objectives; and 2) why they should be awarded this scholarship (including career goals and financial need). U.S. citizenship is not required.

Financial Data The stipend is $2,000 per year.

Duration 1 year; recipients may reapply.

Additional data This program, established in 2005, is supported by the Middle Tennessee Chapter of ASSE.

Number awarded 1 each year.

Deadline November of each year.

[139]
HARRY TABACK 9/11 MEMORIAL SCHOLARSHIP

American Society of Safety Engineers
Attn: ASSE Foundation
1800 East Oakton Street
Des Plaines, IL 60018
(847) 768-3435 Fax: (847) 768-3434
E-mail: agabanski@asse.org
Web: www.asse.org/foundation/scholarships/scholarships.php

Summary To provide financial assistance to upper-division and graduate student members of the American Society of Safety Engineers (ASSE).

Eligibility This program is open to ASSE student members who are working on an undergraduate or graduate degree in occupational safety, health, and environment or a closely-related field (e.g., industrial or environmental engineering, environmental science, industrial hygiene, occupational health nursing). Undergraduates must be full-time students who have completed at least 60 semester hours with a GPA of 3.0 or higher. Graduate students must also be enrolled full time, have completed at least 9 semester hours with a GPA of 3.5 or higher, and have earned a GPA of 3.0 or higher as an undergraduate. Along with their application, they must submit 2 essays of 300 words or less: 1) why they are seeking a degree in occupational safety and health or a closely-related field, a brief description of their current activities, and how those relate to their career goals and objectives; and 2) why they should be awarded this scholarship (including career goals and financial need). U.S. citizenship is required.

Financial Data The stipend is $1,000 per year.

Duration 1 year; recipients may reapply.

Additional data This program was established to honor a victim of the attack on the World Trade Center on September 11, 2001.

Number awarded 1 each year.

Deadline November of each year.

[140]
HARTLEY LORD SCHOLARSHIP

Senior Center at Lower Village
Attn: Scholarship Committee
175 Port Road
Kennebunk, ME 04043
(207) 967-8514 E-mail: deb@seniorcenterkennebunk.org
Web: www.seniorcenterkennebunk.org/scholarships.htm

Summary To provide financial assistance to college students preparing for a career in service to the elderly.

Eligibility This program is open to students working on a degree or certificate in a field that focuses on the well-being and needs of the senior members of society. Those fields include, but are not limited to, community service, eldercare, nursing, or medicine. Applicants must submit essays on why their career choice is consistent with the requirements of the scholarship, extracurricular or community activities in which they have participated, and any awards or other recognition they have received for excellence in scholarship, athletics, or community activities. Selection is based on academic standing, future promise, recommendations, and academic major.

Financial Data The stipend is $1,000. Funds are paid directly to the institution.

Duration 1 year.

Number awarded 1 or more each year.

Deadline April of each year.

[141]
HEALTH CARE FOR MONTANANS SCHOLARSHIP

New West Health Services
130 Neill Avenue
Helena, MT 59601
(406) 457-2200 Toll Free: (888) 500-3355
Fax: (406) 457-2299 E-mail: czipperian@nwhp.com
Web: www.newwesthealth.com/home/about/scholarships

Summary To provide financial assistance to Montana residents who are working on an undergraduate or graduate degree in a health-care related field at designated institutions in the state.

Eligibility This program is open to residents of Montana who are preparing for a career in health care at a designated institution within the state. Applicants must be enrolled in 1) their second year at a 2-year college, 2) their junior or senior year at a 4-year college or university, or 3) a graduate program in public health and/or nursing. They must have a GPA of 3.0 or higher and be able to demonstrate financial need (expected family financial contribution of $7,500 or less). Along with their application, they must submit a 250-word essay on their concept of an ideal health care job in 5 years and how that would fit their vision of what Montana's health care delivery should look like.

Financial Data The stipend for students working on a bachelor's or master's degree is $2,000. The stipend for students working on an associate degree is $1,000.

Duration 1 year; nonrenewable.

Additional data This program was established in 2008. The designated institutions are Montana State University at Bozeman, Montana State University at Billings, Montana State University-Northern, University of Montana at Missoula, Montana Tech of the University of Montana at Butte, Carroll College, University of Great Falls, Rocky Mountain College, Helena College of Technology, and Flathead Valley Community College.

Number awarded Up to 9 each year.

Deadline April of each year.

[142]
HEALTHNET OF JANESVILLE COLLEGE-TO-WORK PROGRAM

Wisconsin Foundation for Independent Colleges, Inc.
Attn: College-to-Work Program
4425 North Port Washington Road, Suite 402
Glendale, WI 53212
(414) 273-5980 Fax: (414) 273-5995
E-mail: wfic@wficweb.org
Web: www.wficweb.org/4.html

Summary To provide financial assistance and work experience to students at member institutions of the Wisconsin Foundation for Independent Colleges (WFIC) who are interested in preparing for a career in health care.

Eligibility This program is open to full-time sophomores, juniors, and seniors at WFIC member colleges and universities. Applicants must be majoring in nursing. They must be interested in a summer internship at HealthNet of Janesville in Janesville, Wisconsin. Along with their application, they must submit a cover letter that describes their career aspirations, explains why this internship would be beneficial to them in their career search and educational pursuits, what they hope to gain from this experience (both personally and professionally), and what made them want to apply for this internship.

Financial Data The stipends are $1,500 for the scholarship and $3,500 for the internship.

Duration 1 year for the scholarship; 10 weeks during the summer for the internship.

Additional data The WFIC member schools are Alverno College, Beloit College, Cardinal Stritch University, Carroll College, Carthage College, Concordia University of Wisconsin, Edgewood College, Lakeland College, Lawrence University, Marian College,

Marquette University, Milwaukee Institute of Art & Design, Milwaukee School of Engineering, Mount Mary College, Northland College, Ripon College, St. Norbert College, Silver Lake College, Viterbo University, and Wisconsin Lutheran College. This program is sponsored by HealthNet of Janesville, Inc.

Number awarded 1 each year.

Deadline Deadline not specified.

[143]
HELEN LAIDLAW FOUNDATION NURSING AND HEALTH CARE SCHOLARSHIPS

Helen Laidlaw Foundation
c/o Nancy E. Huck, President
314 Newman Street
East Tawas, MI 48730-1214
(989) 362-9117   Fax: (989) 362-7675

Summary To provide financial assistance to Michigan residents interested in preparing for a health care-related career at a school in any state.

Eligibility This program is open to high school seniors and students who are currently enrolled full time in an undergraduate or graduate degree or nondegree program at a school in any state. Applicants must be preparing for a career in a health care field. Nursing candidates receive preference. In the selection process, consideration is given first to residents of northeastern Michigan and second to those from the entire state.

Financial Data Stipends range from $500 to $1,500 per year. Funds are paid directly to the recipient's school.

Duration 1 year; may be renewed.

Deadline February of each year.

[144]
HIGHMARK SCHOLARSHIP

Pennsylvania State System of Higher Education Foundation, Inc.
Attn: Director of Scholarship Programs
2986 North Second Street
Harrisburg, PA 17110
(717) 720-4065   Fax: (717) 720-7082
E-mail: eshowers@thePAfoundation.org
Web: www.thepafoundation.org/scholarships/index.asp

Summary To provide financial assistance to freshmen entering institutions of the Pennsylvania State System of Higher Education (PASSHE) who plan to major in a health care-related field.

Eligibility This program is open to freshmen entering 1 of the 14 institutions within the PASSHE. Applicants must be planning to major in a field of health care, including (but not limited to) nursing, pre-physician assistant, pre-medicine, biology, health science, audiology, speech pathology, health services administration, health education, medical imagery, or exercise science. Each PASSHE university establishes its own selection criteria.

Financial Data The stipend is $1,000.

Duration 1 year; nonrenewable.

Additional data This program is sponsored by Highmark Inc.

Number awarded 140 each year: 10 at each PASSHE university.

Deadline Each PASSHE university sets its own deadline.

[145]
H.M. MUFFLY MEMORIAL SCHOLARSHIP

Colorado Nurses Foundation
7400 East Arapahoe Road, Suite 211
Centennial, CO 80112
(303) 694-4728   Fax: (303) 694-4869
E-mail: mail@cnfound.org
Web: www.cnfound.org/scholarships.html

Summary To provide financial assistance to residents of Colorado who are working on a bachelor's or higher degree in nursing at a college or university in the state.

Eligibility This program is open to Colorado residents who have been accepted as a student in an approved nursing program in the state. Applicants must be working on a bachelor's or higher degree. Undergraduates must have a GPA of 3.25 or higher and graduate students must have a GPA of 3.5 or higher. Selection is based on professional philosophy and goals, dedication to the improvement of patient care in Colorado, demonstrated commitment to nursing, critical thinking skills, potential for leadership, involvement in community and professional organizations, recommendations, GPA, and financial need.

Financial Data The stipend is $3,000.

Duration 1 year.

Number awarded 2 each year.

Deadline October of each year.

[146]
HOSA SCHOLARSHIPS

Health Occupations Students of America
6021 Morriss Road, Suite 111
Flower Mound, TX 75028
(972) 874-0062   Toll Free: (800) 321-HOSA
Fax: (972) 874-0063   E-mail: info@hosa.org
Web: www.hosa.org/member/scholar.html

Summary To provide financial assistance for college to members of the Health Occupations Students of America (HOSA).

Eligibility This program is open to high school seniors and current college students who are members of the association and planning to continue their education in the health care field (including nursing). Applicants must submit a 1-page essay describing 3 qualities they have gained through their HOSA experiences and how they plan to use them in their future college, community, and career activities. Selection is based on the essay (26 points), transcripts (20 points), leadership activities and recognition (30 points), community involvement (15 points), and letters of reference (9 points).

Financial Data Stipends range from $1,000 to $7,000.

Duration 1 year.

Additional data Supporters of this program include *Nursing Spectrum*, the National Technical Honor Society, Kaiser Permanente, National Consortium on Health Science Technology Education, and Delmar Learning.

Number awarded Varies each year. Recently, 9 of these scholarships were available: 1 at $7,000, 1 at $4,000, 2 at $2,000, and 5 at $1,000.

Deadline March of each year.

[147]
HOSPICE AND PALLIATIVE NURSES FOUNDATION EDUCATIONAL SCHOLARSHIP

Hospice and Palliative Nurses Foundation
Attn: Director of Development
One Penn Center West, Suite 229
Pittsburgh, PA 15276-0100
(412) 787-9301   Fax: (412) 787-9305
Web: www.hpnf.org/DisplayPage.aspx?Title=Scholarships

Summary To provide financial assistance to members of the Hospice and Palliative Nurses Association (HPNA) who are interested in working on an academic degree.

Eligibility This program is open to HPNA members providing end-of-life care. Applicants must be enrolled in a school of nursing or doctoral program and have successfully completed at least 1 semester of course work. Along with their application, they must submit a 1-page essay on how they would use the funds if they are selected, their career plans following completion of this degree program, and how they plan to use their education to advance end-of-life care.

Financial Data The stipend is $500. Funds may be used for tuition, books, computer software, or supplies related to nursing education.

Duration 1 year; nonrenewable.

Additional data This program began in 2004.

Number awarded 4 each year: 1 in each degree program (associate, bachelor's, master's, doctoral).

Deadline May of each year.

[148]
IDAHO EDUCATION INCENTIVE LOAN FORGIVENESS

Idaho State Board of Education
Len B. Jordan Office Building
650 West State Street, Room 307
P.O. Box 83720
Boise, ID 83720-0037
(208) 332-1574   Fax: (208) 334-2632
E-mail: scholarshiphelp@osbe.idaho.gov
Web: www.boardofed.idaho.gov

Summary To provide scholarship/loans to Idaho students who wish to prepare for a teaching or nursing career in Idaho.

Eligibility Applicants must have graduated from a secondary school in Idaho within the previous 2 years and rank within the upper 15% of their graduating high school class or have earned a cumulative GPA in college of 3.0 or higher. They must enroll as a full time student at an Idaho public college or university, working on a degree that will qualify them to receive an Idaho teaching certificate or write the licensure examination approved by the Board of Nursing for a registered nurse.

Financial Data This is a scholarship/loan program. Loans are forgiven if the recipient pursues a teaching or nursing career within Idaho for at least 2 years.

Duration 1 year; renewable.

Number awarded Approximately 45 each year.

Deadline Deadline not specified.

[149]
IDAHO LEGION AUXILIARY NURSES SCHOLARSHIP

American Legion Auxiliary
Department of Idaho
905 Warren Street
Boise, ID 83706-3825
(208) 342-7066   Fax: (208) 342-7066
E-mail: idalegionaux@msn.com

Summary To provide financial assistance to Idaho veterans and their children who are interested in studying nursing at a school in any state.

Eligibility This program is open to student nurses who are veterans or the children or grandchildren of veterans and have resided in Idaho for 5 years prior to application. Applicants must be attending or planning to attend a school of nursing in any state. They must be between 17 and 35 years of age. Selection is based on financial need, scholarship, and deportment.

Financial Data The stipend is $1,000.

Duration 1 year.

Number awarded 1 each year.

Deadline May of each year.

[150]
IDAHO NURSING SCHOLARSHIP

Idaho Community Foundation
Attn: Scholarship Coordinator
210 West State Street
P.O. Box 8143
Boise, ID 83707
(208) 342-3535   Fax: (208) 342-3577
TDD: (800) 657-5357   E-mail: info@idcomfdn.org
Web: www.idcomfdn.org/pages/schol_general.htm

Summary To provide financial assistance to residents of any state who have been accepted to a nursing program in Idaho.

Eligibility This program is open to students who may be residents of any state but have been accepted to an accredited Idaho nursing program. Applicants must be able to demonstrate financial need. Along with their application, they must submit a brief statement of their educational and career goals and objectives. Preference is given to students in the top third of their class.

Financial Data A stipend is awarded (amount not specified).

Duration 1 year.

Number awarded 1 or more each year.

Deadline April of each year.

[151]
ILLINOIS FARM BUREAU RURAL NURSE PRACTITIONER SCHOLARSHIPS

Illinois Farm Bureau
Attn: Assistant Director of Local Government
1701 North Towanda Avenue
P.O. Box 2901
Bloomington, IL 61702-2901
(309) 557-3151   Fax: (309) 557-3729
E-mail: matherly@ilfb.org
Web: www.ilfb.org/viewdocument.asp?did=13711

Summary To provide scholarship/loans to Illinois residents interested in a career as a rural nurse practitioner.

Eligibility This program is open to residents of Illinois who are registered nurses accepted into an Illinois college or university to become a nurse practitioner. Applicants must agree to practice after completing their degree in 1 of 84 Illinois counties designated as rural for 2 years for each year of support they received.

Financial Data The stipend is $2,000. This is a scholarship/loan program; if the recipients fail to perform their service agreement, they must repay all funds plus interest.

Duration 1 year; may be renewed.

Additional data This program, which began in 1992, is jointly funded by the Illinois Agricultural Association Foundation of the Illinois Farm Bureau and the Rural Illinois Medical Student Assistance Program.

Number awarded 3 each year.

Deadline April of each year.

[152]
ILLINOIS HEALTH IMPROVEMENT ASSOCIATION SCHOLARSHIPS

Illinois Community College System Foundation
401 East Capitol Avenue
Springfield, IL 62701
(217) 789-4230   Fax: (217) 492-5176
E-mail: iccsfoundation@sbcglobal.net
Web: www.iccsfoundation.com/Scholarships.htm

Summary To provide financial assistance to students enrolled in a health care program at an Illinois community college.

Eligibility This program is open to Illinois community college students enrolled in a health care program that provides direct medical care to individuals. Eligible areas of study may include certified nursing assistant, clinical laboratory technician, dental hygienist, electrocardiograph vascular technician, emergency medical technician, mental health associate, mortuary science, nephrology/renal technician, registered and practical nurse, occupational therapist assistant, paramedic, physician assistant, physical therapy aide, psychiatric rehabilitation, radiology technician, respiratory care, pharmacy technician, phlebotomy technician, or surgical technician. Applicants must be committed to practice in Illinois or a city adjacent to the Illinois border where state residents go for primary health care. They must have a GPA of 2.0 or higher and be able to demonstrate financial need.

Financial Data   Stipends range up to $1,000.

Duration   1 year.

Number awarded   Up to 2 each year at each participating Illinois community college.

Deadline   Each college sets its own deadline.

[153]
ILLINOIS LEGION AUXILIARY STUDENT NURSE SCHOLARSHIP

American Legion Auxiliary
Department of Illinois
2720 East Lincoln Street
P.O. Box 1426
Bloomington, IL 61702-1426
(309) 663-9366   Fax: (309) 663-5827
E-mail: staff@ilala.org
Web: illegion.org/auxiliary/scholar.html

Summary   To provide financial assistance to Illinois veterans and their descendants who are attending college in any state to prepare for a career as a nurse.

Eligibility   This program is open to veterans who served during designated periods of war time and their children, grandchildren, and great-grandchildren. Applicants must be currently enrolled at a college or university in any state and studying nursing. They must be residents of Illinois or members of the American Legion Family, Department of Illinois. Along with their application, they must submit a 1,000-word essay on "What my education will do for me." Selection is based on that essay (25%) character and leadership (25%), scholarship (25%), and financial need (25%).

Financial Data   The stipend is $1,000.

Duration   1 year.

Additional data   Applications may be obtained only from a local unit of the American Legion Auxiliary.

Number awarded   1 or more each year.

Deadline   April of each year.

[154]
ILLINOIS NURSES ASSOCIATION CENTENNIAL SCHOLARSHIP

Illinois Nurses Association
Attn: Illinois Nurses Foundation
105 West Adams Street, Suite 2101
Chicago, IL 60603
(312) 419-2900   Fax: (312) 419-2920
E-mail: info@illinoisnurses.com
Web: www.illinoisnurses.com

Summary   To provide financial assistance to nursing undergraduate and graduate students who are members of underrepresented groups.

Eligibility   This program is open to students working on an associate, bachelor's, or master's degree at an accredited NLNAC or CCNE school of nursing. Applicants must be members of a group underrepresented in nursing (African Americans, Hispanics, American Indians, Asians, and males). Undergraduates must have earned a passing grade in all nursing courses taken to date and have a GPA of 2.85 or higher. Graduate students must have completed at least 12 semester hours of graduate work and have a GPA of 3.0 or higher. All applicants must be willing to 1) act as a spokesperson to other student groups on the value of the

scholarship to continuing their nursing education, and 2) be profiled in any media or marketing materials developed by the Illinois Nurses Foundation. Along with their application, they must submit a narrative of 250 to 500 words on how they, as a nurse, plan to affect policy at either the state or national level that impacts on nursing or health care generally, or how they believe they will impact the nursing profession in general.

Financial Data   A stipend is awarded (amount not specified).

Duration   1 year.

Number awarded   1 or more each year.

Deadline   March of each year.

[155]
IMOGENE WARD NURSING SCHOLARSHIP

Florida Association Directors of Nursing Administration/Long
   Term Care
200 Butler Street, Suite 305
West Palm Beach, FL 33407
(561) 659-2167   Fax: (561) 659-1291
E-mail: fadona@fadona.org
Web: www.fadona.org/scholarship-ward.html

Summary   To provide financial assistance to employees of long-term care facilities in Florida who are interested in becoming a registered nurse.

Eligibility   This program is open to employees of long-term care facilities in Florida who are nominated by their employer. If their employer is not a member of Florida Association Directors of Nursing Administration/Long Term Care, the nomination must be endorsed by a member. Nominees must be enrolled at an accredited Florida nursing program and working on certification as an R.N. They must be willing to pledge at least 2 years working full-time in long-term care in Florida. Along with their application, they must submit a 300-word essay on what it takes to be an exceptional nurse. Nominees may be interviewed.

Financial Data   A stipend is awarded (amount not specified).

Duration   1 year.

Number awarded   1 or more each year.

Deadline   October of each year.

[156]
INDIANA HEALTH CARE FOUNDATION SCHOLARSHIP

Indiana Health Care Foundation, Inc.
Attn: Scholarship Committee
One North Capitol Avenue, Suite 100
Indianapolis, IN 46204
(317) 636-6406   Toll Free: (800) 466-IHCA
Fax: (877) 298-3749   E-mail: dhenry@ihca.org
Web: www.ihca.org

Summary   To provide financial assistance to students in Indiana who are interested in working on a degree in long-term care nursing at a school in or near the state.

Eligibility   This program is open to residents of Indiana who have at least a high school degree or GED, have been accepted by a nursing degree program (R.N. or L.P.N.) in Indiana or a bordering state, and have a GPA of 2.5 or higher. Applicants must be preparing for a career working with the elderly in a long-term care environment. Along with their application, they must submit an essay (up to 750 words) on their reasons for applying for this scholarship, their interest in nursing, and their future professional plans and commitment to long-term care. Finalists are interviewed. Special consideration is given to applicants who show a dedication and commitment to working with the elderly in a long-term care environment (nursing homes and/or assisted living facilities). Financial need is not considered in the selection process.

Financial Data Stipends range from $750 to $1,500 per year. Funds are paid directly to the recipient's school and must be used for tuition, fees, or campus housing.

Duration 1 year; recipients may reapply.

Additional data This program was established in 1997.

Deadline May of each year.

[157]
INDIANA LEGION AUXILIARY PAST PRESIDENTS PARLEY NURSING SCHOLARSHIP

American Legion Auxiliary
Department of Indiana
777 North Meridian Street, Room 107
Indianapolis, IN 46204
(317) 630-1390   Toll Free: (888) 723-7999
Fax: (317) 630-1277   E-mail: ala777@sbcglobal.net
Web: www.amlegauxin.org

Summary To provide financial assistance for nursing education to daughters and other female descendants of American Legion Auxiliary members in Indiana.

Eligibility This program is open to daughters, granddaughters, and great-granddaughters of American Legion Auxiliary members (living or deceased). Applicants must be Indiana residents and attending or planning to attend an Indiana institution of higher education. If qualified, they must also be auxiliary members, Selection is based on academic record, interest in the nursing profession, and financial need.

Financial Data The stipend is $500, which is given to the recipient at the time she enters school.

Duration 2 years.

Number awarded 1 or more each year.

Deadline March of each year.

[158]
INDIANA NURSING SCHOLARSHIP FUND PROGRAM

State Student Assistance Commission of Indiana
Attn: Director of Special Programs
150 West Market Street, Suite 500
Indianapolis, IN 46204-2811
(317) 232-2350   Toll Free: (888) 528-4719 (within IN)
Fax: (317) 232-3260   E-mail: special@ssaci.state.in.us
Web: www.in.gov/ssaci/2343.htm

Summary To provide scholarship/loans to Indiana residents who are interested in attending college in the state to prepare for a career as a nurse.

Eligibility Applicants must be Indiana residents, be admitted to an eligible Indiana school as a full- or part-time student to work on a certificate or bachelor's degree in nursing, be able to demonstrate financial need, be U.S. citizens, and have a GPA of 2.0 or higher. They must agree to work as a nurse in Indiana in 1 of the following locations: acute care or specialty hospital, long-term care facility, rehabilitation care facility, home health care entity, hospice program, mental health facility, or a facility located in a shortage area.

Financial Data The stipend is $5,000 per year. Funds may be used only for tuition and fees. Recipients agree in writing to work as a nurse in a health care setting in Indiana for at least the first 2 years after graduation. If they fail to fulfill that service obligation, they will be required to reimburse the state of Indiana.

Duration 1 year; may be renewed up to 3 additional years, but recipients must complete the nursing program within 6 years from the time the first scholarship is awarded.

Additional data This program was created in 1990.

Number awarded Varies each year.

Deadline Deadline not specified.

[159]
INOVA FAIRFAX AUXILIARY SCHOLARSHIP PROGRAM

Inova Health System
Attn: Edelman Nursing Career Development Center
8110 Gatehouse Road, Suite 200 West
Falls Church, VA 22042
(703) 205-2142
E-mail: edelmannursingcareerdevelopmentcenter@inova.org
Web: www.inova.org/working-at-inova/for-nurses/index.jsp

Summary To provide scholarship/loans to nursing students willing to work at Inova Fairfax Hospital after graduation.

Eligibility This program is open to nursing students enrolled full time in the final year of a degree program (A.D.N. or B.S.N.). Applicants must have a GPA of 3.0 or higher and be able to complete their program on time. They must be willing to commit to working at Inova Fairfax Hospital in northern Virginia within 4 months of graduation. Along with their application, they must submit a 1-page narrative explaining their career goals as a registered nurse and why they should be considered for this scholarship. U.S. citizenship or permanent resident status is required.

Financial Data Stipends up to $5,000 are available. Recipients must commit to work full time for at least 2 years within 4 months after graduation as a registered nurse. If they fail to complete the service obligation, they must repay all funds received.

Duration 1 year.

Number awarded 1 each year.

Deadline April of each year.

[160]
INOVA NURSING EXCELLENCE SCHOLARSHIP PROGRAM

Inova Health System
Attn: Edelman Nursing Career Development Center
8110 Gatehouse Road, Suite 200 West
Falls Church, VA 22042
(703) 205-2142
E-mail: edelmannursingcareerdevelopmentcenter@inova.org
Web: www.inova.org/working-at-inova/for-nurses/index.jsp

Summary To provide scholarship/loans to nursing students willing to work in facilities of the Inova Health System after graduation.

Eligibility This program is open to nursing students enrolled full time in the final year of a degree program (A.D.N. or B.S.N.). Applicants must have a GPA of 3.0 or higher and be able to complete their program on time. They must be willing to commit to working at a facility of Inova Health System in northern Virginia within 4 months of graduation. Along with their application, they must submit a 1-page narrative explaining their career goals as a registered nurse and why they should be considered for this scholarship. U.S. citizenship or permanent resident status is required.

Financial Data Stipends up to $5,000 are available. Recipients must commit to work full time for at least 2 years within 4 months after graduation as a registered nurse. If they fail to complete the service obligation, they must repay all funds received.

Duration 1 year.

Number awarded 1 or more each year.

Deadline April of each year.

[161]
INSTITUTE FOR NURSING GENERAL SCHOLARSHIPS

New Jersey State Nurses Association
Attn: Institute for Nursing
1479 Pennington Road
Trenton, NJ 08618-2661
(609) 883-5335   Toll Free: (888) UR-NJSNA
Fax: (609) 883-5343   E-mail: institute@njsna.org
Web: www.njsna.org/displaycommon.cfm?an=5

Summary To provide financial assistance to New Jersey residents who are preparing for a career as a nurse at a school in the state.

Eligibility Applicants must be New Jersey residents currently enrolled in a diploma, associate, baccalaureate, or master's nursing program located in the state. Applicants who are R.N.s must be members of the New Jersey State Nurses Association. Selection is based on financial need, GPA, and leadership potential.

Financial Data The stipend is $1,000.

Duration 1 year.

Number awarded Varies each year; recently, 2 of these scholarships were awarded.

Deadline January of each year.

[162]
IOWA HEALTH CARE ASSOCIATION FOUNDATION SCHOLARSHIP

Iowa Health Care Association
Attn: Iowa Health Care Association Foundation
1775 90th Street
West Des Moines, IA 50266-1563
(515) 978-2204   Toll Free: (800) 422-3106
Fax: (515) 978-2209   E-mail: ihca@iowahealthcare.org
Web: www.iowahealthcare.org

Summary To provide financial assistance to employees of facilities that belong to the Iowa Health Care Association (IHCA) or Iowa Center for Assisted Living (ICAL) who are interested in attending college in any state to prepare for a career in the long-term care field.

Eligibility This program is open to employees of IHCA or ICAL member nursing homes, assisted living residencies, or residential care facilities. Applicants must be interested in attending college in any state to work on a bachelor's or master's degree in nursing (R.N. or L.P.N.), health care administration, physical therapy, or occupational therapy with the goal of employment in the long-term care field. Along with their application, they must submit an essay on their work history in long-term care, their personal qualities that enable them to fulfill the responsibility of providing quality care to facility residents or tenants, the rewards they gain from working in long-term care, and their career plans once their educational goal is achieved. Financial need is not considered in the selection process.

Financial Data The stipend is $1,000. Funds are paid to the recipient's educational institution.

Duration 1 year.

Additional data IHCA and ICAL represent 576 long-term care facilities in Iowa.

Number awarded Up to 25 each year.

Deadline May of each year.

[163]
IOWA LEGION AUXILIARY PAST PRESIDENTS SCHOLARSHIP

American Legion Auxiliary
Department of Iowa
Attn: Education Committee
720 Lyon Street
Des Moines, IA 50309-5457
(515) 282-7987   Fax: (515) 282-7583
E-mail: alasectreas@ialegion.org
Web: ialegion.org/ala/scholarships.htm

Summary To provide financial assistance for nursing education to dependents of Iowa veterans and to veterans who are members of the American Legion.

Eligibility This program is open to members of the American Legion and the American Legion Auxiliary and the children or grandchildren of veterans of World War I, World War II, Korea, Vietnam, Grenada, Lebanon, Panama, or the Persian Gulf. Applicants must reside in Iowa and be enrolled or planning to enroll in a nursing program in that state. Selection is based on character, Americanism, activities, and financial need.

Financial Data The amount of this scholarship depends on the contributions received from past unit, county, district, department, or national presidents.

Duration 1 year.

Number awarded 1 each year.

Deadline May of each year.

[164]
IOWA NURSES FOUNDATION SCHOLARSHIPS

Iowa Nurses Association
Attn: Iowa Nurses Foundation
1501 42nd Street, Suite 471
West Des Moines, IA 50266
(515) 225-0495   Fax: (515) 225-2201
E-mail: info@iowanurses.org
Web: www.iowanurses.org/Default.aspx?tabid=2050

Summary To provide financial assistance to members of the Iowa Nurses Association who are working on an undergraduate or graduate nursing degree at a school in any state.

Eligibility This program is open to practicing R.N.s who are members of the association. Pre-licensure students are not eligible. Applicants must have completed at least 50% of the requirements for a bachelor's degree or at least 12 semester hours of graduate work leading to a master's degree in nursing or doctoral studies in nursing or a related field. They may be attending school in any state but must have a career plan to work in Iowa. Along with their application, they must submit brief essays on their career goals, the areas of nursing practice where they believe they have something special to offer, their interest in that area, how their interest and goals will enhance the delivery of quality health care in Iowa, and how this assistance would impact their ability to meet their educational goals. Financial need is not considered in the selection process.

Financial Data The stipend is $500.

Duration 1 year.

Number awarded 4 each year: 2 to students working on an R.N. to B.S.N. degree and 2 to graduate students.

Deadline February of each year.

[165]
ISABEL HAMPTON ROBB LEADERSHIP AWARD

National Student Nurses' Association
Attn: Isabel Hampton Robb Award
45 Main Street, Suite 606
Brooklyn, NY 11201
(718) 210-0705   Fax: (718) 797-1186
E-mail: nsna@nsna.org
Web: www.nsna.org

Summary To recognize and reward officials of student nurses' associations who demonstrate outstanding leadership.

Eligibility This program is open to current and immediate past state presidents of student nurses' associations who are enrolled in a nursing program. Candidates must be nominated by their state board of directors. Supporting material must include endorsement from the dean/director of the candidates' nursing program, a clinical instructor, and an officer on the current state board; an official transcript; and a list of the candidates' accomplishments during their tenure as state president. Nominees must include a brief essay describing how their accomplishments, professional goals, or vision for the nursing profession recall the life and career of Isabel Hampton Robb (who wrote the first nursing textbook in the United States in 1893).

Financial Data The winner receives a $1,000 cash award plus a copy of the commemorative edition of the 1893 Hampton book.

Duration The award is presented annually.

Additional data This award is sponsored by Elsevier, publisher of Mosby and Saunders Nursing Titles.

Number awarded 1 each year.

Deadline February of each year.

[166]
JACK E. BARGER, SR. MEMORIAL NURSING SCHOLARSHIPS

Pennsylvania State Nurses Association
Attn: Nursing Foundation of Pennsylvania
2578 Interstate Drive, Suite 101
Harrisburg, PA 17110
(717) 692-0542   Toll Free: (888) 707-PSNA
Fax: (717) 692-4540   E-mail: nfp@panurses.org
Web: www.panurses.org/2008/section.cfm?SID=21&ID=4

Summary To provide financial assistance to veterans, military personnel, and their dependents who are studying nursing in Pennsylvania.

Eligibility This program is open to veterans, active-duty military personnel, and the children and spouses of veterans and active-duty military personnel. Applicants must be residents of Pennsylvania and currently enrolled in an undergraduate professional school of nursing in the state. Recipients are selected by lottery from among the qualified applicants.

Financial Data The stipend is $1,000.

Duration 1 year.

Additional data This program is sponsored by the Department of Pennsylvania Veterans of Foreign Wars (VFW). Recipients must attend the VFW Convention to accept the scholarship; travel, meals, and overnight expenses are paid by the VFW.

Number awarded 6 each year.

Deadline April of each year.

[167]
JANEL PARKER CAREER MOBILITY SCHOLARSHIP

American Nephrology Nurses' Association
Attn: ANNA National Office
200 East Holly Avenue
P.O. Box 56
Pitman, NJ 08071-0056
(856) 256-2320   Toll Free: (888) 600-2662
Fax: (856) 589-7463   E-mail: annascholarships@ajj.com
Web: www.annanurse.org

Summary To provide financial assistance to members of the American Nephrology Nurses' Association (ANNA) who are interested in working on a baccalaureate or advanced degree in nursing.

Eligibility Applicants must be current association members, have been members for at least 2 years, be actively involved in nephrology nursing related health care services, and be accepted or enrolled in a baccalaureate or higher degree program in nursing. Along with their application, they must submit a 250-word essay on their career and educational goals that includes the expected time frame for completing their degree, the application of the award to meet expected expenses, and the impact of the completion of the degree program on their nephrology nursing practice.

Financial Data The stipend is $2,500.

Duration 1 year.

Additional data These scholarships, first awarded in 1993, are sponsored by Anthony J. Jannetti, Inc.

Number awarded 1 each year.

Deadline October of each year.

[168]
JESSE BROWN MEMORIAL SCHOLARSHIP

Nurses Organization of Veterans Affairs
Attn: NOVA Foundation
47595 Watkins Island Square
Sterling, VA 20165
(703) 444-5587   Fax: (703) 444-5597
E-mail: nova@vanurse.org
Web: www.vanurse.org/scholarship.html

Summary To provide financial assistance to employees of the U.S. Department of Veterans Affairs (VA) who are working on a baccalaureate degree in nursing.

Eligibility This program is open to VA employees who are enrolled or accepted for enrollment in an NLN-accredited baccalaureate nursing program. Diploma and associate degree programs are not eligible. Selection is based on career goals and professional and civic activities. U.S. citizenship is required.

Financial Data The stipend is $3,000.

Duration 1 year.

Number awarded 1 each year.

Deadline May of each year.

[169]
JESSICA M. BLANDING MEMORIAL SCHOLARSHIP

New England Regional Black Nurses Association, Inc.
P.O. Box 190690
Boston, MA 02119
(617) 524-1951
Web: www.nerbna.org/org/scholarships.html

Summary To provide financial assistance to licensed practical nurses from New England who are working on a degree and have contributed to the African American community.

Eligibility The program is open to residents of the New England states who are licensed practical nurses working on an associate or bachelor's degree in nursing at a school in any state. Applicants must have at least 1 full year of school remaining. Along with their application, they must submit a 3-page essay that covers their career aspirations in the nursing profession; how they have contributed to the African American or other communities of color in such areas as work, volunteering, church, or community outreach; an experience that has enhanced their personal and/or professional growth; and any financial hardships that may hinder them from completing their education.

Financial Data A stipend is awarded (amount not specified).

Duration 1 year.

Number awarded 1 or more each year.

Deadline March of each year.

[170]
JILL LAURA CREEDON SCHOLARSHIP AWARD

ExceptionalNurse.com
Attn: Scholarship Committee
13019 Coastal Circle
Palm Beach Gardens, FL 33410
(561) 627-9872   Fax: (561) 776-9254
TDD: (561) 776-9442   E-mail: ExceptionalNurse@aol.com
Web: www.ExceptionalNurse.com/scholarship.php

Summary To provide financial assistance to nursing students who have a disability.

Eligibility This program is open to students with a documented disability or medical challenge who have applied to, or have already been admitted to, a college or university nursing program on a full-time basis. Applicants must submit an essay on how they plan to contribute to the nursing profession and how their disability will influence their practice as a nurse. Selection is based on the essay, transcripts of high school and/or college courses completed, activities and honors received, 3 letters of recommendation, and financial need.

Financial Data The stipend is $500.

Duration 1 year; nonrenewable.

Additional data This program is funded by the Johnson & Johnson Campaign for Nursing's Future.

Number awarded 1 each year.

Deadline May of each year.

[171]
JOHNSON & JOHNSON SCHOLARSHIP FUND

American Assembly for Men in Nursing
AAMN Foundation
6700 Oporto-Madrid Boulevard
P.O. Box 130220
Birmingham, AL 35213
(205) 956-0146   Fax: (205) 956-0149
E-mail: aamn@aamn.org
Web: www.aamn.org

Summary To provide financial assistance to men working on a pre-R.N. licensure or graduate degree in nursing.

Eligibility This program is open to male students currently enrolled in an accredited pre-R.N. licensure or graduate degree program in nursing. Applicants must have a GPA of 2.75 or higher. Along with their application, they must submit an essay of 250 to 300 words that covers why they want to be a nurse, how they might contribute to the nursing profession, and their current career plans. Financial need is not considered in the selection process.

Financial Data The stipend is $1,000.

Duration 1 year.

Additional data This program was established in 2004 with funding from Johnson & Johnson's Campaign for Nursing's Future.

Number awarded 20 each year: 16 for pre-R.N. licensure students and 4 for graduate students. Of the 20 scholarships, 4 are reserved for minority students.

Deadline March of each year.

[172]
JOSEPH H. ELLINWOOD SCHOLARSHIP

American Legion
Department of Massachusetts
State House
24 Beacon Street, Suite 546-2
Boston, MA 02133-1044
(617) 727-2966   Fax: (617) 727-2969
E-mail: masslegion@verizon.net
Web: www.masslegion.org

Summary To provide financial assistance to the children and grandchildren of members of the American Legion in Massachusetts who plan to study nursing at a school in any state.

Eligibility This program is open to the children and grandchildren of current members in good standing in the American Legion's Department of Massachusetts (or members in good standing at the time of death). Applicants must be under the age of 22, entering their freshman year at a college in any state, in financial need, and preparing for a career as a nurse.

Financial Data The stipend is $1,000. Funds are paid directly to the recipient.

Duration 1 year.

Number awarded 1 each year.

Deadline March of each year.

[173]
JOSH GOTTHEIL MEMORIAL BONE MARROW TRANSPLANT CAREER DEVELOPMENT AWARDS

Oncology Nursing Society
Attn: ONS Foundation
125 Enterprise Drive
Pittsburgh, PA 15275-1214
(412) 859-6100   Toll Free: (866) 257-4ONS
Fax: (412) 859-6163   E-mail: foundation@ons.org
Web: www.ons.org

Summary To provide funding for further education to professional registered nurses who can demonstrate meritorious practice in bone marrow transplant (BMT) nursing.

Eligibility This program is open to professional registered nurses who are interested in pursuing education at the bachelor's or master's degree level. Applicants must be currently employed as a registered nurse working in BMT (at least 75% of time must be devoted to patient care) or in the position of nurse manager, nurse practitioner, clinical nurse specialist, BMT coordinator, or equivalent position. They must have at least 2 years in BMT nursing practice. Candidates are evaluated on the following criteria: 1) clarity of professional goal statement; 2) demonstrated commitment to professional development in BMT nursing; 3) demonstrated commitment to continuing professional practice in BMT nursing; 4) recommendations; and 5) contributions and/or professional nursing practice. Applicants must not have previously received this career development award from the foundation.

Financial Data The stipend is $2,000. Funds may be used to support a continuing education program or to supplement tuition in a bachelor's or master's program.

Duration 1 year.

Additional data These awards were first presented in 1995.

Number awarded 4 each year.

Deadline November of each year.

[174]
JOYCE OLSON ENDOWED SCHOLARSHIP

Kansas State Nurses Association
Attn: Kansas Nurses Foundation
1109 S.W. Topeka Boulevard
Topeka, KS 66612-1602
(785) 233-8638   Fax: (785) 233-5222
E-mail: ksna@ksna.net
Web: www.nursingworld.org/SNAS/KS/Knf.htm

Summary   To provide financial assistance to students in Kansas who are working on a nursing degree at the undergraduate, master's, or doctoral level at a school in the state.

Eligibility   This program is open to residents of Kansas who are working on a nursing degree on the undergraduate or graduate level at a school in the state. Applicants must have a GPA of 3.0 or higher. Along with their application, they must submit a personal narrative describing their anticipated role in nursing in the state of Kansas. Preference is given to full-time students. The following priority is used in awarding scholarships: 1) R.N.s working on B.S.N.s; 2) graduate and postgraduate nursing students; 3) students enrolled in certificate nursing programs (e.g., advanced registered nurse practitioner); and 4) students enrolled in undergraduate nursing programs.

Financial Data   The stipend is $500.

Duration   1 year.

Number awarded   1 each year.

Deadline   June of each year.

[175]
JUDY KNOX SCHOLARSHIP

North Carolina Nurses Association
Attn: North Carolina Foundation for Nursing
103 Enterprise Street
P.O. Box 12025
Raleigh, NC 27605-2025
(919) 821-4250   Toll Free: (800) 626-2153
Fax: (919) 829-5807   E-mail: rns@ncnurses.org
Web: www.ncnurses.org/ncfn.asp

Summary   To provide financial assistance to registered nurses in North Carolina who are interested in working on a bachelor's or master's degree.

Eligibility   This program is open to registered nurses in North Carolina who are working part time on a bachelor's or master's degree at a school in the state. Applicants must have been North Carolina residents for at least 12 months prior to application and have a cumulative GPA of 3.0 or higher. Along with their application, they must submit a 500-word essay on their reasons for pursuing additional education and for doing so on a part-time basis. Selection is based on that essay (25 points), GPA (15 points), professional involvement (20 points), community involvement (5 points), honors (15 points), certifications (15 points), and letters of reference (5 points).

Financial Data   The stipend is $1,000.

Duration   1 year.

Additional data   This program was established in 2009.

Number awarded   1 or more each year.

Deadline   May of each year.

[176]
JULIE EARLE SCHOLARSHIP

Oncology Nursing Society
Attn: ONS Foundation
125 Enterprise Drive
Pittsburgh, PA 15275-1214
(412) 859-6100   Toll Free: (866) 257-4ONS
Fax: (412) 859-6163   E-mail: foundation@ons.org
Web: www.ons.org/Awards/FoundationAwards/Bachelors

Summary   To provide financial assistance to nurses who are currently employed in radiation oncology and are interested in working on a bachelor's degree.

Eligibility   This program is open to nurses who already have a license to practice as a registered nurse (R.N.) and are accepted to or currently enrolled in a bachelor's degree program at an NLN- or CCNE-accredited school of nursing. Applicants must be currently working in radiation oncology. Along with their application, they must submit 1) an essay of 250 words or less on their current role in caring for persons with cancer, and 2) a statement of their professional goals and the relationship of those goals to the advancement of oncology nursing. Financial need is not considered in the selection process.

Financial Data   The stipend is $2,000.

Duration   1 year; nonrenewable.

Additional data   This program was established in 2009. At the end of the year of scholarship participation, recipients must submit a summary describing their educational activities. Applications must be accompanied by a $5 fee.

Number awarded   1 each year.

Deadline   January of each year.

[177]
JUNE GILL NURSING SCHOLARSHIP

New York State Grange
100 Grange Place
Cortland, NY 13045
(607) 756-7553   Fax: (607) 756-7757
E-mail: nysgrange@nysgrange.com
Web: www.nysgrange.com/educationalassistance.html

Summary   To provide financial assistance to members of the Grange in New York and their children who are interested in studying nursing at a school in any state.

Eligibility   This program is open to members of the New York State Grange and the children of members. Applicants must be currently enrolled in a nursing program in any state. Selection is based on academic records, financial need, and a career statement.

Financial Data   The stipend is $1,000 per year.

Duration   1 year; may be renewed 1 additional year.

Additional data   This program was established in 2002.

Number awarded   2 each year.

Deadline   April of each year.

[178]
JUNE GILL NURSING SCHOLARSHIP

New York State Grange
100 Grange Place
Cortland, NY 13045
(607) 756-7553   Fax: (607) 756-7757
E-mail: nysgrange@nysgrange.com
Web: www.nysgrange.com/educationalassistance.html

Summary   To provide financial assistance to members of the Grange in New York and their children who are interested in studying nursing at a school in any state.

Eligibility   This program is open to members of the New York State Grange and the children of members. Applicants must be currently enrolled in a nursing program in any state. Selection is based on academic records, financial need, and a career statement.

Financial Data   The stipend is $1,000 per year.

Duration   1 year; may be renewed 1 additional year.

Additional data   This program was established in 2002.

Number awarded   2 each year.

Deadline   April of each year.

[179]
JUSTINE E. GRANNER MEMORIAL SCHOLARSHIP

Iowa United Methodist Foundation
2301 Rittenhouse Street
Des Moines, IA 50321
(515) 974-8927
Web: www.iumf.org/otherscholarships.html

Summary To provide financial assistance to ethnic minorities in Iowa interested in majoring in a health-related field.

Eligibility This program is open to ethnic minority students preparing for a career in nursing, public health, or a related field at a college or school of nursing in Iowa. Applicants must have a GPA of 3.0 or higher. Preference is given to graduates of Iowa high schools. Financial need is considered in the selection process.

Financial Data The stipend is $1,000.

Duration 1 year.

Number awarded 1 each year.

Deadline March of each year.

[180]
KAISER PERMANENTE NURSING STUDENT SCHOLARSHIPS

KP Pride
Attn: Scholarship Committee
P.O. Box 30573
Oakland, CA 94604-1311
(510) 752-7866   E-mail: info@equalityscholarship.org
Web: www.equalityscholarship.org/apply.htm

Summary To provide financial assistance to nursing students from California who have been involved in the lesbian, gay, bisexual, and transgender (LGBT) community.

Eligibility This program is open to residents of any state who are enrolled or accepted for enrollment in an accredited A.D.N. or B.S.N. nursing program in California. Applicants must be able to provide evidence of involvement in volunteer activities promoting the understanding of and equality for the LGBT community. Students entering a nursing program for the first time must have a high school GPA of 3.0 or higher and a strong emphasis on science and mathematics. All applicants must submit an essay of 2 to 4 pages on why they feel they should receive this scholarship, including how they have demonstrated their support for justice and equality for LGBT people in their community and how being lesbian, gay, bisexual, transgender, or an ally has had an impact on their life. Selection is based on service to the LGBT community, leadership, academic achievement, and hardship or special circumstances.

Financial Data The stipend is $5,000.

Duration 1 year.

Additional data The sponsor, KP Pride, is the Kaiser Permanente Lesbian, Gay, Bisexual and Transgender Association of Northern California and Program Offices.

Number awarded 4 each year.

Deadline April of each year.

[181]
KANSAS HOSPITAL EDUCATION AND RESEARCH FOUNDATION SCHOLARSHIPS

Kansas Hospital Association
Attn: Kansas Hospital Education and Research Foundation
215 S.E. Eighth Avenue
Topeka, KS 66603-3906
(785) 233-7436   Fax: (795) 233-6955
Web: www.kha-net.org

Summary To provide financial assistance to employees of Kansas hospitals and other students in Kansas who are enrolled in a course of study leading to a certificate or degree in a health care program.

Eligibility This program is open to students enrolled or planning to enroll full or part time at an area technical school, 2-year college, or 4-year college or university in Kansas. Applicants must be 1) employees of Kansas hospitals working on a certificate, degree, or credential in an allied health or nursing program that is accredited by its respective governing body; 2) employees of Kansas hospitals working on a master's or doctoral degree in a field of health care; 3) future nursing or allied health education faculty members working on a master's degree or certification; 4) undergraduate or graduate students working on a health care human resources degree; or 5) juniors, seniors, or graduate students working on a degree in health care administration. Priority is given to professions and geographic areas experiencing shortages in Kansas, applicants furthering their knowledge base in health care by working toward a degree or certificate not currently held, students working on a degree to enable them to teach in health care, applicants demonstrating leadership on a project or institutional level, and applicants committed to pursuing their health care career in Kansas.

Financial Data Stipends are $500 for undergraduate hospital employees, $1,000 for graduate hospital employees, $1,000 for students preparing to become a faculty member, $500 for health care human resources students, and $500 for health care administration students.

Duration 1 year.

Additional data Funding for the scholarship in health care human resources is provided by the Kansas Hospital Human Resources' Association. Funding for the scholarships in health care administration is provided by the Kansas Association of Health Care Executives.

Number awarded 16 each year: 6 for undergraduate and graduate students in fields of health care, 3 for students working on a master's degree or a final certification to enable them to teach in a health care field, 1 for a student working on a degree in human resources in health care, and 6 for students working on a degree in health care administration.

Deadline February of each year.

[182]
KANSAS NURSES FOUNDATION GENERAL SCHOLARSHIPS

Kansas State Nurses Association
Attn: Kansas Nurses Foundation
1109 S.W. Topeka Boulevard
Topeka, KS 66612-1602
(785) 233-8638   Fax: (785) 233-5222
E-mail: ksna@ksna.net
Web: www.nursingworld.org/SNAS/KS/Knf.htm

Summary To provide financial assistance to students in Kansas who are working on a nursing degree on the undergraduate, master's, or doctoral level at a school in the state.

Eligibility This program is open to residents of Kansas who are working on a nursing degree on the undergraduate or graduate level at a school in the state. Applicants must have a GPA of 3.0 or higher. Along with their application, they must submit a personal narrative describing their anticipated role in nursing in the state of Kansas. Preference is given to full-time students. The following priority is used in awarding scholarships: 1) R.N.s working on B.S.N.s; 2) graduate and postgraduate nursing students; 3) students enrolled in certificate nursing programs (e.g., advanced registered nurse practitioner); and 4) students enrolled in undergraduate nursing programs.

Financial Data The stipend is $500.

Duration 1 year.

Number awarded 3 each year.

Deadline June of each year.

[183]
KANSAS NURSING SERVICE SCHOLARSHIPS

Kansas Board of Regents
Attn: Student Financial Assistance
1000 S.W. Jackson Street, Suite 520
Topeka, KS 66612-1368
(785) 296-3517   Fax: (785) 296-0983
E-mail: dlindeman@ksbor.org
Web: www.kansasregents.org/financial_aid/nursing.html

Summary To provide scholarship/loans to Kansas residents who are interested in preparing for a nursing career.

Eligibility This program is open to students in Kansas who are committed to practicing nursing (L.P.N. or R.N.) in the state. Applicants must be accepted at a Kansas nursing program (pre-nursing students are ineligible). They must locate a sponsor (defined as a licensed adult care home, psychiatric hospital, medical care facility, home health agency, local health department, or state agency that employs L.P.N.s or R.N.s) that is willing to provide up to half of the scholarship and to provide full-time employment to the recipient after licensure. Financial need is considered if there are more applicants than available funding.

Financial Data Stipends are $2,500 per year for students in L.P.N. programs or $3,500 per year for students in R.N. (associate or bachelor's degree) programs. Sponsors pay from $1,000 to one half of the scholarship and the State of Kansas pays the remaining amount. This is a scholarship/loan program; recipients must work for the sponsor the equivalent of full time for 1 year for each year of scholarship support received. If the recipient changes majors or decides not to work for the sponsor as a nurse, the scholarship becomes a loan, with interest at 5% above the federal PLUS loan rate.

Duration 1 year; may be renewed.

Additional data There is a $10 application fee.

Number awarded Up to 50 awards for L.P.N. students and up to 200 for R.N. students, of which 100 are reserved for applicants whose sponsors are located in rural counties.

Deadline April of each year.

[184]
KATHERINE POPE SCHOLARSHIP

Georgia Nurses Foundation, Inc.
Attn: Scholarship Committee
3032 Briarcliff Road, N.E.
Atlanta, GA 30329-2655
(404) 325-5536   Toll Free: (800) 324-0462
Fax: (404) 325-0407   E-mail: gnf@georgianurses.org
Web: www.georgianurses.org/scholarship_appl.htm

Summary To provide financial assistance to Georgia residents who are working on a nursing degree, at any level, at an accredited school, college, or university.

Eligibility This program is open to residents of Georgia who are currently enrolled (full or part time) in an NLN-accredited program in nursing. Applicants may be working on a degree at any level (including associate, baccalaureate, master's, or doctoral). They must have a GPA of 2.5 or higher and be able to document financial need. Priority is given to applicants who meet the following criteria: enrolled in a Georgia school, plan to practice professional nursing in Georgia following graduation, and a member of a professional organization (e.g., Georgia Association of Nursing Students, Georgia Nurses Association, Georgia Association for Nursing Education).

Financial Data The stipend is at least $500. Funds may be sent directly to the recipient.

Duration 1 year.

Number awarded 1 each year.

Deadline June of each year.

[185]
KATHERINE PORTNOY MATTLESON SCHOLARSHIP

Association of Jewish Registered Nurses
c/o Nona Dorman, Scholarship Chairperson
31 Woodland Street, 6L
Hartford, CT 06105
(860) 724-2323

Summary To provide financial assistance to Jewish residents of Connecticut who are interested in studying at a school of nursing.

Eligibility This program is open to Jewish residents of Connecticut who are enrolled or planning to enroll in an accredited college program in nursing. Selection is based on academic record and community service.

Financial Data The stipend is $800.

Duration 1 year.

Number awarded 1 each year.

Deadline April of each year.

[186]
KATHY WELTER MEMORIAL SCHOLARSHIP

Wisconsin Paralyzed Veterans of America
Attn: Scholarship Committee
2311 South 108th Street
West Allis, WI 53227-1901
(414) 328-8910   Toll Free: (800) 875-WPVA
Fax: (414) 328-8948   E-mail: info@wisconsinpva.org
Web: www.wisconsinpva.org/scholarships.html

Summary To provide financial assistance to nursing students in Wisconsin who are preparing for a career in a spinal cord injury unit or rehabilitation facility.

Eligibility This program is open to 1) students enrolled in the final year of an NLN-accredited nursing program in Wisconsin; and 2) nurses (licensed practical nurses or certified nurse assistants) who have at least 2 years' employment on a spinal cord injury center or floor and are working on an R.N. degree. Applicants must be willing to seek employment in a spinal cord injury unit or rehabilitation facility after graduation. They must be able to demonstrate financial need.

Financial Data The stipend is $1,900.

Duration 1 year.

Additional data Recipients are requested to seek employment in a spinal cord injury unit or rehabilitation facility for 1 year, to be completed within 3 years after graduation.

Number awarded 1 or 2 each year.

Deadline March of each year.

[187]
KEITH BAIN SCHOLARSHIP

American Society of Safety Engineers
Attn: ASSE Foundation
1800 East Oakton Street
Des Plaines, IL 60018
(847) 768-3435   Fax: (847) 768-3434
E-mail: agabanski@asse.org
Web: www.asse.org/foundation/scholarships/scholarships.php

Summary To provide financial assistance to upper-division and graduate student members of the American Society of Safety Engineers (ASSE), especially those in specified categories.

Eligibility This program is open to ASSE student members who are working on an undergraduate or graduate degree in occupational safety, health, and environment or a closely-related field (e.g., industrial or environmental engineering, environmental science, industrial hygiene, occupational health nursing). Priority is given first to members of the Middle Tennessee Chapter of ASSE, second to students at Middle Tennessee State University in Murfreesboro, Tennessee or Murray State University in Murray, Kentucky, and third to residents of ASSE Region VII (Indiana, Kentucky, Michigan, Ohio, Tennessee, or West Virginia). Undergraduates must be full-time students who have completed at least 60 semester hours with a GPA of 3.0 or higher. Graduate students must also be enrolled full time, have completed at least 9 semester hours with a GPA of 3.5 or higher, and have earned a GPA of 3.0 or higher as an undergraduate. Along with their application, they must submit 2 essays of 300 words or less: 1) why they are seeking a degree in occupational safety and health or a closely-related field, a brief description of their current activities, and how those relate to their career goals and objectives; and 2) why they should be awarded this scholarship (including career goals and financial need). U.S. citizenship is not required.

Financial Data   The stipend is $2,000 per year.

Duration   1 year; recipients may reapply.

Additional data   This program, established in 2008, is supported by the Middle Tennessee Chapter of ASSE.

Number awarded   1 each year.

Deadline   November of each year.

[188]
KENTUCKY NURSING INCENTIVE SCHOLARSHIP FUND

Kentucky Board of Nursing
Attn: Nursing Incentive Scholarship Fund
312 Whittington Parkway, Suite 300
Louisville, KY 40222-5172
(502) 429-7180   Toll Free: (800) 305-2042, ext. 7180
Fax: (502) 429-7011
Web: kbn.ky.gov/education/nisf

Summary   To provide scholarship/loans to residents of Kentucky interested in preparing for a career as a nurse and working in the state.

Eligibility   This program is open to Kentucky residents who will be attending approved prelicensure nursing programs (registered nurse or practical nurse) or graduate nursing programs in any state. Applicants must be interested in working as a nurse in Kentucky following graduation. Preference is given to applicants with financial need, licensed practical nurses pursuing registered nursing education, and registered nurses pursuing graduate nursing education.

Financial Data   The stipend is $3,000 per year. This is a scholarship/loan program. Recipients must work as a nurse in Kentucky for 1 year for each academic year funded. If a recipient does not complete the nursing program within the specified time period, or does not complete the required employment, then the recipient is required to repay any monies awarded plus accrued interest at 8%.

Duration   1 year; may be renewed if the recipient maintains normal academic progress (15 credit hours per year for prelicensure and B.S.N. students; 9 credit hours per year for graduate nursing students).

Number awarded   Varies each year.

Deadline   May of each year.

[189]
LAURENCE R. FOSTER MEMORIAL UNDERGRADUATE SCHOLARSHIPS

Oregon Student Assistance Commission
Attn: Grants and Scholarships Division
1500 Valley River Drive, Suite 100
Eugene, OR 97401-2146
(541) 687-7395   Toll Free: (800) 452-8807, ext. 7395
Fax: (541) 687-7414   TDD: (800) 735-2900
E-mail: awardinfo@osac.state.or.us
Web: www.osac.state.or.us/osac_programs.html

Summary   To provide financial assistance to undergraduate students from Oregon who are interested in enrolling at a school in any state to prepare for a public health career.

Eligibility   This program is open to residents of Oregon who are enrolled at least half time at a 4-year college or university in any state to prepare for a career in public health (not private practice). Applicants must be entering the junior or senior year of a health program, including nursing, medical technology, and physician assistant. Preference is given to applicants from diverse environments. Along with their application, they must submit brief essays on 1) what public health means to them; 2) the public health aspect they intend to practice and the health and population issues impacted by that aspect; and 3) their experience living or working in diverse environments.

Financial Data   Stipend amounts vary; recently, they were at least $4,167.

Duration   1 year.

Additional data   This program is administered by the Oregon Student Assistance Commission (OSAC) with funds provided by the Oregon Community Foundation, 1221 S.W. Yamhill, Suite 100, Portland, OR 97205, (503) 227-6846, Fax: (503) 274-7771.

Number awarded   Varies each year; recently, 6 undergraduate and graduate scholarships were awarded.

Deadline   February of each year.

[190]
LAWRENCE OLDENDORF DISTINGUISHED SERVICE AWARD SCHOLARSHIP

American Society of Safety Engineers
Attn: ASSE Foundation
1800 East Oakton Street
Des Plaines, IL 60018
(847) 768-3435   Fax: (847) 768-3434
E-mail: agabanski@asse.org
Web: www.asse.org/foundation/scholarships/scholarships.php

Summary   To provide financial assistance to undergraduate student members of the American Society of Safety Engineers (ASSE).

Eligibility   This program is open to ASSE student members who are working on an undergraduate degree in occupational safety, health, and environment or a closely-related field (e.g., industrial or environmental engineering, environmental science, industrial hygiene, occupational health nursing). Applicants must be full-time students who have completed at least 60 semester hours with a GPA of 3.0 or higher. Along with their application, they must submit 2 essays of 300 words or less: 1) why they are seeking a degree in occupational safety and health or a closely-related field, a brief description of their current activities, and how those relate to their career goals and objectives; and 2) why they should be awarded this scholarship (including career goals and financial need). U.S. citizenship is not required.

Financial Data   The stipend is $2,000 per year.

Duration   1 year; recipients may reapply.

Number awarded   1 each year.

Deadline   November of each year.

[191]
LEADERSHIP SCHOLARSHIPS

Florida Nursing Students Association
c/o Florida Nurses Association
P.O. Box 536985
Orlando, FL 32853-6985
(408) 896-3261   Fax: (408) 896-9042
Web: www.fnsa.net/resource/scholarships

Summary   To provide financial assistance to students from any state and recent graduates of nursing schools in Florida who have been active in the Florida Nursing Students Association (FNSA) and the National Student Nurses' Association (NSNA).

Eligibility This program is open to students from any state who are currently enrolled at a school of nursing in Florida and to recent graduates of those schools. Applicants must have made outstanding individual contributions to FNSA and NSNA. Along with their application, they must submit a 1-page essay on 1) their contributions to and personal gain from NSNA membership, and 2) how they plan to contribute to their professional organizations in the future. Financial need is not considered in the selection process.

Financial Data The stipend is $500.

Duration 1 year.

Additional data This program consists of the following named scholarships: the Heather Scaglione Leadership Scholarship, the Claydell Horne Leadership Scholarship, the Willa Fuller Leadership Scholarship, the Mary Tittle Leadership Scholarship, and the Paula Massey Leadership Scholarship. This program is sponsored by the Florida Nurses Association Foundation.

Number awarded 5 each year.

Deadline October of each year.

[192]
LESLIE GROY SCHOLARSHIP

Public Health Nurses Association of Colorado
Attn: Scholarship Chair
c/o The Alliance
800 Grant Street, Suite 335
Denver, CO 80203
E-mail: gjmiller@jeffco.us
Web: www.phnac.org/index.php?s=18&item=35

Summary To provide financial assistance to members of the Public Health Nurses Association of Colorado (PHNAC) who are interested in working on an undergraduate or advanced degree.

Eligibility This program is open to PHNAC members who are interested in taking courses that will help them attain an undergraduate or advanced degree in public health or public health nursing.

Financial Data The stipend is $1,000. Funds are paid as reimbursement for courses taken, upon receipt of documentation of completion of the course with a passing grade and a short summary paper of the course. Applicants must submit a letter that includes their educational goals and 5-year career goals related to public health nursing in Colorado, a current resume, verification of acceptance to the program, a letter of reference, and an estimate of expenses for the courses to be funded.

Duration 1 academic year.

Number awarded 1 or more each year.

Deadline January or July of each year.

[193]
LIBERTY MUTUAL SCHOLARSHIP

American Society of Safety Engineers
Attn: ASSE Foundation
1800 East Oakton Street
Des Plaines, IL 60018
(847) 768-3435   Fax: (847) 768-3434
E-mail: agabanski@asse.org
Web: www.asse.org/foundation/scholarships/scholarships.php

Summary To provide financial assistance to upper-division student members of the American Society of Safety Engineers (ASSE).

Eligibility This program is open to ASSE student members who are majoring in occupational safety, health, and environment or a closely-related field (e.g., industrial or environmental engineering, environmental science, industrial hygiene, occupational health nursing). Applicants must be full-time students who have completed at least 60 semester hours with a GPA of 3.0 or higher. Along with their application, they must submit 2 essays of 300 words or less: 1) why they are seeking a degree in occupational

safety and health or a closely-related field, a brief description of their current activities, and how those relate to their career goals and objectives; and 2) why they should be awarded this scholarship (including career goals and financial need). U.S. citizenship is not required.

Financial Data The stipend is $3,000 per year.

Duration 1 year; recipients may reapply.

Additional data This program is supported by Liberty Mutual.

Number awarded 2 each year.

Deadline November of each year.

[194]
LILLIAN CAMPBELL MEDICAL SCHOLARSHIP

Wisconsin Veterans of Foreign Wars
214 North Hamilton Street
P.O. Box 1623
Madison, WI 53701-1623
(608) 255-6655   Fax: (608) 255-0652
E-mail: qm@wi.vfwwebmail.com
Web: vfwwebcom.org/wisconsin

Summary To provide financial assistance to students working on a degree in a medical field in Wisconsin who served in the military or are related to a person who did.

Eligibility This program is open to students who have completed at least 1 year of study in Wisconsin in a program in nursing, pharmacy, physician assistant, medical or surgical technology, physical or occupational therapy, dental assisting, radiology, or other related medical profession. Applicants or a member of their immediate family (parent, sibling, child, spouse, or grandparent) must have served in the military. They must have a high school diploma or GED but may be of any age. Along with their application, they must submit a 200-word essay on their goals for studying this medical profession. Financial need is considered in the selection process.

Financial Data The stipend is $1,000.

Duration 1 year.

Number awarded 1 or more each year.

Deadline April of each year.

[195]
LILLIE AND NOEL FITZGERALD MEMORIAL SCHOLARSHIP

New Jersey State Nurses Association
Attn: Institute for Nursing
1479 Pennington Road
Trenton, NJ 08618-2661
(609) 883-5335   Toll Free: (888) UR-NJSNA
Fax: (609) 883-5343   E-mail: institute@njsna.org
Web: www.njsna.org/displaycommon.cfm?an=5

Summary To provide financial assistance to residents of New Jersey who are preparing for a career as a nurse at a school in the state.

Eligibility This program is open to residents of New Jersey who are enrolled in an associate, baccalaureate, or diploma nursing program in the state. Applicants who are R.N.s working on a higher degree in nursing are also eligible if they are members of the New Jersey State Nurses Association. Both high school graduates and adults are eligible. Selection is based on financial need, GPA, and leadership potential.

Financial Data The stipend is $1,000.

Duration 1 year.

Number awarded 1 each year.

Deadline January of each year.

[196]
LINCOLN COMMUNITY FOUNDATION MEDICAL RESEARCH SCHOLARSHIP

Lincoln Community Foundation
215 Centennial Mall South, Suite 100
Lincoln, NE 68508
(402) 474-2345   Toll Free: (888) 448-4668
Fax: (402) 476-8532   E-mail: lcf@lcf.org
Web: www.lcf.org/page29412.cfm

Summary To provide financial assistance to residents of Nebraska who are interested in working on an advanced degree in nursing or another medical field at a school in any state.

Eligibility This program is open to residents of Nebraska who are working on an advanced degree in a medical field (nursing students may apply as undergraduates or graduate students). Applicants must submit an essay explaining their progress toward completing their education, why they have chosen to prepare for a career in a medical field, and their future career goals once they complete their degree. Preference is given to 1) female applicants; 2) students preparing for careers as physicians and nurses; and 3) applicants who demonstrate financial need.

Financial Data Stipends provided by the foundation generally range from $500 to $2,000.

Duration 1 year; may be renewed up to 3 additional years.

Number awarded 1 or more each year.

Deadline May of each year.

[197]
LINDA AND BRAD GILES SCHOLARSHIP

American Society of Safety Engineers
Attn: ASSE Foundation
1800 East Oakton Street
Des Plaines, IL 60018
(847) 768-3435   Fax: (847) 768-3434
E-mail: agabanski@asse.org
Web: www.asse.org/foundation/scholarships/scholarships.php

Summary To provide financial assistance to undergraduate student members of the American Society of Safety Engineers (ASSE).

Eligibility This program is open to ASSE student members who are working on an undergraduate degree in occupational safety, health, and environment or a closely-related field (e.g., industrial or environmental engineering, environmental science, industrial hygiene, occupational health nursing). Applicants must be full-time students who have completed at least 60 semester hours with a GPA of 3.0 or higher. Along with their application, they must submit 2 essays of 300 words or less: 1) why they are seeking a degree in occupational safety and health or a closely-related field, a brief description of their current activities, and how those relate to their career goals and objectives; and 2) why they should be awarded this scholarship (including career goals and financial need). U.S. citizenship is not required. Priority is given to students attending a school with an ASAC/ABET accredited safety program.

Financial Data The stipend is $1,500 per year.

Duration 1 year; recipients may reapply.

Additional data This program was established in 2008.

Number awarded 1 each year.

Deadline November of each year.

[198]
LINDA MOORE SCHOLARSHIP

Epsilon Sigma Alpha International
Attn: ESA Foundation
P.O. Box 270517
Fort Collins, CO 80527
(970) 223-2824   Fax: (970) 223-4456
E-mail: esainfo@esaintl.com
Web: www.esaintl.com/esaf

Summary To provide financial assistance to residents of designated southern states interested in working on a nursing degree at a college in any state.

Eligibility This program is open to residents of Alabama, Arkansas, Florida, Georgia, Kentucky, Louisiana, Maryland, Mississippi, North Carolina, South Carolina, Tennessee, or Virginia. Applicants must be 1) graduating high school seniors with a GPA of 3.0 or higher or with minimum scores of 22 on the ACT or 1030 on the combined critical reading and mathematics SAT; 2) enrolled in college with a GPA of 3.0 or higher; 3) enrolled at a technical school or returning to school after an absence for retraining of job skills or obtaining a degree; or 4) engaged in online study through an accredited college, university, or vocational school. They must be studying or planning to study nursing at a school in any state. Selection is based on character (10%), leadership (20%), service (10%), financial need (30%), and scholastic ability (30%).

Financial Data The stipend is $500.

Duration 1 year; may be renewed.

Additional data Epsilon Sigma Alpha (ESA) is a women's service organization, but scholarships are available to both men and women. Completed applications must be submitted to the ESA state counselor who verifies the information before forwarding them to the scholarship director. A $5 processing fee is required.

Number awarded 1 each year.

Deadline January of each year.

[199]
LOIS HALLBERG NURSE'S SCHOLARSHIP

American Legion Auxiliary
Department of South Dakota
c/o Patricia Coyle, Secretary
P.O. Box 117
Huron, SD 57350-0117
(605) 353-1793   Fax: (605) 352-0336
E-mail: sdlegionaux@msn.com

Summary To provide financial assistance to children of South Dakota veterans who are interested in studying nursing at a school in any state.

Eligibility This program is open to residents of South Dakota between 16 and 22 years of age who are the child or grandchild either of a veteran or a member of the American Legion Auxiliary. Applicants must be attending or planning to attend a school in any state to study nursing. Along with their application, they must submit a statement on "Why I want to be a nurse." Selection is based on character (30%), Americanism (10%), leadership (10%), scholarship (20%), and financial need (30%).

Financial Data The stipend is $500.

Duration 1 year.

Number awarded 2 each year.

Deadline February of each year.

[200]
LOUIE LEFLORE/GRANT FOREMAN SCHOLARSHIP

Choctaw Nation
Attn: Scholarship Advisement Program
16th and Locust
P.O. Box 1210
Durant, OK 74702-1210
(580) 924-8280
Toll Free: (800) 522-6170, ext. 2547 (within OK)
Fax: (580) 920-3122
E-mail: scholarshipadvisement@choctawnation.com
Web: www.choctawnation-sap.com/scholarships.html

Summary To provide financial assistance to members of the Five Civilized Tribes who live in Oklahoma and plan to work on a health-related degree at a school in the state.

Eligibility This program is open to members of the Seminole Nation, Chickasaw Nation, Cherokee Nation, Creek Nation, and Choctaw Nation who reside within the jurisdictional boundaries of their tribe in Oklahoma. Applicants must have been accepted into an accredited program in nursing, pre-health professions, or health professions at a college or university in Oklahoma.

Financial Data A stipend is awarded (amount not specified).

Duration 1 year; may be renewed.

Number awarded 1 each year.

Deadline April of each year.

[201]
LUCY C. AYERS SCHOLARSHIPS

Lucy C. Ayers Foundation, Inc.
The Summit South
300 Centerville Road, Suite 300S
Warwick, RI 02886-0203

Summary To provide financial assistance to nursing students in Rhode Island.

Eligibility This program is open to students enrolled in an accredited Rhode Island nursing program leading to licensure as a registered nurse (R.N.). Applicants may be working on a diploma or an associate, bachelor's, master's, or doctoral degree. They must submit a brief statement describing their reasons for requesting financial aid.

Financial Data The stipend is $1,000.

Duration 1 year.

Additional data This program was established in 1998 with funds from the sale of the Lucy C. Ayers Residence For Nurses, originally chartered in 1926 as the Lucy C. Ayers Home for Nurses. It had served as a residence for retired or temporarily inactive graduate nurses of Rhode Island Hospital and its school of nursing. The program also provides assistance to graduates of the Rhode Island Hospital School of Nursing who need financial aid for continuing education or other purposes.

Number awarded 1 or more per year.

Deadline Deadline not specified.

[202]
M. LOUISE CARPENTER GLOECKNER, M.D. SUMMER RESEARCH FELLOWSHIP

Drexel University College of Medicine
Attn: Director, Archives and Special Collections on Women in Medicine
Hagerty Library
33rd and Market Streets
Philadelphia, PA 19104
(215) 895-6661   Fax: (215) 895-6660
E-mail: archives@drexelmed.edu
Web: archives.drexelmed.edu/fellowship.php

Summary To provide funding to scholars and students interested in conducting research during the summer on the history of women in medicine at the Archives and Special Collections on Women in Medicine at Drexel University in Philadelphia.

Eligibility This program is open to students at all levels, scholars, and general researchers. Applicants must be interested in conducting research utilizing the archives, which emphasize the history of women in medicine, nursing, medical missionaries, the American Medical Women's Association, American Women's Hospital Service, and other women in medicine organizations. Selection is based on research background of the applicant, relevance of the proposed research project to the goals of the applicant, overall quality and clarity of the proposal, appropriateness of the proposal to the holdings of the collection, and commitment of the applicant to the project.

Financial Data The grant is $4,000.

Duration 4 to 6 weeks during the summer.

Number awarded 1 each year.

Deadline January of each year.

[203]
MADELINE PICKETT (HALBERT) COGSWELL NURSING SCHOLARSHIP

National Society Daughters of the American Revolution
Attn: Committee Services Office, Scholarships
1776 D Street, N.W.
Washington, DC 20006-5303
(202) 628-1776
Web: www.dar.org/natsociety/edout_scholar.cfm

Summary To provide financial assistance for nursing education to active members of the Daughters of the American Revolution (DAR) and their descendants.

Eligibility This program is open to undergraduate students currently enrolled in accredited schools of nursing who are members, eligible for membership, or descendants of a member of DAR. Applicants must have completed at least 1 year of nursing school. They must be sponsored by a local chapter of DAR. Selection is based on academic excellence, commitment to field of study, and financial need. U.S. citizenship is required.

Financial Data The stipend is $1,000.

Duration 1 year; nonrenewable.

Number awarded Varies each year.

Deadline February of each year.

[204]
MARGARET A. STAFFORD NURSING SCHOLARSHIP

Delaware Community Foundation
Attn: Executive Vice President
100 West 10th Street, Suite 115
P.O. Box 1636
Wilmington, DE 19899
(302) 571-8004   Fax: (302) 571-1553
E-mail: rgentsch@delcf.org
Web: www.delcf.org/scholarships_guidelines.html

Summary To provide financial assistance to residents of Delaware who are interested in attending college in any state to prepare for a career in nursing.

Eligibility This program is open to Delaware residents who have been accepted into the nursing program at an accredited college or university in any state. Applicants must be beginning or furthering their nursing training. They should be seeking to improve the quality of health care in our society through nursing practices that ensure that patient's needs are a priority. Along with their application, they must submit a 1-page essay on why they desire to undertake a career in nursing. Selection is based on all facets of the applicant's education and activities that point to a successful college experience and nursing career. Preference is given to those students most in need of financial support.

Financial Data The stipend is $1,000.

Duration 1 year; nonrenewable.
Number awarded 1 each year.
Deadline March of each year.

[205]
MARGARET JONES MEMORIAL NURSING FUND

Hawai'i Community Foundation
Attn: Scholarship Department
1164 Bishop Street, Suite 800
Honolulu, HI 96813
(808) 566-5570 Toll Free: (888) 731-3863
Fax: (808) 521-6286 E-mail: scholarships@hcf-hawaii.org
Web: www.hawaiicommunityfoundation.org

Summary To provide financial assistance to Hawaii residents who are interested in preparing for a career in nursing.
Eligibility This program is open to students enrolled as juniors, seniors, or graduate students in 1) a B.S.N. or M.S.N. program in Hawaii, or 2) a Ph.D. program in nursing in Hawaii or on the U.S. mainland. Preference may be given to members of the Hawai'i Nurses Association. Applicants must be residents of the state of Hawaii; be able to demonstrate financial need; be interested in attending an accredited 2- or 4-year college or university as full-time students; and be able to demonstrate academic achievement (3.0 GPA or above).
Financial Data The amounts of the awards depend on the availability of funds and the need of the recipient; recently, stipends averaged $888.
Duration 1 year.
Additional data This fund was established in 1917 to honor Margaret Jones, a nurse killed when the S.S. *Lusitania* was sunk by a German submarine during World War I.
Number awarded Varies each year; recently, 13 of these scholarships were awarded.
Deadline February of each year.

[206]
MARILYN CASEY SCHOLARSHIP

Illinois Community College System Foundation
401 East Capitol Avenue
Springfield, IL 62701
(217) 789-4230 Fax: (217) 492-5176
E-mail: iccsfoundation@sbcglobal.net
Web: www.iccsfoundation.com/Scholarships.htm

Summary To provide financial assistance to students enrolled in a nursing or other health care program at an Illinois community college.
Eligibility This program is open to students at Illinois community colleges who are enrolled in a health care program, especially nursing. Preference is given to students in an A.D.N. program. Applicants must have a GPA of 3.0 or higher and be able to demonstrate financial need.
Financial Data Stipends range up to $2,000 per year.
Duration 1 year; may be renewed 1 additional year.
Additional data This program was established in 2005.
Number awarded 1 or 2 each year at each participating Illinois community college.
Deadline Each college sets its own deadline.

[207]
MARSH RISK CONSULTING SCHOLARSHIP

American Society of Safety Engineers
Attn: ASSE Foundation
1800 East Oakton Street
Des Plaines, IL 60018
(847) 768-3435 Fax: (847) 768-3434
E-mail: agabanski@asse.org
Web: www.asse.org/foundation/scholarships/scholarships.php

Summary To provide financial assistance to upper-division student members of the American Society of Safety Engineers (ASSE).
Eligibility This program is open to ASSE student members who are majoring in occupational safety, health, and environment or a closely-related field (e.g., industrial or environmental engineering, environmental science, industrial hygiene, occupational health nursing). Applicants must be full-time students who have completed at least 60 semester hours with a GPA of 3.0 or higher. Along with their application, they must submit 2 essays of 300 words or less: 1) why they are seeking a degree in occupational safety and health or a closely-related field, a brief description of their current activities, and how those relate to their career goals and objectives; and 2) why they should be awarded this scholarship (including career goals and financial need). U.S. citizenship is not required.
Financial Data The stipend is $1,000 per year.
Duration 1 year; recipients may reapply.
Additional data Funding for this program is provided by Marsh Risk Consulting.
Number awarded 1 each year.
Deadline November of each year.

[208]
MARY BETH HAYWARD SCHOLARSHIP FOR RNS PREPARING TO TEACH NURSING

Ohio Nurses Association
Attn: Ohio Nurses Foundation
4000 East Main Street
Columbus, OH 43213-2983
(614) 237-5414 Fax: (614) 237-6074
E-mail: gharsheymeade@ohnurses.org
Web: www.ohnurses.org

Summary To provide financial assistance to registered nurses in Ohio who are working on a nursing degree as preparation for a career in teaching nursing.
Eligibility This program is open to Ohio residents who have a valid Ohio nursing license. Applicants must have a GPA of 2.5 or higher as an undergraduate or 3.5 or higher if working on a graduate degree. They must be planning to enroll full time at a school in any state to prepare for a career as a teacher in an accredited Ohio nursing program. Along with their application, they must submit a personal statement on why they wish to teach nursing in Ohio. Selection is based on that statement, college academic records, school activities, and community services. Priority is given to members of the Ohio Nurses Association.
Financial Data A stipend is awarded (amount not specified).
Duration 1 year; recipients may reapply for 1 additional year if they maintain a cumulative GPA of 2.5 or higher.
Number awarded 1 or more each year.
Deadline January of each year.

[209]
MARY ELIZA MAHONEY SCHOLARSHIP

New England Regional Black Nurses Association, Inc.
P.O. Box 190690
Boston, MA 02119
(617) 524-1951
Web: www.nerbna.org/org/scholarships.html

Summary To provide financial assistance to high school seniors New England who have contributed to the African American community and are interested in studying nursing at a school in any state.
Eligibility The program is open to seniors graduating from high schools in New England who are planning to enroll full time in an NLN-accredited baccalaureate program in nursing in any state. Applicants must have at least 1 full year of school remaining. Along with their application, they must submit a 3-page essay that

covers their career aspirations in the nursing profession; how they have contributed to the African American or other communities of color in such areas as work, volunteering, church, or community outreach; an experience that has enhanced their personal and/or professional growth; and any financial hardships that may hinder them from completing their education.

Financial Data A stipend is awarded (amount not specified).

Duration 1 year.

Number awarded 1 or more each year.

Deadline March of each year.

[210]
MARY ELLEN HATFIELD SCHOOL NURSING SCHOLARSHIPS

South Carolina Nurses Foundation, Inc.
Attn: Awards Committee Chair
1821 Gadsden Street
Columbia, SC 29201
(803) 252-4781   Fax: (803) 779-3870
E-mail: brownk1@aol.com
Web: www.scnursesfoundation.org/index_files/Page316.htm

Summary To provide financial assistance to school nurses in South Carolina who are interested in working on an associate, bachelor's, or graduate degree in nursing at a school in any state.

Eligibility This program is open to nurses who are currently practicing in a school setting (K-12) in South Carolina and have a valid nursing license. Applicants may be 1) L.P.N.s who are enrolled in an A.D.N. or B.S.N. program and have successfully completed 10 hours of undergraduate work; or 2) R.N.s who are enrolled in a B.S.N. program or a graduate program in nursing or public health and have successfully completed 10 hours of undergraduate work or 12 hours of graduate course work. They must be a current member of a professional organization and have career goals that include making a contribution to school nursing. Along with their application, they must submit a 2-page statement describing what they like about school nursing and how furthering their education will assist them in improving service to school-aged children and youth. Financial need is not considered in the selection process.

Financial Data The stipend is $500.

Duration 1 year.

Additional data These scholarships, first presented in 2006, are offered in conjunction with the South Carolina Department of Health and Environmental Control, Division of Women and Children's Services, Attn: Cathy Young-Jones, Mills/Jarrett Complex, Box 101106, Columbia, SC 29211, (803) 898-0767.

Number awarded 2 each year: 1 to an L.P.N. student and 1 to an R.N. student.

Deadline August of each year.

[211]
MARY OPAL WOLANIN UNDERGRADUATE SCHOLARSHIP

National Gerontological Nurses Association
7794 Grow Drive
Pensacola, FL 32514-7072
(850) 473-1174   Toll Free: (800) 723-0560
Fax: (850) 484-8762   E-mail: ngna@dancyamc.com
Web: www.ngna.org/awards-amp-scholarships.html

Summary To provide financial assistance for undergraduate education to members of the National Gerontological Nurses Association (NGNA).

Eligibility This program is open to members of the association who are full- or part-time nursing students in the junior year of a baccalaureate program or sophomore year of an associate program at a school accredited by the NLN. Applicants must intend to work in a gerontology/geriatric setting after graduation. Along with their application, they must submit 2 letters of recommenda-

tion, a transcript (at least a 3.0 GPA is required), and a 300-word statement of professional and educational goals with emphasis on contributions they expect to make to improve nursing care for older adults.

Financial Data The stipend is $500.

Duration 1 year.

Number awarded 1 or more each year.

Deadline April of each year.

[212]
MARYLAND HOSPITAL ASSOCIATION SCHOLARS PROGRAM

Maryland Hospital Association
Attn: Catherine Crowley, Vice President
6820 Deerpath Road
Elkridge, MD 21075
(410) 379-6200
Web: www.mdhospitals.org

Summary To provide financial assistance to employees and volunteers at hospitals in Maryland who are interested in attending college in the state to work on an undergraduate or graduate degree in a health-related field.

Eligibility This program is open to residents of Maryland who are employees or active volunteers at hospitals in the state. Applicants must be accepted to or enrolled at a college or university in the state in a program leading to an undergraduate or graduate degree or certificate in life sciences, nursing, or allied health. They must be within 1 to 2 years of completing educational requirements and have a GPA of 3.0 or higher.

Financial Data The stipend is $2,500.

Duration 1 year.

Additional data This program, established in 2002, is jointly sponsored by Care First, PRIME, The Chesapeake Registry, and the Maryland Hospital Association.

Number awarded Varies each year. Recently, 17 of these scholarships were awarded: 10 to undergraduate nursing students, 3 to master's degree nursing students, 1 to a doctoral degree nursing student, 2 to students working on an associated degree in allied health, and 1 to a student working on a bachelor's degree in allied health.

Deadline May of each year.

[213]
MARYLAND LEGION AUXILIARY PAST PRESIDENTS' PARLEY NURSING SCHOLARSHIP

American Legion Auxiliary
Department of Maryland
1589 Sulphur Spring Road, Suite 105
Baltimore, MD 21227
(410) 242-9519   Fax: (410) 242-9553
E-mail: hq@alamd.org
Web: www.alamd.org

Summary To provide financial assistance to the female descendants of Maryland veterans who wish to study nursing at a school in any state.

Eligibility This program is open to Maryland residents who are the daughters, granddaughters, great-granddaughters, step-daughters, step-granddaughters, or step-great-granddaughters of ex-servicewomen (or of ex-servicemen, if there are no qualified descendants of ex-servicewomen). Applicants must be interested in attending a school in any state to become a registered nurse and be able to show financial need. They must submit a 300-word essay on the topic "What a Nursing Career Means to Me.".

Financial Data The stipend is $2,000. Funds are sent directly to the recipient's school.

Duration 1 year; may be renewed for up to 3 additional years if the recipient remains enrolled full time.

Number awarded 1 each year.
Deadline April of each year.

[214]
MARYLAND TUITION REDUCTION FOR NONRESIDENT NURSING STUDENTS

Maryland Higher Education Commission
Attn: Office of Student Financial Assistance
839 Bestgate Road, Suite 400
Annapolis, MD 21401-3013
(410) 260-4546   Toll Free: (800) 974-1024, ext. 4546
Fax: (410) 260-3200   TDD: (800) 735-2258
E-mail: tmckelvi@mhec.state.md.us
Web: www.mhec.state.md.us

Summary To provide reduced tuition in exchange for service to residents of states other than Maryland interested in attending Maryland public nursing schools.

Eligibility This program is open to nursing students at Maryland public colleges who are residents of states other than Maryland. Applicants must enroll for at least 6 credits per semester. They are not required to demonstrate financial need.

Financial Data Recipients are entitled to pay the same tuition as if they were Maryland residents. They must agree to work as a full-time nurse in Maryland in an eligible institution or in a home that provides domiciliary, personal, or nursing care for 2 or more unrelated individuals. They must work for 2 years if they attended a 2-year school, for 4 years if they attended a 4-year school, or repay the scholarship with interest. The service obligation must begin within 6 months of graduation.

Duration 1 year; may be renewed for 1 additional year at a 2-year public institution or 3 additional years at a 4-year public institution.

Number awarded Varies each year.

Deadline Each participating Maryland school sets its own deadline.

[215]
MARYLAND WORKFORCE SHORTAGE STUDENT ASSISTANCE GRANT PROGRAM

Maryland Higher Education Commission
Attn: Office of Student Financial Assistance
839 Bestgate Road, Suite 400
Annapolis, MD 21401-3013
(410) 260-4565   Toll Free: (800) 974-1024, ext. 4565
Fax: (410) 260-3200   TDD: (800) 735-2258
E-mail: osfamail@mhec.state.md.us
Web: www.mhec.state.md.us

Summary To provide scholarship/loans to Maryland residents interested in a career in nursing and other specified workforce shortage areas.

Eligibility This program is open to residents of Maryland who are high school seniors, undergraduates, or graduate students. Applicants must be enrolled or planning to enroll at a 2-year or 4-year Maryland college or university. They may major in the following service areas: 1) child development or early childhood education, for students who plan to become full-time employees as a director or senior staff member in a licensed Maryland child care center or as a licensed family day care provider in the state; 2) human services degree programs, for students who plan to become employees of Maryland community-based programs and are interested in working on a degree in aging services, counseling, disability services, mental health, nursing, occupational therapy, physical therapy, psychology, rehabilitation, social work, special education, supported employment, vocational rehabilitation, or other program providing support services to individuals with special needs; 3) education, for students who become teachers in the following areas of certification: technology education (secondary), chemistry (secondary), computer science (secondary),

earth and space science (secondary), English for speakers of other languages (elementary and secondary), foreign languages (German, Italian, Japanese, Latin, or Spanish), mathematics, (secondary), physical science (secondary), physics (secondary), or special education (infant/primary, elementary/middle, secondary/adult, severely and profoundly disabled, hearing impaired, or visually impaired); 4) nursing, for students who become employed as a nurse in a licensed hospital, adult day care center, nursing home, public health agency, home health agency, eligible institution of postsecondary education that awards nursing degrees or diplomas, or other approved organization; 5) physical therapy or occupational therapy, for students who plan to become employed as a therapist or therapy assistant to handicapped children in a public school in Maryland, in an approved non-public education program, or in a state therapeutic hospital; 6) law, for students interested in preparing for a career in providing legal services to low-income residents in the state; 7) social work; or 8) public service, for employment in services in the public or non-profit sectors in which there is a shortage of qualified practitioners to low-income or underserved residents or areas of the state. Applicants are ranked by GPA and then by need within each occupational field. Students with the greatest need within each GPA range are awarded first.

Financial Data Awards are $4,000 per year for full-time undergraduate and graduate students at 4-year institutions, $2,000 per year for part-time undergraduate and graduate students at 4-year institutions, $2,000 per year for full-time students at community colleges, or $1,000 per year for part-time students at community colleges. Within 1 year of graduation, recipients must provide 1 year of service in Maryland in their field of study for each year of financial aid received under this program; failure to comply with that service obligation will require them to repay the scholarship money with interest.

Duration 1 year; may be renewed up to 4 additional years, provided the recipient continues to meet eligibility requirements.

Additional data This program was established in 2007 as a replacement for several programs previously offered by the Maryland Higher Education Commission. Awards in the human services degree programs area are designated the Ida G. and L. Leonard Rubin Scholarship. Awards in the service area of education are designated the Sharon Christa McAuliffe Scholarship. Awards in the service areas of nursing, social work, and public service are designated the Parren J. Mitchell Public Service Scholarship. Awards in the service area of law are designated the William Donald Schaefer Scholarship.

Number awarded Varies each year.

Deadline June of each year.

[216]
MASSACHUSETTS EDUCATIONAL REWARDS GRANT PROGRAM

Massachusetts Office of Student Financial Assistance
454 Broadway, Suite 200
Revere, MA 02151
(617) 727-9420   Fax: (617) 727-0667
E-mail: osfa@osfa.mass.edu
Web: www.osfa.mass.edu

Summary To provide financial assistance for college to Massachusetts residents who are working in low-income jobs and interested in obtaining additional training to transition to employment in nursing and other targeted high-demand occupations.

Eligibility This program is open to 1) dislocated workers and 2) incumbent workers whose income is at or below 200% of the federal poverty level (currently, $21,660 for a family of 1, rising to $74,020 for a family of 8). Applicants must have been residents of Massachusetts for at least 1 year and be able to demonstrate financial need. They must be enrolled full or part time in a certificate or degree program in Massachusetts that will provide training in a high-demand occupational field. U.S. citizenship or permanent resident status is required.

Financial Data Awards range from $200 to $3,000 per year, depending on the need of the recipient. The award may include up to 30% of the students calculated cost of living.

Duration 1 year; may be renewed.

Additional data The eligible high-demand occupational fields includes specific areas of health care (e.g., dental hygienists, medical and clinical laboratory technicians, licensed practical and vocational nurses, occupational therapy assistants, physical therapy assistants, and registered nurses); life, physical, and social science (e.g., biological technicians, environmental science and protection technicians); personal care and service (e.g., hairdressers, cosmetologists); office and administrative support (e.g., legal secretaries, desktop publishers); installation, maintenance, and repair (e.g., automotive service technicians and mechanics, telecommunications equipment installers and repairers); architecture, engineering, and computers (e.g., architectural and civil drafters, engineering technicians, computer specialists); construction and production (e.g., carpenters, electricians, glaziers); and other industries (e.g., paralegals and legal assistants, broadcast technicians, travel agents). For a complete list, contact the sponsor.

Number awarded Varies each year.

Deadline September of each year.

[217]
MASSACHUSETTS LABOR RELATIONS SCHOLARSHIPS

Massachusetts Nurses Association
Attn: Massachusetts Nurses Foundation
340 Turnpike Street
Canton, MA 02021
(781) 830-5745   Toll Free: (800) 882-2056, ext. 745
Fax: (781) 821-4445   E-mail: cmessia@mnarn.org
Web: www.massnurses.org/about-man/mns/scholarships

Summary To provide financial assistance to members of the Massachusetts Nurses Association (MNA) who are working on an undergraduate or graduate degree in nursing, labor relations, or a related field.

Eligibility This program is open to MNA members who are registered nurses or health care professionals with at least 1 year of professional experience. Applicants must have been accepted into an NLN-accredited baccalaureate or master's degree program in nursing or a baccalaureate or master's degree program in labor relations or a related field. Along with their application, they must submit a 500-word essay on their career goals, how education will enhance those goals, and their contribution to the profession of nursing or health care through practice, education, research, and/or labor relations. Selection is based on the essay, professional development activities, community work, and 2 professional references. Minorities are specifically encouraged to apply.

Financial Data The stipend is $1,000.

Duration 1 year.

Number awarded 2 each year.

Deadline May of each year.

[218]
MASSACHUSETTS NURSES ASSOCIATION UNIT 7 SCHOLARSHIPS

Massachusetts Nurses Association
Attn: Massachusetts Nurses Foundation
340 Turnpike Street
Canton, MA 02021
(781) 830-5745   Toll Free: (800) 882-2056, ext. 745
Fax: (781) 821-4445   E-mail: cmessia@mnarn.org
Web: www.massnurses.org/about-man/mns/scholarships

Summary To provide financial assistance to registered nurses and health care professionals who are members of the Massachusetts Nurses Association (MNA) and planning to work on an undergraduate or graduate degree.

Eligibility This program is open to MNA members in Unit 7 who are either registered nurses or other health care professionals with at least 2 years of professional experience. Applicants must have been accepted into an NLN-accredited undergraduate or graduate degree program in their respective field. Along with their application, they must submit a 500-word essay on their career goals, how education will enhance those goals, and their contribution to their profession. Selection is based on the essay, 2 professional references, community work, and professional development activities. Minorities are specifically encouraged to apply.

Financial Data The stipend is $1,000.

Duration 1 year.

Additional data Unit 7 is a bargaining unit that represents registered nurses, public health nurses, nurse practitioners, nursing instructors, community psychiatric mental health nurses, community mental health nursing advisers, health care facility inspectors, psychologists, physical therapists, occupational therapists, and audiologists.

Number awarded 2 each year: 1 to a nurse and 1 to a health care professional.

Deadline May of each year.

[219]
MAUD BYRD WINDHAM SCHOLARSHIP

Alabama-West Florida United Methodist Foundation, Inc.
170 Belmont Drive
P.O. Box 8066
Dothan, AL 36304
(334) 793-6820   Fax: (334) 794-6480
E-mail: foundation@alwfumf.org
Web: www.alwfumf.org

Summary To provide financial assistance for college to students from the Alabama-West Florida Conference of the United Methodist Church who are interested in preparing for a career in nursing and other designated fields.

Eligibility This program is open to members of United Methodist Churches within the Alabama-West Florida Conference. Applicants must be enrolled or planning to enroll in college in order to prepare for a career in a church-related vocation, nursing, or medicine. They must submit an essay on why they feel they should receive this scholarship and documentation of financial need.

Financial Data The stipend is $500.

Duration 1 year.

Number awarded 1 or more each year.

Deadline June of each year.

[220]
MAXINE V. FENNELL MEMORIAL SCHOLARSHIP

New England Regional Black Nurses Association, Inc.
P.O. Box 190690
Boston, MA 02119
(617) 524-1951
Web: www.nerbna.org/org/scholarships.html

Summary To provide financial assistance to licensed practical nurses from New England who are studying to become a registered nurse (R.N.) and have contributed to the African American community.

Eligibility The program is open to residents of the New England states who are licensed practical nurses and currently enrolled in an NLN-accredited R.N. program (diploma, associate, baccalaureate) at a school in any state. Applicants must have at least 1 full year of school remaining. Along with their application, they must submit a 3-page essay that covers their career aspirations in the nursing profession; how they have contributed to the African

American or other communities of color in such areas as work, volunteering, church, or community outreach; an experience that has enhanced their personal and/or professional growth; and any financial hardships that may hinder them from completing their education.

Financial Data A stipend is awarded (amount not specified).

Duration 1 year.

Number awarded 1 or more each year.

Deadline March of each year.

[221]
MCKESSON SCHOLARSHIPS

National Student Nurses' Association
Attn: Foundation
45 Main Street, Suite 606
Brooklyn, NY 11201
(718) 210-0705   Fax: (718) 797-1186
E-mail: nsna@nsna.org
Web: www.nsna.org

Summary To provide financial assistance to nursing students enrolled in programs leading to licensure as a registered nurse (R.N.).

Eligibility This program is open to students currently enrolled in state-approved schools of nursing and working on an associate degree, baccalaureate degree, or diploma leading to licensure as an R.N. Graduating high school seniors are not eligible. Applicants must submit a 200-word description of their professional and educational goals and how this scholarship will help them achieve those goals. Selection is based on academic achievement, financial need, and involvement in student nursing organizations and community health activities. U.S. citizenship or permanent resident status is required.

Financial Data Stipends range from $1,000 to $2,500.

Duration 1 year.

Additional data This program is sponsored by the McKesson Foundation. Applications must be accompanied by a $10 processing fee.

Number awarded Varies each year. Recently, 15 of these scholarships were awarded.

Deadline January of each year.

[222]
MCLEAN SCHOLARSHIP FOR NURSING AND PHYSICIAN ASSISTANT MAJORS

Association of Independent Colleges and Universities of
   Pennsylvania
101 North Front Street
Harrisburg, PA 17101-1405
(717) 232-8649   Fax: (717) 233-8574
E-mail: info@aicup.org
Web: www.aicup.org

Summary To provide financial assistance to students from any state at member institutions of the Association of Independent Colleges and Universities of Pennsylvania (AICUP) who are enrolled in a nursing or physician assistant program.

Eligibility This program is open to undergraduate students from any state enrolled full time at AICUP colleges and universities. Applicants must be enrolled in a nursing or physician assistant program and have a GPA of 3.0 or higher. Along with their application, they must submit a 2-page essay on how they chose their major, the steps they are taking to ensure that they succeed in their major, what they plan to do after graduation, the volunteer and extracurricular activities in which they participate, and how those activities relate to their major. Selection is based on their GPA (30%), steps taken to ensure success in their major (10%), career goals (10%), volunteer work (25%), relationship of volunteer and extracurricular activities to their major (10%), and extent of their leadership activities (15%). Applications must be submit-

ted to the financial aid office at the AICUP college or university that the student attends.

Financial Data The stipend is $2,500.

Duration 1 year.

Additional data The AICUP includes 83 private colleges and universities in Pennsylvania. For a list of those institutions, contact AICUP. This program was established in 1998 by the McLean Contributionship of Bryn Mawr, Pennsylvania.

Number awarded Varies each year. Recently, 7 of these scholarships were awarded.

Deadline April of each year.

[223]
M.D. "JACK" MURPHY MEMORIAL NURSES TRAINING FUND

American Legion
Department of Missouri
P.O. Box 179
Jefferson City, MO 65102-0179
(573) 893-2353   Toll Free: (800) 846-9023
Fax: (573) 893-2980   E-mail: info@missourilegion.org
Web: www.missourilegion.org

Summary To provide financial assistance to residents of Missouri who are the descendants of veterans and interested in studying nursing at a school in any state.

Eligibility This program is open to residents of Missouri who are high school seniors or current college students working on or planning to work on a program of training to become a registered nurse. Applicants must graduate in the top 40% of their high school class. They must be 1) the child, grandchild, or great-grandchild of a veteran who served 90 days on active duty in the Air Force, Army, Coast Guard, Marine Corps, or Navy of the United States and received an honorable discharge; 2) unmarried; 3) under 21 years of age; and 4) attending or planning to attend an accredited college or university in any state as a full-time student. Financial need is considered in the selection process.

Financial Data The stipend is $750 per year, payable in 2 equal installments.

Duration 1 year; may be renewed for 1 additional year.

Number awarded 1 each year.

Deadline April of each year.

[224]
MEDICAL ENLISTED COMMISSIONING PROGRAM

U.S. Navy
Attn: Navy Medicine Manpower, Personnel, Education and
   Training Command
Code OG3
8901 Wisconsin Avenue, 16th Floor, Tower 1
Bethesda, MD 20889-5611
(301) 319-4520   Fax: (301) 295-1783
E-mail: beverly.kemp@med.navy.mil
Web: www.med.navy.mil

Summary To provide Navy and Marine enlisted personnel with an opportunity to earn a bachelor's degree in nursing while continuing to receive their regular pay and allowances.

Eligibility This program is open to enlisted personnel who are serving on active duty in any rating of the U.S. Navy, U.S. Marine Corps, Naval Reserve (including the Training and Administration of the Reserve Program), and the Marine Corps Reserve (including the Active Reserve Program). Applicants must have completed at least 30 semester or credit hours of college work (with a cumulative GPA of 2.5 or higher) so they can complete a bachelor's degree in nursing (B.S.N.) within 36 months. They must have SAT scores of at least 1000 (500 mathematics and 500 critical reading) or ACT scores of at least 42 (21 mathematics and 21 English). If they have a B.S.N. from a non-accredited institution, or can complete both a B.S.N. and M.S.N. within 36 months, they may apply for that option. At the time of commissioning, they must be younger than 42 years of age. U.S. citizenship is required.

Financial Data Participants receive full pay and allowances for their enlisted pay grade and are eligible for advancement while in college. They are responsible for tuition, fees, books, and other expenses. If eligible, they may use the Montgomery GI Bill or the Veterans Educational Assistance Program (VEAP) educational benefits, but they may not participate in the Navy Tuition Assistance Program.

Duration Up to 36 months of full-time, year-round study, until completion of a B.S.N. degree.

Additional data Following graduation, participants are commissioned as ensigns in the Nurse Corps and attend Officer Indoctrination School. They incur an 8-year service obligation, of which at least 4 years must be served on active duty.

Number awarded Varies each year.

Deadline September of each year.

[225]
MEDICAL PROFESSIONS SCHOLARSHIPS OF STRAIGHTFORWARD MEDIA

StraightForward Media
508 Seventh Street, Suite 202
Rapid City, SD 57701
(605) 348-3042   Fax: (605) 348-3043
E-mail: info@straightforwardmedia.com
Web: www.straightforwardmedia.com

Summary To provide financial assistance to students working on a degree in a medical-related profession.

Eligibility This program is open to students who are working on or planning to work on a degree in a medical-related profession (including physicians, technicians, physician's assistants, nurses, therapists, and other health professionals). Applicants must submit online essays (no minimum or maximum word limit) on 1) why they chose a medical profession over other educational opportunities and what contribution they will make to the medical world, and 2) how this scholarship will help them meet their educational and professional goals. Financial need is not considered in the selection process.

Financial Data The stipend is $500. Funds are paid directly to the student.

Duration 1 year.

Number awarded 4 each year: 1 for each award cycle.

Deadline February, May, August, or November of each year.

[226]
MEDICAL-SURGICAL NURSES CAREER MOBILITY SCHOLARSHIP

Academy of Medical-Surgical Nurses
Attn: Foundation
200 East Holly Avenue
P.O. Box 56
Pitman, NJ 08071-0056
Toll Free: (866) 877-AMSN   E-mail: AMSN@ajj.com
Web: www.medsurgnurse.org

Summary To provide financial assistance to members of the Academy of Medical-Surgical Nurses (AMSN) who are interested in furthering their education.

Eligibility This program is open to AMSN members who are enrolled or planning to enroll in a program of additional training, including L.P.N. to R.N., R.N. to B.S.N., R.N. to M.S.N., or M.S.N. to doctorate. Applicants must submit a brief statement describing how additional education will enhance their care of adult medical-surgical patients.

Financial Data The stipend is $1,000.

Duration 1 year; nonrenewable.

Number awarded 1 each year.

Deadline May of each year.

[227]
MEDINA SCHOLARSHIP FOR HISPANICS IN SAFETY

American Society of Safety Engineers
Attn: ASSE Foundation
1800 East Oakton Street
Des Plaines, IL 60018
(847) 768-3435   Fax: (847) 768-3434
E-mail: agabanski@asse.org
Web: www.asse.org/foundation/scholarships/scholarships.php

Summary To provide financial assistance to Hispanic upper-division and graduate student members of the American Society of Safety Engineers (ASSE).

Eligibility This program is open to ASSE student members who are working on an undergraduate or graduate degree in occupational safety, health, and environment or a closely-related field (e.g., industrial or environmental engineering, environmental science, industrial hygiene, occupational health nursing). Applicants must be bilingual (Spanish-English); Hispanic ethnicity is preferred. Students attending an ABET-accredited school also receive preference. Undergraduates must be full-time students who have completed at least 60 semester hours with a GPA of 3.0 or higher. Graduate students must also be enrolled full time, have completed at least 9 semester hours with a GPA of 3.5 or higher, and have earned a GPA of 3.0 or higher as an undergraduate. Along with their application, they must submit 2 essays of 300 words or less: 1) why they are seeking a degree in occupational safety and health or a closely-related field, a brief description of their current activities, and how those relate to their career goals and objectives; and 2) why they should be awarded this scholarship (including career goals and financial need). U.S. citizenship is not required.

Financial Data The stipend is $3,000 per year.

Duration 1 year; recipients may reapply.

Additional data This program was established in 2005.

Number awarded 1 each year.

Deadline November of each year.

[228]
MERRILL N. AND JULIA H. BRADLEY SURGERY SCHOLARSHIP FUND

St. Vincent's Health System
Attn: St. Vincent's Foundation
De Paul Building
2800 University Building, Suite 101
Birmingham, AL 35233
(205) 939-7296
Web: www.stvhs.com/foundations/bham/Scholarship.asp

Summary To provide scholarship/loans to students interested in working at St. Vincent's Hospital as a surgical nurse in Birmingham, Alabama following certification as an R.N.

Eligibility This program is open to students working full time on an associate (A.D.N.) or bachelor's (B.S.N.) degree in surgical nursing. Applicants must commit to working at St. Vincent's Hospital in Birmingham, Alabama following completion of their degree and certification as an R.N. Along with their application, they must submit a statement of their personal philosophy and how it relates to the mission of the Daughters of Charity and St. Vincent's Hospital. Selection is based on that statement; grades; recommendations from their supervisor in surgery, a surgeon, and another surgery associate; and financial need.

Financial Data The stipend is $2,500 per year. This is a scholarship/loan program. Recipients are required to work full time at St. Vincent's for 2 years or repay all assistance received.

Duration 1 year; may be renewed 1 additional year.

Number awarded 1 each year.
Deadline April of each year.

[229]
MICHIGAN LEGION AUXILIARY MEDICAL CAREER SCHOLARSHIP

American Legion Auxiliary
Department of Michigan
212 North Verlinden Avenue
Lansing, MI 48915
(517) 267-8809   Fax: (517) 371-3698
E-mail: scholarships@michalaux.org
Web: www.michalaux.org/scholarships.htm

Summary To provide financial assistance for college to Michigan veterans' descendants who are interested in preparing for careers in nursing, physical therapy, or respiratory therapy at a school in the state.

Eligibility This program is open to the children, grandchildren, great-grandchildren, or stepchildren of honorably-discharged or deceased veterans who served in designated periods of war time. Applicants must be in the top quarter of their class, in financial need, and residents of Michigan at the time of application and for 1 year preceding the date of the award. They must be interested in training as a registered nurse, licensed practical nurse, physical therapist, or respiratory therapist at a school in Michigan.

Financial Data The stipend is $500. The grant, paid directly to the recipient's school, may be used for tuition, room and board, fees, books, and supplies for the first year of study at a Michigan school of nursing, physical therapy, or respiratory therapy.

Duration 1 year; nonrenewable.

Number awarded 3 each year: 1 each for nursing, physical therapy, and respiratory therapy.

Deadline March of each year.

[230]
MICHIGAN NURSES FOUNDATION SCHOLARSHIP PROGRAM

Michigan Nurses Association
Attn: Michigan Nurses Foundation
2310 Jolly Oak Road
Okemos, MI 48864-4599
(517) 349-5640, ext. 213   Toll Free: (888) MI-NURSE
Fax: (517) 349-5818   E-mail: Pam.Wojtowicz@minurses.org
Web: www.michigannursesfoundation.org/awards.shtml

Summary To provide financial assistance to undergraduate or graduate nursing students at schools in Michigan.

Eligibility This program is open to students enrolled at a Michigan school of nursing that grants a certificate for practical nursing or an associate, baccalaureate, or higher degree in nursing. Applicants must submit brief statements on their vision of their future nursing practice and how they intend to use the scholarship monies if awarded. Selection is based on community involvement, financial need, and participation in the Michigan Nursing Student Association or Michigan Nurses Association.

Financial Data The stipend is $500.

Duration 1 year.

Number awarded At least 4 each year.

Deadline July of each year.

[231]
MILDRED COLLINS NURSING/HEALTH SCIENCE/ MEDICINE SCHOLARSHIP

African-American/Caribbean Education Association, Inc.
P.O. Box 1224
Valley Stream, NY 11582-1224
(718) 949-6733   E-mail: aaceainc@yahoo.com
Web: www.aaceainc.com/Scholarships.html

Summary To provide financial assistance to high school seniors of African American or Caribbean heritage who plan to study a field related to nursing, health science, or medicine in college.

Eligibility This program is open to graduating high school seniors who are U.S. citizens of African American or Caribbean heritage. Applicants must be planning to attend a college or university and major in a field related to nursing, health science, or medicine. They must have completed 4 years of specified college preparatory courses with a grade of 90 or higher and have an SAT score of at least 1790. They must also have completed at least 200 hours of community service during their 4 years of high school, preferably in the field that they plan to study in college. Financial need is not considered in the selection process. New York residency is not required, but applicants must be available for an interviews in the Queens, New York area.

Financial Data The stipend ranges from $1,000 to $2,500. Funds are paid directly to the recipient.

Duration 1 year.

Number awarded 1 each year.

Deadline April of each year.

[232]
MILDRED NUTTING NURSING SCHOLARSHIP

National Society Daughters of the American Revolution
Attn: Committee Services Office, Scholarships
1776 D Street, N.W.
Washington, DC 20006-5303
(202) 628-1776
Web: www.dar.org/natsociety/edout_scholar.cfm

Summary To provide financial assistance to undergraduate students working on a degree in nursing.

Eligibility This program is open to undergraduate students currently enrolled in accredited schools of nursing who have completed at least 1 year. Applicants must be sponsored by a local chapter of the Daughters of the American Revolution (DAR). Preference is given to applicants from the greater Lowell, Massachusetts area. Selection is based on academic excellence, commitment to field of study, and financial need. U.S. citizenship is required.

Financial Data The stipend is $1,000.

Duration 1 year; nonrenewable.

Number awarded Varies each year.

Deadline February of each year.

[233]
MINNESOTA LEGION AUXILIARY PAST PRESIDENTS PARLEY HEALTH CARE SCHOLARSHIP

American Legion Auxiliary
Department of Minnesota
State Veterans Service Building
20 West 12th Street, Room 314
St. Paul, MN 55155-2069
(651) 224-7634   Toll Free: (888) 217-9598
Fax: (651) 224-5243   E-mail: deptoffice@mnala.org
Web: www.mnala.org/ala/scholarship.asp

Summary To provide financial assistance for education in health care fields to members of the American Legion Auxiliary in Minnesota.

Eligibility This program is open to residents of Minnesota who have been members of the American Legion Auxiliary for at least 3 years. Applicants must have a GPA of 2.0 or higher and be planning to study in Minnesota. Their proposed major may be in any phase of health care, including nursing assistant, registered nursing, licensed practical nurse, X-ray or other technician, physical or other therapist, dental hygienist, or dental assistant.

Financial Data The stipend is $1,000. Funds are sent directly to the recipient's school after satisfactory completion of the first quarter.
Duration 1 year.
Number awarded Up to 10 each year.
Deadline March of each year.

[234]
MINNESOTA NURSES ASSOCIATION BACCALAUREATE SCHOLARSHIP

Minnesota Nurses Association
Attn: Minnesota Nurses Association Foundation
1625 Energy Park Drive, Suite 200
St. Paul, MN 55108
(651) 414-2822   Toll Free: (800) 536-4662, ext. 122
Fax: (651) 695-7000   E-mail: linda.owens@mnnurses.org
Web: www.mnnurses.org

Summary To provide financial assistance to members of the Minnesota Nurses Association (MNA) and the Minnesota Student Nurses Association (MSNA) who are interested in working on a baccalaureate degree in nursing.
Eligibility This program is open to MNA and MSNA members who are enrolled or entering a baccalaureate program in nursing in Minnesota. Applicants must submit: a current transcript; a short essay describing their interest in nursing, their long-range career goals, and how their continuing education will have an impact on the profession of nursing in Minnesota; a description of their financial need; and 2 letters of support.
Financial Data The stipend is $2,000 per year.
Duration 1 year; may be renewed.
Number awarded 1 or more each year.
Deadline May of each year.

[235]
MIRIAM FAY FURLONG GRANT

Alpha Tau Delta
Attn: Lynn Zeman, Scholarship Chair
1904 Poinsettia Avenue
Manhattan Beach, CA 90266
E-mail: bilynzeman@yahoo.com
Web: www.atdnursing.org/awards.htm

Summary To provide financial assistance for undergraduate education in nursing to members of Alpha Tau Delta (a national fraternity for professional nurses).
Eligibility This program is open to members in good standing of the fraternity who are entering their junior or senior year of study and can demonstrate financial need. Selection is based on merit and service to the organization.
Financial Data Stipends range from $100 to $1,000.
Duration 1 year.
Number awarded 1 each year.
Deadline April of each year.

[236]
MISSISSIPPI NURSES FOUNDATION SCHOLARSHIP

Mississippi Nurses Association
Attn: Mississippi Nurses Foundation
31 Woodgreen Place
Madison, MS 39110
(601) 898-0850   Fax: (601) 898-0190
E-mail: foundation@msnurses.org
Web: msnursesfoundation.com/scholarships

Summary To provide financial assistance to members of the Mississippi Association of Student Nurses who are enrolled in a registered nursing program in the state.

Eligibility This program is open to members of the association who have been admitted to a basic professional registered nursing program in Mississippi. Applicants must submit an essay of 500 to 1,000 words that begins with the phrase, "The nursing profession will be better in the next decade, because my goals and ambitions includeÖ" Selection is based on that essay, leadership potential, involvement in professional activities, and academic performance.
Financial Data The stipend is $1,000.
Duration 1 year.
Number awarded 1 each year.
Deadline September of each year.

[237]
MISSISSIPPI NURSING EDUCATION LOAN/ SCHOLARSHIP PROGRAM-BSN

Mississippi Office of Student Financial Aid
3825 Ridgewood Road
Jackson, MS 39211-6453
(601) 432-6997   Toll Free: (800) 327-2980 (within MS)
Fax: (601) 432-6527   E-mail: sfa@ihl.state.ms.us
Web: www.mississippi.edu/riseupms/financialaid-state.php

Summary To provide scholarship/loans to Mississippi residents who are interested in working on a bachelor's degree in nursing.
Eligibility This program is open to Mississippi residents working on a B.S.N. degree as a full- or part-time junior or senior at an accredited school of nursing in the state. Applicants must have earned a GPA of 2.5 or higher on all previous college work. They must agree to employment in professional nursing (patient care) in Mississippi.
Financial Data Scholarship/loans are $4,000 per academic year for up to 2 years or a total of $8,000 (prorated over 3 years for part-time participants). For each year of service in Mississippi as a professional nurse (patient care), 1 year's loan will be forgiven. For nurses who received prorated funding over 3 years, the length of service required is 2 years. In the event the recipient fails to fulfill the service obligation, repayment of principal and interest is required.
Duration 1 year; may be renewed up to 1 additional year of full-time study or 2 years of part-time study, provided the recipient maintains a GPA of 2.5 or higher each semester.
Additional data The service requirement may not be deferred to work on a master's degree.
Number awarded Varies each year, depending on the availability of funds; awards are granted on a first-come, first-served basis.
Deadline March of each year.

[238]
MISSISSIPPI NURSING EDUCATION LOAN/ SCHOLARSHIP PROGRAM-RN TO BSN

Mississippi Office of Student Financial Aid
3825 Ridgewood Road
Jackson, MS 39211-6453
(601) 432-6997   Toll Free: (800) 327-2980 (within MS)
Fax: (601) 432-6527   E-mail: sfa@ihl.state.ms.us
Web: www.mississippi.edu/riseupms/financialaid-state.php

Summary To provide scholarship/loans to registered nurses in Mississippi who are interested in working on a bachelor's degree.
Eligibility This program is open to residents of Mississippi who have a current nursing license (R.N.). Applicants must be working on a baccalaureate degree in nursing (B.S.N.) as a full- or part-time student at an accredited school of nursing in Mississippi and have earned a GPA of 2.5 or higher on all previous college work. They must agree to employment in professional nursing (patient care) in Mississippi or teaching at an accredited school of nursing in the state.

Financial Data Scholarship/loans are $4,000 per academic year for up to 2 years or a total of $8,000 (prorated over 3 years for part-time participants). For each year of service in Mississippi as a professional nurse (patient care) or teacher at an accredited school of nursing, 1 year's loan will be forgiven. For nurses who received prorated funding over 3 years, the time of service required is 2 years. In the event the recipient fails to fulfill the service obligation, repayment of principal and interest is required.

Duration 1 year; may be renewed up to 1 additional year of full-time study or 2 years of part-time study provided the recipient maintains a GPA of 2.5 or higher each semester.

Number awarded Varies each year, depending on the availability of funds; awards are granted on a first-come, first-served basis.

Deadline March of each year.

[239]
MISSISSIPPI UNDERGRADUATE CAR TAG STIPEND PROGRAM

Mississippi Nurses Association
Attn: Mississippi Nurses Foundation
31 Woodgreen Place
Madison, MS 39110
(601) 898-0850   Fax: (601) 898-0190
E-mail: foundation@msnurses.org
Web: msnursesfoundation.com/scholarships

Summary To provide scholarship/loans to residents of Mississippi who are working on an undergraduate degree in nursing at a school in the state and have a license plate for nursing on their car.

Eligibility This program is open to residents of Mississippi who have a current registered nurse (R.N.) license and are currently enrolled full time in an associate or baccalaureate nursing program in the state. Applicants must have a special nursing license plate on their personal vehicle at the time of application and during receipt of funding. They must have a GPA of 3.0 or higher. Along with their application, they must submit a 500-word essay on the value of nursing to the nursing student, Mississippi, and the patient. Selection is based on that essay, transcripts, school of nursing activities, community activities, awards and honors, and 3 letters of reference.

Financial Data The stipend is $6,000. Funds are paid directly to students at the rate of $500 per month for 12 months. Students must sign a contract to work in Mississippi within the first 2 years following completion of the program. If they fail to comply with that contract, they must repay all funds received, plus interest.

Duration 1 year.

Number awarded Varies each year. Recently, 4 of these stipends were awarded: 2 to associate degree students and 2 to baccalaureate students.

Deadline June of each year.

[240]
MISSOURI NURSES ASSOCIATION FOUNDATION SCHOLARSHIPS

Missouri Nurses Association
Attn: Missouri Nurses Association Foundation
1904 Bubba Lane
P.O. Box 105228
Jefferson City, MO 65110-5228
(573) 636-4623   Fax: (573) 636-9576
E-mail: info@missourinurses.org
Web: www.missourinurses.org/programs/foundation.html

Summary To provide financial assistance to students working on a bachelor's degree in nursing at a school in Missouri.

Eligibility This program is open to Missouri residents enrolled full time as juniors or seniors at an accredited school of nursing in the state. Applicants must be working on a baccalaureate degree

in nursing and have a GPA of 3.0 or higher. Along with their application, they must submit a transcript, a letter of reference, a 1-page personal statement describing why they chose a career in nursing, and a 2-page resume that covers their extracurricular activities, leadership roles, honors, and community service. Financial need is not considered in the selection process.

Financial Data The stipend is $500.

Duration 1 year.

Number awarded 3 every other year.

Deadline March of odd-numbered years.

[241]
MLN/MCNEA NURSING STUDENT SCHOLARSHIP AWARDS

Michigan League for Nursing
Attn: Director
2410 Woodlake Drive
Okemos, MI 48864
(517) 347-8091   Fax: (517) 347-4096
E-mail: cstacy@mhc.org
Web: www.michleaguenursing.org/ViewPage.cfm?NavID=21

Summary To provide financial assistance to undergraduate nursing students in Michigan.

Eligibility This program is open to students who are currently enrolled in a licensed practical nurse, associate degree, or bachelor's degree nursing program in Michigan, have completed at least 1 nursing course with a clinical component, and have at least a 2.0 GPA. Applicants must submit a 500-word essay on a nursing-related topic. Selection is based on academic record, financial need, contributions, and quality of the essay.

Financial Data The stipend is $1,000.

Duration 1 year.

Additional data This program is jointly sponsored by the Michigan League for Nursing (MLN) and the Michigan Council of Nursing Education Administrators (MCNEA).

Number awarded Varies each year; recently, 7 of these scholarships were awarded.

Deadline February of each year.

[242]
MOLLIE C. AND LARENE B. WOODARD NURSING SCHOLARSHIP

Louisiana State Nurses Association
Attn: Louisiana Nurses Foundation
5713 Superior Drive, Suite A-6
Baton Rouge, LA 70816
(225) 201-0993   Fax: (225) 201-0971
E-mail: lsna@lsna.org
Web: www.lsna.org/Woodard-scholarship.html

Summary To provide financial assistance to residents of Louisiana who are attending college in that state or a bordering state to prepare for a career as a registered nurse (R.N.).

Eligibility This program is open to residents of Louisiana who are currently enrolled full time in the clinical component of a program that prepares them for a career as an R.N. Applicants must be attending a school in Louisiana or a state that borders it (Arkansas, Mississippi, or Texas). They must have a GPA of 3.0 or higher and be able to demonstrate financial need. Along with their application, they must submit a 250-word statement describing their motivation for choosing nursing as a career.

Financial Data The stipend is $5,000 per year.

Duration 1 year; may be renewed, provided the recipient maintains a GPA of 2.7 or higher.

Number awarded 1 or more each year.

Deadline June of each year.

[243]
MOLN MEMBER SCHOLARSHIPS

Minnesota Organization of Leaders in Nursing
1821 University Avenue West, Suite S256
St. Paul, MN 55104
(651) 999-5344   Fax: (651) 917-1835
E-mail: office@moln.org
Web: www.moln.org/sections/scholarships.php

Summary To provide financial assistance to members of the Minnesota Organization of Leaders in Nursing (MOLN) who are interested in returning to school to earn an additional degree in nursing.

Eligibility This program is open to MOLN members (must have been voting members for at least 12 months) who are currently enrolled or have been admitted to a relevant bachelor's, master's, or doctoral degree program. Applicants must have a GPA of 3.0 or higher in their current academic work. Along with their application, they must submit a 2-page essay on their goals in returning to school to complete a degree, how attainment of this degree will facilitate their professional development as a leader in nursing, and how their educational and career goals relate to the goals of MOLN. Selection is based on the essay, a letter of recommendation, and transcripts. Financial need is not considered.

Financial Data The stipend is $500.
Duration 1 year.
Number awarded Up to 6 each year.
Deadline June of each year.

[244]
MOLN RN STUDENT EDUCATIONAL SCHOLARSHIP

Minnesota Organization of Leaders in Nursing
1821 University Avenue West, Suite S256
St. Paul, MN 55104
(651) 999-5344   Fax: (651) 917-1835
E-mail: office@moln.org
Web: www.moln.org/sections/scholarships.php

Summary To provide financial assistance to students who have been admitted to an R.N. nursing program in Minnesota.

Eligibility This program is open to students who have been admitted to an R.N. nursing program (associate or bachelor's degree) in Minnesota. Applicants must have a GPA of 3.0 or higher and be recommended by a member of Minnesota Organization of Leaders in Nursing (MOLN). Along with their application, they must submit a 1-page essay on their goals in preparing for a nursing career and their perception of the concept that every nurse is a leader. Selection is based on the essay and demonstrated leadership potential.

Financial Data The stipend is $500.
Duration 1 year.
Number awarded 1 each year.
Deadline June of each year.

[245]
MONSTER.COM NURSING DEGREE SCHOLARSHIP FOR EMERGENCY DEPARTMENT EMPLOYEES

Emergency Nurses Association
Attn: ENA Foundation
915 Lee Street
Des Plaines, IL 60016-6569
(847) 460-4100   Toll Free: (800) 900-9659, ext. 4100
Fax: (847) 460-4004   E-mail: foundation@ena.org
Web: www.ena.org

Summary To provide financial assistance to emergency department personnel working on an undergraduate degree in nursing.

Eligibility This program is open to hospital emergency department employees (e.g., emergency medical technicians, clerical coordinators, CNAs, registration clerks) who are working on an associate or baccalaureate degree in nursing. Applicants must submit a letter from their supervisor verifying their interest in emergency nursing and at least 1 year of emergency department employment. They are not required to be a member of the Emergency Nurses Association (ENA), but they are must submit a letter of reference from an ENA member. Along with their application, they must submit a 1-page statement on their professional and educational goals and how this scholarship will help them attain those goals. Selection is based on content and clarity of the goal statement (45%), professional association involvement (35%), presentation of the application (10%), and letters of reference (10%).

Financial Data The stipend is $2,000.
Duration 1 year.
Additional data This program is supported by Monster.com.
Number awarded 1 each year.
Deadline May of each year.

[246]
MONSTER.COM UNDERGRADUATE SCHOLARSHIP

Emergency Nurses Association
Attn: ENA Foundation
915 Lee Street
Des Plaines, IL 60016-6569
(847) 460-4100   Toll Free: (800) 900-9659, ext. 4100
Fax: (847) 460-4004   E-mail: foundation@ena.org
Web: www.ena.org

Summary To provide financial assistance for baccalaureate study to nurses who are members of the Emergency Nurses Association (ENA).

Eligibility This program is open to nurses (R.N., L.P.N., L.V.N.) who are working on a bachelor's degree. Applicants must have been members of the association for at least 12 months and have a GPA of 3.0 or higher. They must submit a 1-page statement on their professional and educational goals and how this scholarship will help them attain those goals. Selection is based on content and clarity of the goal statement (45%), professional association involvement (35%), presentation of the application (10%), and letters of reference (10%).

Financial Data The stipend is $4,000.
Duration 1 year; nonrenewable.
Additional data This program is supported by Monster.com.
Number awarded 2 each year.
Deadline May of each year.

[247]
MORGAN-SANDERS ENDOWED SCHOLARSHIP

Kansas State Nurses Association
Attn: Kansas Nurses Foundation
1109 S.W. Topeka Boulevard
Topeka, KS 66612-1602
(785) 233-8638   Fax: (785) 233-5222
E-mail: ksna@ksna.net
Web: www.nursingworld.org/SNAS/KS/Knf.htm

Summary To provide financial assistance to students in Kansas who are working on an undergraduate or graduate degree in nursing at a school in the state.

Eligibility This program is open to residents of Kansas who have a GPA of 3.0 or higher. The award is given according to the following priorities, in descending order: 1) R.N.s working on a B.S.N. degree; 2) graduate students in nursing education, nursing administration, or adult education programs (with priority given to master's and then doctoral level); 3) nonacademic nursing or nursing-related programs leading to a certificate; 4) students enrolled in undergraduate B.S.N. programs; and 5) students enrolled in undergraduate A.D.N. programs. Students enrolled in graduate or certificate program preparation for clinical nurse specialists, nurse practitioners, nurse midwives, and nurse anesthetists are not eligible. Preference is given to students engaged in full-time study. Along with their application, they must submit a personal narrative describing their anticipated role in nursing in the state.

Financial Data   The stipend is $500.

Duration   1 year.

Number awarded   1 each year.

Deadline   June of each year.

[248]
NADONA OF NORTH DAKOTA NURSING SCHOLARSHIP

NADONA of North Dakota
c/o Julie Hanson, President
750 Main Street East
Mayville, ND 58277
(701) 786-3401   Fax: (701) 789-9022
E-mail: jhanson-lhm@polarcomm.com
Web: www.ndnadona.org

Summary   To provide financial assistance to employees of long-term care facilities in North Dakota who are interested in working on a degree in nursing at a school in any state.

Eligibility   This program is open to employees of long-term care facilities in North Dakota that also have a member of NADONA of North Dakota on the staff. Applicants must be a licensed R.N., L.P.N., or certified nursing assistant. They must be planning to attend a school in any state to work on to work on an R.N. or L.P.N. in nursing management or gerontology or a master's degree in nursing, health care administration, or nurse practitioner. Along with their application, they must submit brief statements on 1) their future professional plans and interests unique to long-term care; and 2) any personal or professional experiences in long-term care that have led to their decision to prepare for a career in long-term care administration and the challenges they believe the long-term care profession holds.

Financial Data   A stipend is awarded (amount not specified).

Duration   1 year.

Additional data   The sponsor is the North Dakota affiliate of National Association Directors of Nursing Administration in Long Term Care (NADONA).

Number awarded   1 or more each year.

Deadline   August of each year.

[249]
NATIONAL AMERICAN ARAB NURSES ASSOCIATION SCHOLARSHIPS

National American Arab Nurses Association
P.O. Box 43
Dearborn Heights, MI 48127
(313) 680-5049   E-mail: info@n-aana.org
Web: www.n-aana.org/scholarship/index.asp

Summary   To provide financial assistance to nursing students who are members of the National American Arab Nurses Association (NAANA).

Eligibility   This program is open to NAANA members who are studying nursing at the associate degree, bachelor's degree, master's degree, or R.N. to B.S.N. levels. Applicants must have a GPA of 3.5 or higher and a record of leadership in academic, professional, and/or student organizations. Along with their application, they must submit a 1-page essay on their career goals, leadership activities, and why they deserve the award. Financial need is not considered in the selection process. U.S. citizenship or permanent resident status is required.

Financial Data   Stipends are $1,000 or $500.

Duration   1 year.

Additional data   Until 2006, NAANA was named the American Arab Nurses Association.

Number awarded   Varies each year.

Deadline   May of each year.

[250]
NATIONAL ASSOCIATION OF HISPANIC NURSES MICHIGAN CHAPTER SCHOLARSHIPS

National Association of Hispanic Nurses-Michigan Chapter
c/o Dottie Rodriquez, Scholarship Committee
769 Fox River Drive
Bloomfield Township, MI 48304
(313) 282-8471
Web: michiganhispanicnurses.org

Summary   To provide financial assistance to Hispanic undergraduate nursing students enrolled in a program in Michigan.

Eligibility   This program is open to undergraduate Hispanic students working on a generic nursing degree or certificate (A.D.N., B.S.N., or L.P.N.) at a school in Michigan; L.P.N. to R.N. and R.N. to B.S.N. students are not eligible. Applicants must have completed at least 1 year of their program and have a GPA of 2.5 or higher. Along with their application, they must submit a 2-page essay that includes personal background information, school involvement, community service, and goals after graduation. Financial need is not considered in the selection process.

Financial Data   The stipend is $500.

Duration   1 year; nonrenewable.

Additional data   Recipients must agree to perform 10 to 20 hours of volunteer service to the sponsor within 1 year of receipt of this scholarship.

Number awarded   6 each year.

Deadline   October of each year.

[251]
NATIONAL ASSOCIATION OF SCHOOL NURSES DIRECTED RESEARCH GRANTS

National Association of School Nurses
Attn: NASN Research Committee
8484 Georgia Avenue, Suite 420
Silver Spring, MD 20910
(240) 821-1130   Toll Free: (866) 627-6767
Fax: (301) 585-1791   E-mail: nasn@nasn.org
Web: www.nasn.org/Default.aspx?tabid=371

Summary   To provide funding to members of the National Association of School Nurses (NASN) who are interested in conducting research on specified school nursing issues.

Eligibility   This program is open to qualified professional school nurses who have been members of the association for at least 1 year. Applicants must be 1) engaged in the practice of school nursing, the education of school nurses, or the study of school nursing as a graduate or undergraduate student; or 2) retired from school nursing. They must be interested in conducting research on 1 of several topics that are selected annually by the association as research priorities. Recently, the topics were: impact of school nursing services on student health and academic outcomes, effectiveness of health promotion and disease prevention, cost effectiveness of school health services, and predictors of successful outcomes for students needing health interventions. Selection is based on research question and purpose (5%), study aim and hypothesis (10%), background/review of literature/theoretical discussion (15%), methodology (35%), significance to school nursing (15%), qualifications of the researcher (15%), and overall quality of application (5%).

Financial Data   Grants range up to $5,000 and average $2,500.

Duration   1 year.

Additional data   This program, originally called the Carol Costante Research Grant, began in 1998.

Number awarded   1 to 3 each year.

Deadline   February of each year.

[252]
NATIONAL ASSOCIATION OF SCHOOL NURSES RESEARCH GRANTS

National Association of School Nurses
Attn: NASN Research Committee
8484 Georgia Avenue, Suite 420
Silver Spring, MD 20910
(240) 821-1130   Toll Free: (866) 627-6767
Fax: (301) 585-1791   E-mail: nasn@nasn.org
Web: www.nasn.org/Default.aspx?tabid=371

Summary To provide funding to members of the National Association of School Nurses (NASN) who are interested in conducting research on a school nursing issue.

Eligibility This program is open to qualified professional school nurses who have been members of the association for at least 1 year. Applicants must be 1) engaged in the practice of school nursing, the education of school nurses, or the study of school nursing as a graduate or undergraduate student; or 2) retired from school nursing. They must be interested in conducting a research project on any topic that has an impact on student health and well being. Selection is based on research question and purpose (5%), study aim and hypothesis (10%), background/review of literature/theoretical discussion (15%), methodology (35%), significance to school nursing (15%), qualifications of the researcher (15%), and overall quality of application (5%).

Financial Data Grants range up to $5,000 and average $2,500.

Duration 1 year.

Additional data This program was established in 1997 by combining 3 prior programs: the Lillian Wald Research Award, established in 1982 for research impacting the health of children; the Pauline Fenelon Research Award, established in 1987 for research in school nurse practice issues; and the Lina Rogers Award, established in 1990 for research impacting school nursing services for students.

Number awarded 1 or more each year.

Deadline February of each year.

[253]
NATIONAL STUDENT NURSES' ASSOCIATION GENERAL SCHOLARSHIPS

National Student Nurses' Association
Attn: Foundation
45 Main Street, Suite 606
Brooklyn, NY 11201
(718) 210-0705   Fax: (718) 797-1186
E-mail: nsna@nsna.org
Web: www.nsna.org

Summary To provide financial assistance to nursing or pre-nursing students.

Eligibility This program is open to students currently enrolled in state-approved schools of nursing or pre-nursing associate degree, baccalaureate, diploma, generic master's, generic doctoral, R.N. to B.S.N., R.N. to M.S.N., or L.P.N./L.V.N. to R.N. programs. Graduating high school seniors are not eligible. Support for graduate education is provided only for a first degree in nursing. Applicants must submit a 200-word description of their professional and educational goals and how this scholarship will help them achieve those goals. Selection is based on academic achievement, financial need, and involvement in student nursing organizations and community health activities. U.S. citizenship or permanent resident status is required.

Financial Data Stipends range from $1,000 to $2,500. A total of approximately $125,000 is awarded each year by the foundation for all its scholarship programs.

Duration 1 year.

Additional data This program includes the following named scholarships: the Anne Merin Memorial Scholarship, the Eileen Bowden Memorial Scholarship, the Alice Robinson Memorial Scholarship, the Jeannette Collins Memorial Scholarship, the Cleo Doster Memorial Scholarship, and the Mary Ann Tuft Scholarships. Sponsors include 3M Health Care, Bank of America, Catholic Healthcare West, Chi Eta Phi Sorority, Delmar Cengage Learning, Elsevier, HSBC Bank USA, Johnson & Johnson, Kaiser Permanente, Landau Uniforms, Pfizer, Sigma Theta Tau International, and United Healthcare. Applications must be accompanied by a $10 processing fee.

Number awarded Varies each year; recently, 63 of these scholarships were awarded.

Deadline January of each year.

[254]
NATIONAL STUDENT NURSES' ASSOCIATION SPECIALTY SCHOLARSHIPS

National Student Nurses' Association
Attn: Foundation
45 Main Street, Suite 606
Brooklyn, NY 11201
(718) 210-0705   Fax: (718) 797-1186
E-mail: nsna@nsna.org
Web: www.nsna.org

Summary To provide financial assistance to nursing students in designated specialties.

Eligibility This program is open to students currently enrolled in state-approved schools of nursing or pre-nursing associate degree, baccalaureate, diploma, generic master's, generic doctoral, R.N. to B.S.N., R.N. to M.S.N., or L.P.N./L.V.N. to R.N. programs. Graduating high school seniors are not eligible. Support for graduate education is provided only for a first degree in nursing. Applicants must designate their intended specialty, which may be anesthesia nursing, critical care, emergency, gerontology, informatics, nephrology, nurse educator, oncology, orthopedic, or perioperative. Along with their application, they must submit a 200-word description of their professional and educational goals and how this scholarship will help them achieve those goals. Selection is based on academic achievement, financial need, and involvement in student nursing organizations and community activities related to health care. U.S. citizenship or permanent resident status is required.

Financial Data Stipends range from $1,000 to $2,500. A total of approximately $125,000 is awarded each year by the foundation for all its scholarship programs.

Duration 1 year.

Additional data Funding for this program is provided in partnership with other nursing organizations, including the American Association of Nurse Anesthetists, the American Association of Critical-Care Nurses, the American Nephrology Nurses' Association, the American Organization of Nurse Executives, Decision Critical, Inc., the Emergency Nurses Association, the Infusion Nurses Society, and the Oncology Nursing Society. Applications must be accompanied by a $10 processing fee.

Number awarded Varies each year; recently 16 of these scholarships were awarded.

Deadline January of each year.

[255]
NAVY ADVANCED EDUCATION VOUCHER PROGRAM

U.S. Navy
Naval Education and Training Command
Center for Personal and Professional Development
Attn: AEV Program Office
6490 Saufley Field Road
Pensacola, FL 32509-5204
(850) 452-7271   Fax: (850) 452-1272
E-mail: rick.cusimano@navy.mil
Web: www.navycollege.navy.mil/aev/aev_home.cfm

Summary To provide financial assistance to Navy enlisted personnel who are interested in earning an undergraduate or graduate degree during off-duty hours.
Eligibility This program is open to senior enlisted Navy personnel in ranks E-7 and E-8. Applicants should be transferring to, or currently on, shore duty with sufficient time ashore to complete a bachelor's or master's degree. Personnel at rank E-7 may have no more than 16 years time in service and at E-8 no more than 18 years. The area of study must be certified by the Naval Postgraduate School as Navy-relevant.
Financial Data This program covers 100% of education costs (tuition, books, and fees). For a bachelor's degree, the maximum is $6,700 per year or a total of $20,000 per participant. For a master's degree, the maximum is $20,000 per year or a total of $40,000 per participant.
Duration Up to 36 months from the time of enrollment for a bachelor's degree; up to 24 months from the time of enrollment for a master's degree.
Additional data Recently approved majors for bachelor's degrees included human resources, construction management, information technology, emergency and disaster management, paralegal, engineering, business administration, leadership and management, nursing, strategic foreign languages, and electrical/electronic technology. Approved fields of study for master's degrees included business administration, education and training management, emergency and disaster management, engineering and technology, homeland defense and security, human resources, information technology, leadership and management, project management, and systems analysis. Recipients of this assistance incur an obligation to remain on active duty following completion of the program for a period equal to 3 times the number of months of education completed, to a maximum obligation of 36 months.
Number awarded Varies each year. Recently, 20 of these vouchers were awarded: 15 for bachelor's degrees and 5 for master's degrees.
Deadline February of each year.

[256]
NAVY NURSE CANDIDATE PROGRAM

U.S. Navy
Attn: Navy Medicine Manpower, Personnel, Education and
  Training Command
Code OH
8901 Wisconsin Avenue, Building 1, Tower 13, Room 13132
Bethesda, MD 20889-5611
(301) 295-1217   Toll Free: (800) USA-NAVY
Fax: (301) 295-1811   E-mail: OH@med.navy.mil
Web: www.med.navy.mil

Summary To provide financial assistance for nursing education to students interested in serving in the Navy.
Eligibility This program is open to full-time students in a bachelor of science in nursing program who are U.S. citizens under 40 years of age. Prior to or during their junior year of college, applicants must enlist in the U.S. Navy Nurse Corps Reserve. Following receipt of their degree, they must be willing to serve on active duty as a nurse in the Navy.
Financial Data This program pays a $10,000 initial grant upon enlistment (paid in 2 installments of $5,000 each) and a stipend of $1,000 per month. Students are responsible for paying all school expenses.
Duration Up to 24 months.
Additional data Students who receive support from this program for 1 to 12 months incur an active-duty service obligation of 4 years; students who receive support for 13 to 24 months have a service obligation of 5 years.
Number awarded Varies each year.
Deadline Deadline not specified.

[257]
NAVY NURSE CORPS NROTC SCHOLARSHIP PROGRAM

U.S. Navy
Attn: Naval Education and Training Command
NSTC OD2
250 Dallas Street, Suite A
Pensacola, FL 32508-5268
(850) 452-4941, ext. 25166
Toll Free: (800) NAV-ROTC, ext. 25166
Fax: (850) 452-2486
E-mail: PNSC_NROTC.scholarship@navy.mil
Web: www.nrotc.navy.mil/nurse.aspx

Summary To provide financial assistance to graduating high school seniors who are interested in joining Navy ROTC and majoring in nursing in college.
Eligibility Eligible to apply for these scholarships are graduating high school seniors who have been accepted at a college with a Navy ROTC unit on campus or a college with a cross-enrollment agreement with such a college. Applicants must be U.S. citizens between the ages of 17 and 23 who plan to study nursing in college and are willing to serve for 4 years as active-duty Navy officers in the Navy Nurse Corps following graduation from college. They must not have reached their 27th birthday by the time of college graduation and commissioning; applicants who have prior active-duty military service may be eligible for age adjustments for the amount of time equal to their prior service, up to a maximum of 36 months. They must have minimum SAT scores of 530 in critical reading and in 520 mathematics or minimum ACT scores of 22 in English and 21 in mathematics.
Financial Data This scholarship provides payment of full tuition and required educational fees, as well as $375 per semester for textbooks, supplies, and equipment. The program also provides a stipend for 10 months of the year that is $250 per month as a freshman, $300 per month as a sophomore, $350 per month as a junior, and $400 per month as a senior.
Duration 4 years.
Number awarded Varies each year.
Deadline January of each year.

[258]
NEBRASKA NURSES ASSOCIATION SCHOLARSHIPS

Nebraska Nurses Association
P.O. Box 82086
Lincoln, NE 68501-2086
E-mail: admin@nebraskanurses.org
Web: www.nebraskanurses.org

Summary To provide financial assistance to Nebraska residents working on a nursing degree at a school in the state.
Eligibility This program is open to residents of Nebraska who have completed more than 50% of the required degree courses at an accredited nursing program in the state. Applicants must have a GPA of 3.0 or higher. Along with their application, they must submit a 500-word essay on why they chose nursing as a career and their career goals. Selection is based on that essay, GPA, and 2 letters of recommendation.
Financial Data The stipend is $500.
Duration 1 year.
Additional data This program is sponsored by the Arthur L. Davis Publishing Agency.
Number awarded 2 each year.
Deadline September.

[259]
NED CARTER SCHOLARSHIPS

Association of Fire Districts of the State of New York
c/o Frank A. Nocerino, Secretary/Treasurer
948 North Bay Avenue
North Massapequa, NY 11758-2581
(516) 799-8575   Toll Free: (800) 520-9594
Fax: (516) 799-2516   E-mail: FNOC@aol.com
Web: www.firedistnys.com/scholarships.html

Summary To provide financial assistance to relatives of fire fighters affiliated with the Association of Fire Districts of New York State who plan to prepare for a career in nursing or another field related to community service at a school in any state.

Eligibility This program is open to high school seniors who are related to a fire fighter in an affiliated member organization of the association. Applicants must be planning to attend a 2- or 4-year college or university in any state to prepare for a career in a community service-related field (e.g., fire service, nursing, social work, health-related services, teaching, library science). Financial need is considered in the selection process.

Financial Data The stipend is $1,500.

Duration 1 year.

Number awarded 3 each year: 1 in each region (central, east, and west) of the state.

Deadline February of each year.

[260]
NEONATAL NURSING ACADEMIC SCHOLARSHIP AWARD

Academy of Neonatal Nursing
2270 Northpoint Parkway
Santa Rosa, CA 95407-7398
(707) 568-2168   Fax: (707) 569-0786
Web: www.academyonline.org/awards_scholarships.html

Summary To provide financial assistance to members of the Academy of Neonatal Nursing (ANN) who are working on an undergraduate or graduate degree in neonatal nursing or a related nursing major.

Eligibility This program is open to ANN members who have been in good standing for at least 2 years. Applicants must have at least 2 years of neonatal practice experience with at least 1 of those years completed in the past 18 months. They must be enrolled in a nursing academic degree program or a neonatal graduate program in which they have completed at least 2 degree-required courses with a GPA of 3.0 or higher. Only professionally-active neonatal nurses are eligible, i.e., currently engaged in a clinical, research, or educational role that contributes directly to the health care of neonates or to the nursing profession and taking 15 contact hours of continuing education a year. Along with their application, they must submit a 200-word essay on why they are pursuing their education and how attainment of this degree will benefit them in their professional role. Financial need is not considered in the selection process.

Financial Data The stipend is $1,000. Funds are paid directly to the recipient and the educational program.

Duration 1 year; recipients are not eligible for another scholarship for 5 years.

Number awarded 1 each year.

Deadline May of each year.

[261]
NEPHROLOGY NURSES CAREER MOBILITY SCHOLARSHIPS

American Nephrology Nurses' Association
Attn: ANNA National Office
200 East Holly Avenue
P.O. Box 56
Pitman, NJ 08071-0056
(856) 256-2320   Toll Free: (888) 600-2662
Fax: (856) 589-7463   E-mail: annascholarships@ajj.com
Web: www.annanurse.org

Summary To provide financial assistance to members of the American Nephrology Nurses' Association (ANNA) who are interested in working on a baccalaureate or advanced degree in nursing.

Eligibility Applicants must be current association members, have been members for at least 2 years, be actively involved in nephrology nursing-related health care services, and be accepted or enrolled in a baccalaureate or higher degree program in nursing. Along with their application, they must submit a 250-word essay on their career and educational goals that includes the expected time frame for completing their degree, the application of the award to meet expected expenses, and the impact of the completion of the degree program on their nephrology nursing practice.

Financial Data The stipend is $2,000.

Duration 1 year.

Additional data These scholarships were first awarded in 1993.

Number awarded 5 each year.

Deadline October of each year.

[262]
NEPHROLOGY NURSING CERTIFICATION COMMISSION CAREER MOBILITY SCHOLARSHIPS

American Nephrology Nurses' Association
Attn: ANNA National Office
200 East Holly Avenue
P.O. Box 56
Pitman, NJ 08071-0056
(609) 256-2320   Toll Free: (888) 600-2662
Fax: (856) 589-7463   E-mail: annascholarships@ajj.com
Web: www.annanurse.org

Summary To provide financial assistance to members of the American Nephrology Nurses' Association (ANNA) who are Certified Nephrology Nurses or Certified Dialysis Nurses and are interested in working on a baccalaureate or graduate degree in nursing to enhance their nephrology nursing practice.

Eligibility Applicants must have a current credential as a Certified Nephrology Nurse (CNN) or Certified Dialysis Nurse (CDN) administered by the Nephrology Nursing Certification Commission (NNCC), be current association members, have been members for at least 2 years, be actively involved in nephrology nursing related health care services, and be accepted or enrolled in a baccalaureate or higher degree program in nursing. Along with their application, they must submit a 250-word essay on their career and educational goals that includes the expected time frame for completing their degree, the application of the award to meet expected expenses, and the impact of the completion of the degree program on their nephrology nursing practice.

Financial Data The stipend is $2,000.

Duration 1 year.

Additional data Funds for this program, established in 1993, are supplied by the NNCC.

Number awarded 3 each year.

Deadline October of each year.

[263]
NEW ENGLAND AREA FUTURE LEADERSHIP AWARD

American Society of Safety Engineers
Attn: ASSE Foundation
1800 East Oakton Street
Des Plaines, IL 60018
(847) 768-3435   Fax: (847) 768-3434
E-mail: agabanski@asse.org
Web: www.asse.org/foundation/scholarships/scholarships.php

Summary To provide financial assistance to upper-division and graduate student members of the American Society of Safety Engineers (ASSE). especially those from the Northeast.

Eligibility This program is open to ASSE student members who are working on an undergraduate or graduate degree in occupational safety, health, and environment or a closely-related field (e.g., industrial or environmental engineering, environmental science, industrial hygiene, occupational health nursing). Undergraduates must be full-time students who have completed at least 60 semester hours with a GPA of 3.0 or higher. Graduate students must also be enrolled full time, have completed at least 9 semester hours with a GPA of 3.5 or higher, and have earned a GPA of 3.0 or higher as an undergraduate. Along with their application, they must submit 2 essays of 300 words or less: 1) why they are seeking a degree in occupational safety and health or a closely-related field, a brief description of their current activities, and how those relate to their career goals and objectives; and 2) why they should be awarded this scholarship (including career goals and financial need). Priority is given first to residents of New England, and second to residents of the ASSE Region VIII (which covers the 6 New England states plus New York, New Jersey, and Pennsylvania). U.S. citizenship is not required.

Financial Data The stipend is $1,000 per year.

Duration 1 year; recipients may reapply.

Additional data This program was established in 2008.

Number awarded 1 each year.

Deadline November of each year.

[264]
NEW ENGLAND NAVY NURSE CORPS ASSOCIATION SCHOLARSHIP

New England Navy Nurse Corps Association
c/o Maria K. Carroll, Scholarship Committee
22 William Drive
Middletown, RI 02842-5266

Summary To provide financial assistance to registered nurses (R.N.s) and nursing students working on a bachelor's or master's degree at a college or university in New England.

Eligibility This program is open to R.N.s and nursing students in the New England states. Applicants must be working on a bachelor's or master's degree in nursing and have a GPA of 2.3 or higher. They must have completed at least 1 clinical nursing course. Along with their application, they must submit a 500-word essay on why they are qualified for this scholarship, their career goals, and their potential for contribution to the profession.

Financial Data The stipend is $1,000.

Duration 1 year.

Number awarded 2 each year.

Deadline May of each year.

[265]
NEW HAMPSHIRE CHAPTER ACEP NURSING SCHOLARSHIP

American College of Emergency Physicians-New Hampshire
  Chapter
Attn: Joy Potter
7 North State Street
Concord, NH 03301
(603) 224-7083   E-mail: joy.potter@nhms.org
Web: www.nhacep.org/scholarships.htm

Summary To provide financial assistance to New Hampshire residents who are working on a degree in nursing at an institution in the state.

Eligibility This program is open to students enrolled or planning to enroll full or part time in an accredited New Hampshire nursing degree program. Applicants must have been residents of the state for at least 3 years. Along with their application, they must submit brief essays on why they want to be a nurse, the qualities and special skills they bring to nursing, their professional goals, and where they see themselves in nursing in 5 years.

Financial Data The stipend is $500.

Duration 1 year.

Number awarded 1 or more each year.

Deadline May of each year.

[266]
NEW HAMPSHIRE WORKFORCE INCENTIVE PROGRAM FORGIVABLE LOANS

New Hampshire Postsecondary Education Commission
Attn: Financial Aid Programs Coordinator
3 Barrell Court, Suite 300
Concord, NH 03301-8543
(603) 271-2555, ext. 360   Fax: (603) 271-2696
TDD: (800) 735-2964
E-mail: cynthia.capodestria@pec.state.nh.us
Web: www.nh.gov/postsecondary/financial/wip.html

Summary To provide scholarship/loans to New Hampshire residents who are interested in attending college in the state to prepare for careers in nursing and other designated professions.

Eligibility This program is open to residents of New Hampshire who wish to prepare for careers in fields designated by the commission as shortage areas. Currently, the career shortage areas are education (chemistry, general science, mathematics, physical sciences, physics, special education, and world languages), and nursing (L.P.N. through graduate). Applicants must be enrolled as a junior, senior, or graduate student at a college in New Hampshire and able to demonstrate financial need.

Financial Data Stipends are determined by the institution; recently, they averaged $1,200 per year. This is a scholarship/loan program; recipients must agree to pursue, within New Hampshire, the professional career for which they receive training. Recipients of loans for 1 year have their notes cancelled upon completion of 1 year of full-time service; repayment by service must be completed within 3 years from the date of licensure, certification, or completion of the program. Recipients of loans for more than 1 year have their notes cancelled upon completion of 2 years of full-time service; repayment by service must be completed within 5 years from the date of licensure, certification, or completion of the program. If the note is not cancelled because of service, the recipient must repay the loan within 2 years.

Duration 1 year; may be renewed.

Additional data The time for repayment of the loan, either in cash or through professional service, is extended while the recipient is 1) engaged in a course of study, at least on a half-time basis, at an institution of higher education; 2) serving on active duty as a member of the armed forces of the United States, or as a member of VISTA, the Peace Corps, or AmeriCorps, for a period up to 3 years; 3) temporarily totally disabled for a period up to 3 years; or 4) unable to secure employment because of the need to care for a disabled spouse, child, or parent for a period up to 12 months. The repayment obligation is cancelled if the recipient is unable to work because of a permanent total disability, receives relief under federal bankruptcy laws, or dies. This program went into effect in 1999.

Number awarded Varies each year; recently, 45 of these loans were awarded.

Deadline May of each year for fall semester; December of each year for spring semester.

[267]
NEW JERSEY GOVERNOR'S NURSING SCHOLARSHIPS

New Jersey State Nurses Association
Attn: Institute for Nursing
1479 Pennington Road
Trenton, NJ 08618-2661
(609) 883-5335   Toll Free: (888) UR-NJSNA
Fax: (609) 883-5343   E-mail: institute@njsna.org
Web: www.njsna.org/displaycommon.cfm?an=5

Summary To provide financial assistance to residents of New Jersey who are applying to or enrolled in a nursing program in the state.

Eligibility This program is open to New Jersey residents who are high school graduates or adults. Applicants must be currently enrolled in a diploma, associate degree, or bachelor's degree program in nursing at a school in the state. R.N.s working on a degree in nursing are also eligible if they are members of the New Jersey State Nurses Association. Selection is based on financial need, GPA, and leadership potential.

Financial Data The stipend is $1,000.

Duration 1 year.

Number awarded 3 each year.

Deadline January of each year.

[268]
NEW JERSEY HFMA MEMBER SCHOLARSHIP

Healthcare Financial Management Association-New Jersey
   Chapter
Attn: Laura A. Hess
P.O. Box 6422
Bridgewater, NJ 08807
Toll Free: (888) 652-4362   Fax: (908) 722-8775
E-mail: njhfma@aol.com
Web: www.hfmanj.org/Scholarship-Information.page

Summary To provide financial assistance to members of the New Jersey Chapter of the Healthcare Financial Management Association (HFMA) and their families who are interested in working on a degree related to health care administration at a school in any state.

Eligibility Applicants must have been a member of the chapter for at least 2 years or the spouse or dependent of a 2-year member. They must be enrolled in an accredited college, university, nursing school, or other allied health professional school in any state. Preference is given to applicants working on a degree in finance, accounting, health care administration, or a field of study related to health care. Along with their application, they must submit an essay describing their educational and professional goals and the role of this scholarship in helping achieve those. Selection is based on the essay, merit, academic achievement, civic and professional activities, course of study, and content of the application. Financial need is not considered.

Financial Data The stipend ranges up to $3,000.

Duration 1 year.

Number awarded 1 or more each year.

Deadline March of each year.

[269]
NEW JERSEY LEGION AUXILIARY PAST PRESIDENTS' PARLEY NURSES SCHOLARSHIPS

American Legion Auxiliary
Department of New Jersey
c/o Lucille M. Miller, Secretary/Treasurer
1540 Kuser Road, Suite A-8
Hamilton, NJ 08619
(609) 581-9580   Fax: (609) 581-8429
E-mail: newjerseyala@juno.com
Web: www.alanj.org

Summary To provide financial assistance to New Jersey residents who are the descendants of veterans and interested in studying nursing at a school in any state.

Eligibility This program is open to the children, grandchildren, and great-grandchildren of veterans who served in the U.S. armed forces during specified periods of war time. Applicants must be graduating high school seniors who have been residents of New Jersey for at least 2 years. They must be planning to study nursing at a school in any state. Along with their application, they must submit a 1,000-word essay on a topic that changes annually; recently, students were asked to write on the topic, "Honoring Our Promise Everyday-How I Can Serve My Country and Our Veterans." Selection is based on academic achievement (40%), character (15%), leadership (15%), Americanism (15%), and financial need (15%).

Financial Data A stipend is awarded (amount not specified).

Duration 1 year.

Number awarded 1 or more each year.

Deadline April of each year.

[270]
NEW MEXICO LEGION AUXILIARY PAST PRESIDENTS PARLEY SCHOLARSHIPS

American Legion Auxiliary
Department of New Mexico
1215 Mountain Road, N.E.
Albuquerque, NM 87102
(505) 242-9918   Fax: (505) 247-0478
E-mail: alauxnm@netscape.com

Summary To provide financial assistance to residents of New Mexico who are the children of veterans and studying nursing or a related medical field at a school in any state.

Eligibility This program is open to New Mexico residents who are attending college in any state. Applicants must be the children of veterans who served during specified periods of war time. They must be studying nursing or a related medical field. Selection is based on scholarship, character, leadership, Americanism, and financial need.

Financial Data A stipend is awarded (amount not specified).

Deadline April of each year.

[271]
NEW MEXICO NURSE EDUCATOR LOAN-FOR-SERVICE PROGRAM

New Mexico Higher Education Department
Attn: Financial Aid Division
2048 Galisteo Street
Santa Fe, NM 87505-2100
(505) 476-8411   Toll Free: (800) 279-9777
Fax: (505) 476-8454   E-mail: Theresa.acker@state.nm.us
Web: hed.state.nm.us

Summary To provide loans-for-service to nursing education students from New Mexico who are willing to work in the state after graduation.

Eligibility This program is open to residents of New Mexico interested in working on a bachelor's, master's, or doctoral degree to prepare for a career as a nursing educator. Applicants must have been accepted by a New Mexico public postsecondary institution in a program that will enable them to enhance or gain employment in a nursing faculty position at a public college or university in the state. Along with their application, they must submit an essay explaining their need for this assistance and why they are interested in becoming a nurse educator in New Mexico. U.S. citizenship or eligible non-citizen status is required.

Financial Data The loan is $5,000 per year for enrollment in 9 credit hours and above, $3,000 per year for enrollment in 6 to 8 credit hours, or $1,500 per year for enrollment in 5 credit hours or less. This is a loan-for-service program; for every year of service as a nursing faculty member in New Mexico, a portion of the loan is forgiven. If the entire service agreement is fulfilled, 100% of the loan is eligible for forgiveness. Penalties may be assessed if the service agreement is not satisfied.

Duration 1 year; may be renewed.

Number awarded Varies each year, depending on the availability of funds.

Deadline June of each year.

[272]
NEW MEXICO NURSING LOAN-FOR-SERVICE PROGRAM

New Mexico Higher Education Department
Attn: Financial Aid Division
2048 Galisteo Street
Santa Fe, NM 87505-2100
(505) 476-8411   Toll Free: (800) 279-9777
Fax: (505) 476-8454   E-mail: Theresa.acker@state.nm.us
Web: hed.state.nm.us

Summary To provide loans-for-service to nursing students from New Mexico willing to work in underserved areas of the state after graduation.

Eligibility This program is open to residents of New Mexico interested in preparing for a career as a nurse (including a licensed practical nursing certificate, associate degree in nursing, bachelor of science in nursing, master of science in nursing, or advanced practice nurse). Applicants must be enrolled or accepted in an accredited program at a New Mexico public postsecondary institution. As a condition of the loan, they must declare an intent to practice in a designated shortage area of New Mexico for at least 1 year after completing their education. Along with their application, they must submit a brief essay on why they want to enter the field of nursing and obligate themselves to a rural practice in New Mexico. U.S. citizenship or eligible non-citizen status is required.

Financial Data The loan depends on the financial need of the recipient, to a total of $12,000 per year. This is a loan-for-service program; for every year of service as a nurse in New Mexico, a portion of the loan is forgiven. If the entire service agreement is fulfilled, 100% of the loan is eligible for forgiveness. Penalties may be assessed if the service agreement is not satisfied.

Duration 1 year; may be renewed up to 3 additional years.

Number awarded Varies each year, depending on the availability of funds.

Deadline June of each year.

[273]
NEW YORK STATE ENA SEPTEMBER 11 SCHOLARSHIP FUND

Emergency Nurses Association
Attn: ENA Foundation
915 Lee Street
Des Plaines, IL 60016-6569
(847) 460-4100   Toll Free: (800) 900-9659, ext. 4100
Fax: (847) 460-4004   E-mail: foundation@ena.org
Web: www.ena.org

Summary To provide financial assistance to rescue workers enrolled in an undergraduate degree in nursing.

Eligibility This program is open to pre-hospital care providers, fire fighters, and police officers who are working on an associate or baccalaureate nursing degree. Rescue workers from all states are eligible. Applicants must have a GPA of 3.0 or higher and be a member of a state or national professional EMT, fire fighter, or police officer association. They are not required to be a member of the Emergency Nurses Association (ENA), but they are must submit a letter of reference from an ENA member. Along with their application, they must submit a 1-page statement on their professional and educational goals and how this scholarship will help them attain those goals. Selection is based on content and clarity of the goal statement (45%), professional association involvement (35%), presentation of the application (10%), and letters of reference (10%).

Financial Data The stipend is $2,500.

Duration 1 year.

Additional data This program is sponsored by the New York ENA State Council.

Number awarded 2 each year.

Deadline May of each year.

[274]
NEWARK CITY HOSPITAL SCHOOL OF NURSING ALUMNI ASSOCIATION SCHOLARSHIP

New Jersey State Nurses Association
Attn: Institute for Nursing
1479 Pennington Road
Trenton, NJ 08618-2661
(609) 883-5335   Toll Free: (888) UR-NJSNA
Fax: (609) 883-5343   E-mail: institute@njsna.org
Web: www.njsna.org/displaycommon.cfm?an=5

Summary To provide financial assistance to residents of New Jersey who are applying to or enrolled in a nursing program in the state.

Eligibility This program is open to New Jersey residents who are high school graduates or adults. Applicants must be applying to or currently enrolled in a diploma, associate degree, or bachelor's degree program in nursing at a school in New Jersey. R.N.s working on a degree in nursing are also eligible if they are members of the New Jersey State Nurses Association. Selection is based on financial need, GPA, and leadership potential.

Financial Data The stipend is $1,000.

Duration 1 year.

Number awarded 1 each year.

Deadline January of each year.

[275]
NICOLE MARIE GOULART MEMORIAL SCHOLARSHIP

Luso-American Education Foundation
Attn: Administrative Director
7080 Donlon Way, Suite 202
P.O. Box 2967
Dublin, CA 94568
(925) 828-3883   Fax: (925) 828-3883
E-mail: odom@luso-american.org
Web: www.luso-american.org

Summary To provide financial assistance to undergraduate students with a Portuguese connection who are majoring in designated fields.

Eligibility This program is open to U.S. residents who are sophomores, juniors, and seniors at 4-year colleges and universities and are of Portuguese descent or who took Portuguese language classes in high school. Applicants must be majoring in medicine/health, neurology, nursing, pharmacology, emergency medical technology, or protective services. They must have a GPA of 3.5

or higher. Selection is based on promise of success in college, financial need, leadership, vocational promise, and sincerity of purpose.

Financial Data A stipend is awarded (amount not specified).
Duration 1 year; renewable.
Number awarded 1 each year.
Deadline February of each year.

[276]
NJADONA SCHOLARSHIPS

New Jersey Association of Directors of Nursing
  Administration/Long Term Care, Inc.
Attn: Scholarship Committee
195 Carriage Hill Circle
Mantua, NJ 08051-1161
(865) 468-9869   Fax: (865) 468-9865
E-mail: njadona@aol.com
Web: www.njadona.org

Summary To provide financial assistance to employees of member facilities of the New Jersey Association of Directors of Nursing Administration/Long Term Care (NJADONA) who are interested in obtaining a degree in nursing.

Eligibility This program is open to employees in good standing of NJADONA member facilities who are attending school to become an L.P.N. or R.N. or to obtain a degree in nursing or nursing administration. Applicants must submit a 200-word statement explaining why they chose long-term care and how this scholarship will help them reach their professional goals.

Financial Data The stipend is $500.
Duration 1 year.
Number awarded 1 or more each year.
Deadline March of each year.

[277]
NORTH CAROLINA ASSOCIATION OF HEALTH CARE RECRUITERS SCHOLARSHIPS

North Carolina Association of Health Care Recruiters
c/o Beverly Barnett, President
Novant Health
3333 Silas Creek Parkway
Winston-Salem, NC 27103
(336) 277-1910   Fax: (336) 277-1902
E-mail: bnbarnet@novanthealth.org
Web: www.ncahcr.org/scholarships.htm

Summary To provide financial assistance to residents of North Carolina who are interested in working on a degree in nursing or allied health at a school in the state.

Eligibility This program is open to residents of North Carolina who are enrolled or planning to enroll full time at an accredited institution in the state. Applicants must be interested in working on an associate or baccalaureate degree in nursing or allied health. Along with their application, they must submit a statement of their reasons for applying for a scholarship.

Financial Data The stipend is $500.
Duration 1 year.
Number awarded 1 or more each year.
Deadline Deadline not specified.

[278]
NORTH CAROLINA NURSE EDUCATION SCHOLARSHIP LOAN PROGRAM

North Carolina State Education Assistance Authority
Attn: Nurse Education Scholarship Loan Program
10 T.W. Alexander Drive
P.O. Box 13663
Research Triangle Park, NC 27709-3663
(919) 549-8614   Toll Free: (800) 700-1775
Fax: (919) 248-4687   E-mail: information@ncseaa.edu
Web: www.ncseaa.edu/NESLP.htm

Summary To provide loans-for-service to residents of North Carolina enrolled at institutions in the state who wish to prepare for a career in nursing.

Eligibility This program is open to students at any of the 56 North Carolina Community Colleges, the 11 constituent institutions of the University of North Carolina, or the 4 private colleges and universities in North Carolina that offer nursing education instruction. Applicants must be preparing for licensure in North Carolina as a Licensed Practical Nurse (L.P.N.) or a Registered Nurse (R.N.). U.S. citizenship and North Carolina residency are required. Selection is based on academic performance, student's willingness to practice full time as an L.P.N. or R.N. in North Carolina following completion of the education program, student's willingness to comply with the rules and regulations of this program, and financial need.

Financial Data Scholarship/loans range from $2,000 to $5,000. The maximum for students enrolled in Associate Degree Nursing (A.D.N.) and practical nurse education (L.P.N.) programs is $3,000 per year; the maximum award for students enrolled in a baccalaureate (B.S.N.) program is $5,000 per year. This is a loan-for-service program; recipients are required to provide 1 year of service as a nurse in North Carolina for each year of support received. Loans not repaid in service must be repaid in cash plus 10% interest from the date of disbursement. Recipients have up to 7 years to repay loans with service or 10 years to repay in cash.

Duration 1 year. Students in an A.D.N. program may renew the scholarship for 1 additional year. Students in a B.S.N. program may renew the scholarship for 3 additional years. Scholarships for L.P.N. programs are nonrenewable.

Additional data Information and applications are available at the financial aid office of the participating North Carolina college or university offering the level of nursing instruction desired. This program was first funded in 1989.

Number awarded Varies each year; recently, a total of 484 students were receiving $1,041,569 in support through this program.
Deadline Deadline not specified.

[279]
NORTH CAROLINA STATE CONTRACTUAL SCHOLARSHIP FUND PROGRAM

North Carolina State Education Assistance Authority
Attn: Grants, Training, and Outreach Department
10 T.W. Alexander Drive
P.O. Box 13663
Research Triangle Park, NC 27709-3663
(919) 549-8614   Toll Free: (800) 700-1775
Fax: (919) 248-4687   E-mail: information@ncseaa.edu
Web: www.ncseaa.edu/SCSF.htm

Summary To provide financial assistance to residents of North Carolina enrolled at private colleges and universities in the state.

Eligibility This program is open to North Carolina residents who are enrolled full or part time at approved North Carolina private colleges and universities. Applicants must normally be undergraduates, although they may have a bachelor's degree if they are enrolled in a licensure program for teachers or nurses. Students enrolled in a program of study in theology, divinity, religious education, or any other program of study designed primarily for career preparation in a religious vocation are not eligible. Financial need is considered in the selection process.

Financial Data Stipends depend on the need of the recipient and the availability of funds. Recently, they averaged more than $2,600 per year.

Duration 1 year.

Additional data Recipients are selected by the financial aid offices of the eligible private institutions in North Carolina. This program was established in 1971.

Number awarded Varies each year; recently, a total of 16,137 students received $42,992,813 through this program.

Deadline Deadline not specified.

[280]
NORTH CAROLINA STUDENT LOAN PROGRAM FOR HEALTH, SCIENCE, AND MATHEMATICS

North Carolina State Education Assistance Authority
Attn: Health, Science, and Mathematics Program
10 T.W. Alexander Drive
P.O. Box 13663
Research Triangle Park, NC 27709-3663
(919) 549-8614   Toll Free: (800) 700-1775
Fax: (919) 248-4687   E-mail: information@ncseaa.edu
Web: www.ncseaa.edu/HSM.htm

Summary To provide forgivable loans to North Carolina residents who are interested in preparing for a career as a primary care physician, allied health professional, or science and mathematics educator.

Eligibility This program is open to North Carolina residents who have been accepted as full-time students in an accredited associate, baccalaureate, master's, or doctoral program leading to a degree in 1 of the following areas: audiology, cardiology, chiropractic medicine, clinical psychology, communications assistant, cytotechnology, dental hygiene, dentistry, mathematics education, medical social work, medical technology, nurse midwifery, nursing, nursing administration, nursing anesthetist, nursing family practitioner, nutritional sciences, occupational therapy/assistant, oncology, optometry, osteopathic medicine, pharmacy, physician assistant in primary care, physical therapy/assistant, podiatry, primary care physician, radiological technology, respiratory therapy/technician, science education, speech language pathology, or veterinary medicine. Applicants must be enrolled or planning to enroll full time at a college or university in North Carolina unless they are working on a degree in a field not offered at a North Carolina institution (i.e., chiropractic medicine, optometry, osteopathic medicine, or podiatry). Selection is based on major, academic capability, and financial need.

Financial Data Maximum loans are $3,000 per year for associate degree and certificate programs, $5,000 per year for baccalaureate degree/certificate programs, $6,500 per year for master's degree programs, or $8,500 per year for health- professional doctoral programs. The interest rate is 4% while the borrowers are attending school and 10% after they leave school. Loans (including accrued interest) are forgiven if the recipients work in North Carolina in their professional area for 1 year for each year of support received; primary care physicians and some allied health professionals must work in designated shortage areas in the state to qualify for loan forgiveness.

Duration 1 year; renewable for 1 additional year for diploma, associate, certificate, and master's degree programs, for 2 additional years for baccalaureate degree programs, or for 3 additional years for doctoral programs.

Additional data This program, formerly known as the North Carolina Medical Student Loan Program, was established in 1945.

Number awarded Varies each year; recently, a total of 390 students were receiving $2,578,178 in support through this program.

Deadline April of each year.

[281]
NORTH CAROLINA UNDERGRADUATE NURSE SCHOLARS PROGRAM

North Carolina State Education Assistance Authority
Attn: Nurse Scholars Program
10 T.W. Alexander Drive
P.O. Box 13663
Research Triangle Park, NC 27709-3663
(919) 549-8614   Toll Free: (800) 700-1775
Fax: (919) 248-4687   E-mail: information@ncseaa.edu
Web: www.ncseaa.edu/NSP.htm

Summary To provide loans-for-service to residents of North Carolina who wish to attend school in the state to prepare for a career in nursing.

Eligibility This program is open to high school seniors, high school graduates, or currently-enrolled college students who are U.S. citizens, North Carolina residents, and interested in becoming a nurse. Applicants must be enrolled or planning to enroll full time at a North Carolina college, university, or hospital that prepares them for licensure as a registered nurse. They must have a GPA of 3.0 or higher. Selection is based on academic achievement, leadership potential, and the promise of service as a registered nurse in North Carolina; financial need is not considered.

Financial Data Annual stipends are $3,000 for candidates for an associate degree, $3,000 for candidates for a diploma in nursing, $5,000 for full-time students in a B.S.N. program, or $2,500 for part-time students in a B.S.N. program. This is a loan-for-service program; 1 year of full-time work as a nurse in North Carolina cancels 1 year of support under this program. Recipients who fail to honor the work obligation must repay the balance plus 10% interest. They have up to 7 years to repay the loan in service or 10 years to repay in cash.

Duration 1 year; may be renewed 1 additional year by candidates for an associate degree, registered nurses completing a B.S.N. degree, and community college transfer students and juniors in a B.S.N. program, or for 3 additional years by freshmen and nontraditional students in a B.S.N. program.

Additional data The North Carolina General Assembly created this program in 1989; the first recipients were funded for the 1990-91 academic year.

Number awarded Varies; generally, up to 450 new undergraduate degree awards are made each year. Recently, a total of 679 students were receiving $3,061,750 through this program.

Deadline February of each year for B.S.N. programs; May of each year for A.D.N. and diploma students.

[282]
NORTH DAKOTA NURSING EDUCATION LOAN PROGRAM

North Dakota Board of Nursing
919 South Seventh Street, Suite 504
Bismarck, ND 58504-5881
(701) 328-9777   Fax: (701) 328-9785
Web: www.ndbon.org

Summary To provide forgivable loans to students in North Dakota who are working on an undergraduate degree, graduate degree, or continuing education program in nursing.

Eligibility This program is open to 1) students enrolled in a North Dakota board-approved or recognized undergraduate nursing education program for practical nurses or registered nurses; 2) nurses who have a current North Dakota license and have been accepted into or are currently enrolled in a graduate program that is acceptable to the Board of Nursing, and 3) nurses who are residents of North Dakota and interested in taking refresher courses. All applicants must demonstrate financial need. Along with their application, they must submit official transcripts, co-signer information, 3 letters of reference, personal financial information, a financial aid inquiry form (except for graduate students), and a student status form verifying their acceptance and expected enrollment date in the nursing program or major.

Financial Data   Students in a licensed practical nurse program who plan to complete studies for an associate degree in nursing may receive up to $1,000 per year. Students in a registered nurse program who plan to complete a baccalaureate degree in nursing may receive up to $1,500 per year. Graduate students may receive up to $2,500 to complete their master's degree in nursing. Graduate students working on a doctoral degree in nursing may receive up to $5,000. Licensed practical nurses or registered nurses may receive up to the cost of a continuing education/refresher course. This is a scholarship/loan program. Recipients must agree to work as a nurse in North Dakota after graduation; the repayment rate will be $1 for each hour of employment. If employment in North Dakota is terminated before the loan is canceled, or the recipient does not work in North Dakota, or the recipient does not pass the NCLEX examination within 180 days of graduation, the loan must be repaid. The interest rate charged is approximately 9%.

Duration   2 years for students in a licensed practical nurse program; the last 2 years for students in a baccalaureate nursing degree program.

Additional data   Recipients may request a deferment of payment if they proceed directly to the next level of education. There is a $15 application fee. The spouse of an applicant is not acceptable as the co-signer of the note. The co-signer should be a North Dakota resident. If the co-signer is not a North Dakota resident, the applicant must provide a letter of explanation. Proof of majority of the co-signer (18 years or older) may be required. Undergraduate recipients must be enrolled in school in a minimum of 6 credits per semester or 12 credits per year.

Number awarded   30 to 35 each year.

Deadline   June of each year.

[283]
NORTH FLORIDA CHAPTER SAFETY EDUCATION SCHOLARSHIP

American Society of Safety Engineers
Attn: ASSE Foundation
1800 East Oakton Street
Des Plaines, IL 60018
(847) 768-3435   Fax: (847) 768-3434
E-mail: agabanski@asse.org
Web: www.asse.org/foundation/scholarships/scholarships.php

Summary   To provide financial assistance to undergraduate and graduate student members of the American Society of Safety Engineers (ASSE) from Florida.

Eligibility   This program is open to undergraduate and graduate students who are working on a degree in occupational safety, health, and environment or a closely-related field (e.g., industrial or environmental engineering, environmental science, industrial hygiene, occupational health nursing). Priority is given first to part- and full-time students who belong to the ASSE North Florida Chapter; second to full-time students at any Florida college or university; and third to full-time students at an ASAC/ABET accredited program in any state. Undergraduates must have completed at least 60 semester hours with a GPA of 3.0 or higher. Graduate students must have completed at least 9 semester hours with a GPA of 3.5 or higher and have earned a GPA of 3.0 or higher as an undergraduate. Full-time students must be ASSE student members; part-time students must be ASSE general or professional members. Along with their application, they must submit 2 essays of 300 words or less: 1) why they are seeking a degree in occupational safety and health or a closely-related field, a brief description of their current activities, and how those relate to their career goals and objectives; and 2) why they should be awarded this scholarship (including career goals and financial need). U.S. citizenship is not required.

Financial Data   The stipend is $1,000 per year.

Duration   1 year; recipients may reapply.

Additional data   This program is sponsored by the ASSE North Florida Chapter.

Number awarded   1 each year.

Deadline   November of each year.

[284]
NOVA FOUNDATION SCHOLARSHIPS

Nurses Organization of Veterans Affairs
Attn: NOVA Foundation
47595 Watkins Island Square
Sterling, VA 20165
(703) 444-5587   Fax: (703) 444-5597
E-mail: nova@vanurse.org
Web: www.vanurse.org/scholarship.html

Summary   To provide financial assistance to employees of the U.S. Department of Veterans Affairs (VA) who are working on an undergraduate or graduate degree in nursing.

Eligibility   This program is open to VA employees who are enrolled or accepted for enrollment in an NLN-accredited baccalaureate, master's, post-master's, or doctoral degree program in nursing. Diploma and associate degree programs are not eligible. Selection is based on career goals, professional and civic activities, academic performance, and recommendations. U.S. citizenship is required.

Financial Data   The stipend is $1,500.

Duration   1 year.

Number awarded   8 each year.

Deadline   May of each year.

[285]
NSNA MOBILITY SCHOLARSHIPS

National Student Nurses' Association
Attn: Foundation
45 Main Street, Suite 606
Brooklyn, NY 11201
(718) 210-0705   Fax: (718) 797-1186
E-mail: nsna@nsna.org
Web: www.nsna.org

Summary   To provide financial assistance to nurses interested in pursuing additional education.

Eligibility   This program is open to 1) registered nurses enrolled in programs leading to a baccalaureate or master's degree in nursing or 2) licensed practical and vocational nurses enrolled in programs leading to licensure as a registered nurse. Graduating high school seniors are not eligible. Applicants must submit a 200-word description of their professional and educational goals and how this scholarship will help them achieve those goals. Selection is based on academic achievement, financial need, and involvement in student nursing organizations and community activities related to health care. U.S. citizenship or permanent resident status is required.

Financial Data   Stipends range from $1,000 to $2,500. A total of approximately $155,000 is awarded each year by the foundation for all its scholarship programs.

Duration   1 year.

Additional data   Applications must be accompanied by a $10 processing fee.

Number awarded   Varies each year. Recently, 2 of these scholarships were awarded, both sponsored by Anthony J. Jannetti, Inc.

Deadline   January of each year.

[286]
NSNA/NURSING SPECTRUM NURSE WEEK ESSAY CONTEST

National Student Nurses' Association
Attn: Nursing Spectrum Writing Contest
45 Main Street, Suite 606
Brooklyn, NY 11201
(718) 210-0705   Fax: (718) 797-1186
E-mail: nsna@nsna.org
Web: www.nsna.org

Summary   To recognize and reward members of the National Student Nurses' Association (NSNA) who submit outstanding essays on a topic related to nursing as a career.

Eligibility   This contest is open members of the association who are enrolled in a nursing program. Contestants are invited to submit an essay, up to 1,000 words, on a topic that changes annually. Recently, applicants were invited to write on the question: "During this drastic shortage of nurse educators, what is the importance of increasing promotion of such a career and how can it be done?" Essays are judged on the basis of relevance to theme, writing style, originality, creativity, grammar, and spelling.

Financial Data   The grand prize winner receives $500 and complimentary registration to the NSNA national convention. Other prizes are $125 for first and $100 for second.

Duration   The competition is held annually.

Additional data   This competition, first held in 2003, is jointly sponsored by NSNA and *Nursing Spectrum,* in which the grand prize essay is published. All winning essays are also published in *Imprint* and posted on both organization's web sites.

Number awarded   3 each year.

Deadline   March of each year.

[287]
NURSE CORPS OPTION OF THE SEAMAN TO ADMIRAL-21 PROGRAM

U.S. Navy
Attn: Commander, Naval Service Training Command
250 Dallas Street, Suite A
Pensacola, FL 32508-5268
(850) 452-9563   Fax: (850) 452-2486
E-mail: PNSC_STA21@navy.mil
Web: www.sta-21.navy.mil

Summary   To allow outstanding enlisted Navy personnel to complete a bachelor's degree and receive a commission in the Nurse Corps.

Eligibility   This program is open to U.S. citizens who are currently serving on active duty in the U.S. Navy or Naval Reserve, including Full Time Support (FTS), Selected Reserves (SEL-RES), and Navy Reservists on active duty except for those on active duty for training (ACDUTRA). Applicants must be high school graduates (or GED recipients) who are able to complete requirements for a baccalaureate degree in nursing in 36 months or less. They must have completed at least 30 semester units in undergraduate nursing prerequisite courses with a GPA of 2.5 or higher. They must be at least 18 years of age and able to complete degree requirements and be commissioned prior to age 42. Within the past 3 years, they must have taken the SAT (and achieved scores of at least 500 on the mathematics section and 500 on the critical reading section) or the ACT (and achieved a score of 41 or higher, including at least 21 on the mathematics portion and 20 on the English portion).

Financial Data   Awardees continue to receive their regular Navy pay and allowances while they attend college on a full-time basis. They also receive reimbursement for tuition, fees, and books up to $10,000 per year. If base housing is available, they are eligible to live there. Participants are not eligible to receive benefits under the Navy's Tuition Assistance Program (TA), the

Montgomery GI Bill (MGIB), the Navy College Fund, or the Veterans Educational Assistance Program (VEAP).

Duration   Selectees are supported for up to 36 months of full-time, year-round study or completion of a bachelor's degree, as long as they maintain a GPA of 2.5 or higher.

Additional data   This program was established in 2001 as a replacement for the Fleet Accession to Naval Reserve Officer Training Corps (NROTC) Nurse Option. Upon acceptance into the program, selectees attend the Naval Science Institute (NSI) in Newport, Rhode Island for an 8-week program in the fundamental core concepts of being a naval officer (navigation, engineering, weapons, military history and justice, etc.). They then enter an NROTC affiliated college or university with a nursing program that confers an accredited baccalaureate degree in nursing to pursue full-time study. They become members of and drill with the NROTC unit. When they complete their bachelor's degree in nursing, they are commissioned as ensigns in the United States Naval Reserve and assigned to initial training as an officer in the Nurse Corps. After commissioning, 5 years of active service are required.

Number awarded   Varies each year.

Deadline   June of each year.

[288]
NURSE EDUCATORS OF ILLINOIS UNDERGRADUATE SCHOLARSHIPS

Nurse Educators of Illinois
Attn: Scholarships
P.O. Box 695
Morton Grove, IL 60053
(847) 983-0954   E-mail: neionline@neionline.org
Web: www.neionline.org/NEI%20Scholarship.htm

Summary   To provide financial assistance to undergraduate members of Nurse Educators of Illinois who are enrolled in an accredited B.S.N., A.D.N., or diploma program in nursing.

Eligibility   This program is open to full- or part-time (half-time or more) students who are attending an accredited undergraduate or R.N. diploma nursing program. Applicants must be enrolled at the senior level (B.S.N.) or in their final year of an R.N. diploma or A.D.N. program at the time of the award. They must have a GPA of 3.5 or higher (official transcript is required), an above-average level of clinical achievement, leadership in an organization and/or community service, and evidence of verbal and written communication skills. Nurse Educators of Illinois membership on an individual or program level is required.

Financial Data   The stipend is $1,000.

Duration   1 year.

Additional data   Nurse Educators of Illinois was founded in 2004 as a successor to the Illinois League for Nursing.

Number awarded   Varies each year.

Deadline   June of each year.

[289]
NURSE ONEITA DONGIEUX AWARD FOR EXCELLENCE

Mississippi Nurses Association
Attn: Mississippi Nurses Foundation
31 Woodgreen Place
Madison, MS 39110
(601) 898-0850   Fax: (601) 898-0190
E-mail: foundation@msnurses.org
Web: msnursesfoundation.com/scholarships

Summary   To provide financial assistance to students enrolled at Mississippi schools of nursing.

Eligibility   This program is open to residents of Mississippi currently enrolled at a public school of nursing in the state. Applicants must have a GPA of 3.0 or higher. Along with their application, they must submit a 2-page essay on who or what inspired their interest in nursing. Selection is based on that essay, school of nursing activities, community activities, and awards and honors.

Financial Data The stipend is $500.

Duration 1 year.

Number awarded 1 each year.

Deadline January of each year.

[290]
NURSES FOUNDATION OF WISCONSIN SCHOLARSHIP

Wisconsin Nurses Association
Attn: Nurses Foundation of Wisconsin, Inc.
6117 Monona Drive, Suite 1
Madison, WI 53716
(608) 221-0383   Fax: (608) 221-2788
E-mail: info@wisconsinnurses.org
Web: www.wisconsinnurses.org

Summary To provide financial assistance to registered nurses in Wisconsin who are interested in continuing their education at a school in any state.

Eligibility This program is open to registered nurses in Wisconsin who are interested in working on a bachelor's or advanced degree in nursing at a school in any state. Applicants must be members of the Wisconsin Nurses Association. They must submit a copy of their Wisconsin Certificate of Registration, a copy of their association membership card, a letter that identifies their professional goals, a summary of their financial need, and 2 letters of support. Selection is based on financial need and potential to make a contribution to nursing in Wisconsin.

Financial Data The stipend is $1,000.

Duration 1 year.

Number awarded Varies each year; recently, 2 of these scholarships were awarded.

Deadline April of each year.

[291]
NURSING EDUCATION ASSISTANCE LOAN PROGRAM

South Dakota Board of Nursing
4305 South Louise Avenue, Suite 201
Sioux Falls, SD 57106-3115
(605) 362-2760   Fax: (605) 362-2768
Web: doh.sd.gov/boards/nursing/loan.aspx

Summary To provide forgivable loans to South Dakota residents interested in preparing for a career as a nurse.

Eligibility This program is open to South Dakota residents who have been accepted into an approved nursing education program (for licensed practical nurses, registered nurses, or advanced practice nurses). Applicants must be planning to work on a diploma, associate degree, baccalaureate, master's degree, or doctorate. They must be able to demonstrate financial need. U.S. citizenship is required.

Financial Data The amount of each loan is determined annually by the South Dakota Board of Nursing, up to a maximum of $1,000 per full academic year. Funds may be used only for direct educational expenses (e.g., tuition, books, and fees), not for room or board. Recipients may elect to repay the loan either in full (within 5 years) or by employment in nursing in the state at the conversion rate of $1 per hour.

Duration 1 year; recipients may reapply. Loans must be repaid within 5 years (either in cash or by service as a nurse in South Dakota).

Additional data The South Dakota Legislature authorized this program in 1989. Monies to fund the program are generated by a $10 fee charged to all LPNs and RNs in South Dakota at the time of license renewal.

Number awarded Varies each year.

Deadline May of each year for students in registered nursing and advanced practice nursing programs; September of each year for students in licensed practical nursing programs.

[292]
NURSING FOUNDATION OF RHODE ISLAND STUDENT SCHOLARSHIPS

Nursing Foundation of Rhode Island
Attn: Scholarship Committee
P.O. Box 41702
Providence, RI 02940
(401) 223-9680   E-mail: nfri@rinursingfoundation.org
Web: www.rinursingfoundation.org/scholarships.htm

Summary To provide financial assistance to students currently enrolled in nursing schools in Rhode Island.

Eligibility This program is open to students enrolled in a nursing program who have demonstrated financial need, have maintained at least a 3.0 GPA for registered nurses (R.N.s) or 2.0 for practical nurses, and have demonstrated clinical proficiency, enthusiasm, and motivation in their studies. Applicants must submit an essay of 2 to 3 paragraphs about the reasons why they need the scholarship to complete their nursing program. Preference is given to students who are in the latter half of their nursing program, full-time students, residents of Rhode Island, and students enrolled in a Rhode Island nursing program.

Financial Data The stipend ranges from $500 to $1,000. Checks are written jointly to the recipient and the recipient's school.

Duration 1 year.

Additional data This program includes several named scholarships: the Sabinne Cunningham Scholarship, the Elsie Drew Scholarship, the Kathleen Dwyer Scholarship, the Helen Enright Scholarship, the Ethel Ferrara Scholarship, the Mulvey Family Scholarship, the Betsy Nield Scholarship, and the Frank Sherman Scholarship.

Number awarded Varies each year; recently, 23 of these scholarships were awarded.

Deadline April of each year for practical nursing students; May of each year for R.N. students.

[293]
ODONA L.P.N. TO R.N. SCHOLARSHIPS

Ohio Directors of Nursing Administration in Long Term Care
Attn: Scholarship Committee
190 East Pacemont Road
Columbus, OH 43202
Toll Free: (866) 226-3662
Web: www.odonaltc.org/pages/scholarships.asp

Summary To provide financial assistance to licensed practical nurses (L.P.N.s) whose supervisors are members of Ohio Directors of Nursing Administration in Long Term Care (ODONA) and who are studying to become a registered nurse (R.N.) at a school in the state.

Eligibility This program is open to L.P.N.s enrolled in R.N. nursing programs in Ohio who have been working in long-term care for at least 1 year. Applicants must be currently employed at a facility where the director of nursing (DON) or assistant director of nursing (ADON) is a member of ODONA. Along with their application, they must submit a narrative of at least 100 words on why they wish to become an R.N. and be considered for a scholarship and how it will impact their practice.

Financial Data Stipends range from $500 to $1,500.

Duration 1 year.

Number awarded Up to 5 each year: 1 in each of Ohio's 5 regions.

Deadline January of each year.

[294]
ODONA NURSING ASSISTANT SCHOLARSHIPS

Ohio Directors of Nursing Administration in Long Term Care
Attn: Scholarship Committee
190 East Pacemont Road
Columbus, OH 43202
Toll Free: (866) 226-3662
Web: www.odonaltc.org/pages/scholarships.asp

Summary To provide financial assistance for additional training to nursing assistants whose supervisors are members of Ohio Directors of Nursing Administration in Long Term Care (ODONA).

Eligibility This program is open to students enrolled in nursing programs in Ohio who have been working in long-term care for at least 1 year. Applicants must be currently employed at a facility where the director of nursing (DON) or assistant director of nursing (ADON) is a member of ODONA. Along with their application, they must submit a narrative of at least 100 words on why they wish to be considered for a scholarship and how it will impact their practice.

Financial Data Stipends range from $500 to $1,500.

Duration 1 year.

Number awarded 1 each year.

Deadline January of each year.

[295]
ODONA SCHOLARSHIPS

Ohio Directors of Nursing Administration in Long Term Care
Attn: Scholarship Committee
190 East Pacemont Road
Columbus, OH 43202
Toll Free: (866) 226-3662
Web: www.odonaltc.org/pages/scholarships.asp

Summary To provide financial assistance for additional training to members of Ohio Directors of Nursing Administration in Long Term Care (ODONA).

Eligibility This program is open to ODONA members who have been working in long-term care for at least 1 year as directors of nursing (DON) or assistant directors of nursing (ADON). Applicants must be planning to enroll in a formal educational program related to their work at a school of nursing in any state. Along with their application, they must submit a narrative of at least 100 words on why they wish to be considered for a scholarship and how it will impact their practice.

Financial Data Stipends range from $500 to $1,500.

Duration 1 year.

Number awarded Up to 5 each year: 1 in each of Ohio's 5 regions.

Deadline January of each year.

[296]
OHIO LEGION AUXILIARY PAST PRESIDENTS' PARLEY SCHOLARSHIPS

American Legion Auxiliary
Department of Ohio
1100 Brandywine Boulevard, Building D
P.O. Box 2760
Zanesville, OH 43702-2760
(740) 452-8245   Fax: (740) 452-2620
E-mail: ala_katie@rrohio.com

Summary To provide financial assistance to Ohio residents who are dependents or descendants of veterans and interested in attending school in any state to studying nursing.

Eligibility This program is open to the wives, children, stepchildren, grandchildren, adopted children, or great-grandchildren of veterans who are interested in working on a degree in nursing at a school in any state, are sponsored by a unit of the American Legion Auxiliary, and are residents of Ohio. The qualifying veteran must be disabled, deceased, or in financial need. Selection is based on character, scholastic standing, qualifications for the nursing profession, and financial need.

Financial Data Stipends are either $750 or $300. Funds are paid directly to the recipients upon proof of enrollment.

Duration 1 year.

Number awarded Varies each year. Recently, 17 of these scholarships were awarded: 2 at $750 and 15 at $300.

Deadline May of each year.

[297]
OHIO NURSE EDUCATION ASSISTANCE LOAN PROGRAM FOR NURSES

Ohio Board of Regents
Attn: State Grants and Scholarships
30 East Broad Street, 36th Floor
Columbus, OH 43215-3414
(614) 466-4818   Toll Free: (888) 833-1133
Fax: (614) 466-5866
E-mail: nealp_admin@regents.state.oh.us
Web: regents.ohio.gov/sgs/nealp/students.php

Summary To provide scholarship/loans to students in Ohio who intend to study nursing.

Eligibility This program is open to Ohio residents who are enrolled at least half time in an approved nursing education program in Ohio. Applicants must demonstrate financial need and intend to engage in direct clinical practice as a registered nurse or licensed practical nurse following graduation. U.S. citizenship or permanent resident status is required.

Financial Data The maximum award is currently $1,500 per year. This is a scholarship/loan program; up to 100% of the loan may be forgiven at the rate of 20% per year if the recipient serves as a nurse under specified conditions for up to 5 years. If the loan is not repaid with service, it must be repaid in cash with interest at the rate of 8% per year.

Duration 1 year; renewable for up to 3 additional years.

Additional data This program, established in 1990, is administered by the Ohio Board of Regents with assistance from the Ohio Board of Nursing.

Number awarded Varies each year; recently, 35 students received benefits through this program.

Deadline July of each year.

[298]
OHIO NURSES FOUNDATION TRADITIONAL NURSING STUDENT SCHOLARSHIP

Ohio Nurses Association
Attn: Ohio Nurses Foundation
4000 East Main Street
Columbus, OH 43213-2983
(614) 237-5414   Fax: (614) 237-6074
E-mail: gharsheymeade@ohnurses.org
Web: www.ohnurses.org

Summary To provide financial assistance to residents of Ohio who are interested in working on a degree in nursing at a school in any state.

Eligibility This program is open to residents of Ohio interested in attending college in any state to prepare for a career as a nurse. Applicants must be attending or have attended a high school in the state. If still in high school, they must have a cumulative GPA of 3.5 or higher at the end of their junior year. If out of high school, they may not have had a break of more than 2 years between high school and enrollment in a nursing program. Along with their application, they must submit a 100-word personal statement on how they will advance the profession of nursing in Ohio. Selection is based on that statement, high school or college academic records, school activities, and community services.

Financial Data The stipend is $1,000 per year.

Duration 1 year; recipients may reapply for 1 additional year if they remain enrolled full time and maintain a cumulative GPA of 2.5 or higher.

Number awarded 1 or more each year.

Deadline January of each year.

[299]
OKLAHOMA NURSING STUDENT ASSISTANCE PROGRAM

Physician Manpower Training Commission
Attn: Nursing Program Coordinator
5500 North Western Avenue, Suite 201
Oklahoma City, OK 73118
(405) 843-5667　　　　　　　　　Fax: (405) 843-5792
E-mail: michelle.cecil@pmtc.state.ok.us
Web: www.pmtc.state.ok.us/nsap.htm

Summary To provide scholarship/loans to nursing students from Oklahoma who are interested in practicing in rural communities in the state.

Eligibility This program is open to residents of Oklahoma who have been admitted to an accredited program of nursing in any state at the L.P.N., A.D.N., B.S.N., or M.S.N. level. Applicants must be interested in practicing nursing in Oklahoma communities, especially rural communities. They may apply either for direct funding from the state or with matching support from a health institution in the state, such as a hospital, nursing home, or other health care entity. Along with their application, they must submit ACT scores, high school and/or college GPA, and documentation of financial need. U.S. citizenship is required.

Financial Data The minimum scholarship/loan provided by the state for all levels is $500 per year. The maximum is $1,750 per year for L.P.N. students, $2,000 per year for A.D.N. students, or $2,500 per year for B.S.N. or M.S.N. students. The loan is forgiven if the nurse fulfills a work obligation at an approved health institution in Oklahoma of 1 year for each year of financial assistance received; participants in the matching program must work for their sponsor. Nurses who decide not to fulfill their work obligation are required to repay the principal amount plus 12% interest and a possible penalty of up to 98% of the principal.

Duration Funding is available for completion of an L.P.N. program, for 2 years for an A.D.N. program, or the final 2 years of a B.S.N. or M.S.N. program.

Additional data This program was established in 1982.

Number awarded Between 250 and 300 of these awards are granted each year. Since the program began, more than 5,250 nursing students have received support.

Deadline June of each year.

[300]
OLIVER JOEL AND ELLEN PELL DENNY HEALTHCARE SCHOLARSHIP FUND

Winston-Salem Foundation
Attn: Student Aid Department
860 West Fifth Street
Winston-Salem, NC 27101-2506
(336) 725-2382　　　　　　Toll Free: (866) 227-1209
Fax: (336) 727-0581　　　　E-mail: info@wsfoundation.org
Web: www.wsfoundation.org/students

Summary To provide financial assistance to residents of North Carolina working on a degree or certificate in fields related to health care at a college or university in the state.

Eligibility This program is open to North Carolina residents working on a certificate, diploma, or bachelor's or associate degree in health care fields, including (but not limited to) registered nursing, licensed practical nursing, nuclear medicine, radiography, and respiratory therapy. Applicants must be attending or planning to attend a 2- or 4-year college or university in North Carolina as a traditional or nontraditional student. They must have

a cumulative GPA of 2.5 or higher in health care classes and be able to demonstrate financial need. Preference is given to residents of Davidson, Davie, Forsyth, Stokes, Surry, and Yadkin counties. Some of the scholarships are set aside for eligible non-citizens.

Financial Data The stipend is $1,200 per year.

Duration 1 year; may be renewed.

Additional data There is a $20 application fee (waived if the applicant is unable to pay).

Number awarded 1 or more each year, including 5 scholarships set aside for eligible non-citizens.

Deadline August of each year.

[301]
ONCOLOGY NURSING CERTIFICATION CORPORATION BACHELOR'S SCHOLARSHIPS

Oncology Nursing Society
Attn: ONS Foundation
125 Enterprise Drive
Pittsburgh, PA 15275-1214
(412) 859-6100　　　　　　Toll Free: (866) 257-4ONS
Fax: (412) 859-6163　　　　E-mail: foundation@ons.org
Web: www.ons.org/Awards/FoundationAwards/Bachelors

Summary To provide financial assistance to nurses and other students who are interested in working on a bachelor's degree in oncology nursing.

Eligibility This program is open to students who are accepted to or currently enrolled in a bachelor's degree program at an NLN- or CCNE-accredited school of nursing. Applicants must be able to demonstrate an interest in and commitment to oncology nursing. They may 1) already have a current license to practice as a registered nurse (R.N.); 2) currently have a postsecondary degree at some level but not be an R.N.; or 3) have only a high school diploma. Along with their application, they must submit 1) an essay of 250 words or less on their role or interest in caring for persons with cancer, and 2) a statement of their professional goals and the relationship of those goals to the advancement of oncology nursing. Non-R.N. applicants must be in the nursing component of the B.S.N. program. High school students and individuals in the liberal arts component of a B.S.N. program are not eligible. Financial need is not considered in the selection process.

Financial Data The stipend is $2,000.

Duration 1 year; nonrenewable.

Additional data This program, supported by the Oncology Nursing Certification Corporation, awarded its first scholarships in 1992. At the end of the year of scholarship participation, recipients must submit a summary describing their educational activities. Applications must be accompanied by a $5 fee.

Number awarded Varies each year; recently, 10 of these scholarships were awarded.

Deadline January of each year.

[302]
ONCOLOGY PRACTICE ALLIANCE SCHOLARSHIP

Oncology Nursing Society
Attn: ONS Foundation
125 Enterprise Drive
Pittsburgh, PA 15275-1214
(412) 859-6100　　　　　　Toll Free: (866) 257-4ONS
Fax: (412) 859-6163　　　　E-mail: foundation@ons.org
Web: www.ons.org/Awards/FoundationAwards/Bachelors

Summary To provide financial assistance to residents of Ohio and West Virginia who are interested in working on a bachelor's degree in oncology nursing.

Eligibility This program is open to residents of Ohio and West Virginia who are currently enrolled in the nursing component of a bachelor's degree program at an NLN-accredited school of nursing. Applicants must be able to demonstrate an interest in and commitment to oncology nursing. Along with their application, they must submit 1) an essay of 250 words or less on their interest in caring for persons with cancer, and 2) a statement of their professional goals and the relationship of those goals to the advancement of oncology nursing. High school students and individuals in the liberal arts component of a B.S.N. program are not eligible. Financial need is not considered in the selection process.

Financial Data The stipend is $2,000.

Duration 1 year; nonrenewable.

Additional data This program is supported by the Oncology Practice Alliance, Inc. At the end of the year of scholarship participation, recipients must submit a summary describing their educational activities. Applications must be accompanied by a $5 fee.

Number awarded 1 each year.

Deadline January of each year.

[303]
ONF-SMITH EDUCATION SCHOLARSHIP

Oregon Nurses Association
Attn: Oregon Nurses Foundation
18765 S.W. Boones Ferry Road, Suite 200
Tualatin, OR 97062-8498
(503) 293-0011   Fax: (503) 293-0013
E-mail: tangedal@oregonrn.org
Web: www.oregonrn.org

Summary To provide financial assistance to residents of any state who are working on an undergraduate or graduate degree in nursing at a school in Oregon.

Eligibility This program is open to students from any state who are currently enrolled in an accredited bachelor's or graduate program in nursing in Oregon and have a GPA of 3.0 or higher. Applicants who are already registered nurses must be a member of the Oregon Nurses Association; applicants who are not yet registered nurses must be a member of an Oregon affiliate of the National Student Nurses Association. Selection is based on leadership abilities and experiences (35%); experiences with other cultures, minority groups, and underserved populations (30%); career plans in nursing (30%); and reasons for needing this funding (5%).

Financial Data The stipend is $1,000. Funds are paid directly to the recipient's school.

Duration 1 year.

Number awarded 1 or more each year.

Deadline February of each year.

[304]
OREGON LEGION AUXILIARY DEPARTMENT NURSES SCHOLARSHIP

American Legion Auxiliary
Department of Oregon
30450 S.W. Parkway Avenue
P.O. Box 1730
Wilsonville, OR 97070-1730
(503) 682-3162   Fax: (503) 685-5008
E-mail: alaor@pcez.com

Summary To provide financial assistance to the wives, widows, and children of Oregon veterans who are interested in studying nursing at a school in any state.

Eligibility This program is open to Oregon residents who are the wives or children of veterans with disabilities or the widows of deceased veterans. Applicants must have been accepted by an accredited hospital or university school of nursing in any state. Selection is based on ability, aptitude, character, determination, seriousness of purpose, and financial need.

Financial Data The stipend is $1,500.

Duration 1 year; may be renewed.

Number awarded 1 each year.

Deadline May of each year.

[305]
OREGON NURSES FOUNDATION CENTENNIAL EDUCATION SCHOLARSHIP

Oregon Nurses Association
Attn: Oregon Nurses Foundation
18765 S.W. Boones Ferry Road, Suite 200
Tualatin, OR 97062-8498
(503) 293-0011   Fax: (503) 293-0013
E-mail: tangedal@oregonrn.org
Web: www.oregonrn.org

Summary To provide financial assistance to students accepted to a nursing program in Oregon to work on an associate or bachelor's degree.

Eligibility This program is open to students who are enrolled or planning to enroll in an accredited nursing program in Oregon. Applicants must have a GPA of 3.0 or higher and be planning to earn an associate or bachelor's degree in nursing. Selection is based on leadership abilities and experiences (35%); experiences with other cultures, minority groups, and underserved populations (30%); career plans in nursing (30%); and reasons for needing this funding (5%).

Financial Data The stipend is $1,000.

Duration 1 year.

Additional data This program was established in 2003.

Number awarded 1 or more each year.

Deadline March, June, September, or December of each year.

[306]
PALMETTO GOLD SCHOLARSHIPS

South Carolina Nurses Foundation, Inc.
Attn: Palmetto Gold Committee
1821 Gadsden Street
Columbia, SC 29201
(803) 252-4781   Fax: (803) 779-3870
E-mail: info@scpalmettogold.org
Web: www.scpalmettogold.org

Summary To provide financial assistance to students enrolled in a registered nurse training program in South Carolina.

Eligibility This program is open to students who are nominated by the dean of a registered nurse program in South Carolina. Nominees must 1) display caring and commitment to patients, families, and colleagues; 2) demonstrate leadership and assistance to others to grow and develop; 3) promote the profession of nursing in a positive way; and 4) show promise of excellence by achieving a high level of academic success (at least a 3.0 GPA). They must submit a 200-word essay describing their career goals in nursing.

Financial Data The stipend is $1,000.

Duration 1 year.

Additional data This program began in 2002.

Number awarded 23 each year: 1 at each registered nurse training program in South Carolina.

Deadline Nominations must be submitted by October of each year.

[307]
PATSY QUINT OCCUPATIONAL HEALTH NURSES ENDOWED SCHOLARSHIP

Kansas State Nurses Association
Attn: Kansas Nurses Foundation
1109 S.W. Topeka Boulevard
Topeka, KS 66612-1602
(785) 233-8638   Fax: (785) 233-5222
E-mail: ksna@ksna.net
Web: www.nursingworld.org/SNAS/KS/Knf.htm

Summary To provide financial assistance to nurses in Kansas interested in working on a degree in occupational health at a school in the state.

Eligibility This program is open to residents of Kansas who are either 1) R.N.s currently in occupational health and working on a baccalaureate degree, or 2) occupational health nurses working on a master's or doctoral degree with an emphasis on occupational health. Applicants must have a GPA of 3.0 or higher. Along with their application, they must submit a personal narrative on their anticipated role in nursing in Kansas.

Financial Data The stipend is $500.

Duration 1 year.

Number awarded 1 each year.

Deadline June of each year.

[308]
PAULINE THOMPSON NURSING EDUCATION SCHOLARSHIP

Pennsylvania State Nurses Association
Attn: Nursing Foundation of Pennsylvania
2578 Interstate Drive, Suite 101
Harrisburg, PA 17110
(717) 692-0542   Toll Free: (888) 707-PSNA
Fax: (717) 692-4540   E-mail: nfp@panurses.org
Web: www.panurses.org/2008/section.cfm?SID=21&ID=4

Summary To provide financial assistance to undergraduate nursing students in Pennsylvania.

Eligibility Applicants must be enrolled in a baccalaureate, associate degree, or R.N. to B.S.N. competition nursing program located in Pennsylvania that is accredited by the National League for Nursing. Baccalaureate students must be in their junior or senior year (application may be made at the end of the sophomore or junior year). Associate degree students must be in their final year (application may be made at the end of the first year). Registered nurses must have been accepted into a baccalaureate program. All applicants must be Pennsylvania residents. They must be in good academic standing (GPA of 3.0 or higher) and able to show both leadership qualities and involvement in community service. Applicants must be members of the Student Nurses Association of Pennsylvania, unless there is no school chapter; applicants who are R.N.s must be members of the Pennsylvania State Nurses Association. Financial need is not considered in the selection process.

Financial Data The stipend is $1,000.

Duration 1 year; nonrenewable.

Additional data The recipient must attend the foundation's annual banquet to receive the scholarship. The recipient will be the guest of the foundation at the banquet and financial support for travel and overnight accommodations will be provided if necessary.

Number awarded 1 or more each year.

Deadline May of each year.

[309]
PENN HOSA SCHOLARSHIPS

Pennsylvania Health Occupations Students of America
Attn: PENN HOSA Foundation, Inc.
c/o Executive Director
200 North Third Street
P.O. Box 678
Harrisburg, PA 17109
(717) 652-9377   Fax: (717) 231-4463
E-mail: hheidelbau@verizon.net
Web: pahosa.org/scholarship.htm

Summary To provide financial assistance to student members of the Health Occupations Students of America (HOSA) in Pennsylvania who are interested in working on a degree in the health field.

Eligibility This program is open to HOSA student members in secondary, postsecondary, and collegiate chapters in Pennsylvania. Applicants must be enrolled or planning to enroll in a course of study in the health field at a technical school, college, or university. Selection is based on academic performance, interest and goals, leadership qualities, citizenship, school activities, and financial need. Most awards are for nursing, but other health fields (e.g., occupational therapy, pre-medical, veterinary technician, medical imaging, radiology, physician assistant, physical therapy, massage therapy, athletic trainer) also qualify.

Financial Data Stipends are $2,000 or $1,500.

Duration 1 year.

Number awarded Varies each year. Recently, 40 of these scholarships were awarded: 30 at $2,000 and 10 at $1,500.

Deadline February of each year.

[310]
PENNSYLVANIA ASSOCIATION OF SCHOOL NURSES AND PRACTITIONERS CERTIFIED SCHOOL NURSE SCHOLARSHIP

Pennsylvania Association of School Nurses and Practitioners
c/o Michelle Ficca, Scholarship Chair
Bloomsburg University of Pennsylvania
3136 MCHS
Bloomsburg, PA 17815
(570) 389-4000   E-mail: pasnapweb@pasnap.org
Web: www.pasnap.org/education/scholarships.html

Summary To provide financial assistance to students in Pennsylvania preparing for a career as a school nurse.

Eligibility This program is open to 1) nursing and nurse practitioner students in Pennsylvania intending to practice school nursing and enrolled or accepted in a B.S.N. or school nurse certification program; and 2) certified school nurses working on a graduate degree in nursing in Pennsylvania. Applicants must submit a 1-page letter outlining their goals in school nursing, a copy of their acceptance letter or official transcript, a current resume, and a copy of their current nursing license. Selection is based on a random drawing from all qualified applications; financial need is not considered.

Financial Data The stipend is $1,000. Funds are paid directly to the financial aid office in the recipient's institution.

Duration 1 year.

Number awarded 2 each year.

Deadline March of each year.

[311]
PENNSYLVANIA ASSOCIATION OF SCHOOL NURSES AND PRACTITIONERS FUTURE NURSE SCHOLARSHIP

Pennsylvania Association of School Nurses and Practitioners
c/o Nancy Kaminski, Membership Chair
1300 Crest Lane
Oakdale, PA 15071
(412) 881-4940, ext. 2345   E-mail: pasnapweb@pasnap.org
Web: www.pasnap.org/education/scholarships.html

Summary   To provide financial assistance to high school seniors in Pennsylvania planning to attend college in any state to prepare for a career as a nurse.

Eligibility   This program is open to seniors graduating from high schools in Pennsylvania. Applicants must be planning to attend an institution of higher education in any state to work on a bachelor's degree in nursing. Along with their application, they must submit 1) a copy of their current high school transcript, including their SAT/ACT scores and class rank; 2) a list of their co-curricular and extracurricular activities; 3) a 1-page personal statement on why they are choosing nursing and what they think nursing will add to their life; and 4) 2 letters of reference. Financial need is not considered in the selection process.

Financial Data   The stipend is $1,000. Funds are paid directly to the financial aid office in the recipient's institution.

Duration   1 year.

Additional data   This program was established in 2008 in memory of Richard Berritini, a Certified School Nurse at Port Allegheny High School who lost his life while serving in the National Guard in Afghanistan.

Number awarded   1 each year.

Deadline   April of each year.

[312]
PENNSYLVANIA RAINBOW NURSING SCHOLARSHIP

Pennsylvania Masonic Youth Foundation
Attn: Educational Endowment Fund
1244 Bainbridge Road
Elizabethtown, PA 17022-9423
(717) 367-1536   Toll Free: (800) 266-8424 (within PA)
Fax: (717) 367-0616   E-mail: pyf@pagrandlodge.org
Web: www.pagrandlodge.org/pyf/scholar/index.html

Summary   To provide financial assistance to members of Rainbow Girls in Pennsylvania who are attending nursing school in any state.

Eligibility   This program is open to active Pennsylvania Rainbow Girls in good standing. Applicants must have completed at least 1 year at an accredited nursing school in any state.

Financial Data   The stipend depends on the availability of funds.

Duration   1 year; may be renewed.

Number awarded   Varies each year, depending on the availability of funds.

Deadline   Requests for applications must be submitted by January of each year. Completed applications are due by the end of February.

[313]
PENNSYLVANIA SCITECH SCHOLARSHIPS

Pennsylvania Higher Education Assistance Agency
Attn: State Grant and Special Programs
1200 North Seventh Street
P.O. Box 8114
Harrisburg, PA 17105-8114
(717) 720-2800   Toll Free: (800) 692-7392
TDD: (800) 654-5988   E-mail: nets@pheaa.org
Web: www.pheaa.org

Summary   To provide scholarship/loans to residents of Pennsylvania who are interested in studying approved science or technology fields at a public or private college or university in the state and then working in the state after graduation.

Eligibility   This program is open to residents of Pennsylvania who graduated from a high school in the state and are currently enrolled full time as at least a sophomore at an approved Pennsylvania public or private college or university. Applicants must be working on a bachelor's degree in an approved science or technology field and have a GPA of 3.0 or higher. They must apply for a federal Pell Grant and a Pennsylvania State Grant, but financial need is not considered in the selection process. Funds are awarded on a first-come, first-served basis.

Financial Data   Scholarships provide up to $3,000 per year.

Duration   Up to 3 years, provided the recipient maintains a GPA of 3.0 or higher and full-time enrollment.

Additional data   This program, established in 1999 as part of the New Economy Technology Scholarship (NETS) program, is administered jointly by the Pennsylvania Department of Education (PDE) and the Pennsylvania Higher Education Assistance Agency (PHEAA). The PDE designates the approved fields of study in consultation with the Team Pennsylvania State Workforce Investment Board. Recently, the approved fields included pre-veterinary studies, nutrition sciences, pre-medical studies, pre-nursing, computer typography and composition equipment operator, computer programmer, quality control technology, nuclear engineering, physician assistant, pre-pharmacy studies, and industrial and physical pharmacy and cosmetic sciences. Recipients are required to 1) complete an approved internship or relevant work experience in a technology-intensive field with a Pennsylvania company prior to receiving a degree; and 2) begin full-time employment in the state within 1 year after completion of studies, 1 year for each year that the grant was awarded. If the student fails to satisfy both of those requirements, the scholarship grant reverts to a loan and must be repaid with interest.

Number awarded   Varies each year.

Deadline   December of each year for first-time applicants; September of each year for renewal applicants.

[314]
PENNSYLVANIA TECHNOLOGY SCHOLARSHIPS

Pennsylvania Higher Education Assistance Agency
Attn: State Grant and Special Programs
1200 North Seventh Street
P.O. Box 8114
Harrisburg, PA 17105-8114
(717) 720-2800   Toll Free: (800) 692-7392
TDD: (800) 654-5988   E-mail: nets@pheaa.org
Web: www.pheaa.org

Summary   To provide scholarship/loans to residents of Pennsylvania who are interested in studying approved science or technology fields at a college or technical institute in the state and then working in the state after graduation.

Eligibility   This program is open to residents of Pennsylvania who graduated from a high school in the state and are currently enrolled at an approved Pennsylvania 2- or 4-year college or licensed technical institute. Applicants must be enrolled in an approved science or technology program of less than 4 years in length and have a GPA of 3.0 or higher. They must apply for a federal Pell Grant and a Pennsylvania State Grant, but financial need is not considered in the selection process. Funds are awarded on a first-come, first-served basis.

Financial Data   For full-time students, scholarships provide up to $1,000 per year. Part-time students receive up to 20% of their tuition and mandatory fees or $1,000, whichever is less.

Duration   1 year; may be renewed for 1 additional year, provided the recipient maintains a GPA of 3.0 or higher.

Additional data   This program, established in 1999 as part of the New Economy Technology Scholarship (NETS) program, is administered jointly by the Pennsylvania Department of Education (PDE) and the Pennsylvania Higher Education Assistance Agency (PHEAA). The PDE designates the approved fields of study in consultation with the Team Pennsylvania State Workforce Investment Board. Recently, the approved fields included aeronautics/aviation/aerospace science and technology, pre-veterinary studies, computer typography and composition equipment operator, computer programmer, pre-medical studies, pre-pharmacy studies, pre-nursing, quality control technology, industrial mechanics and maintenance technology, and science technologies and technicians. Recipients are required to begin full-time employment in the state within 1 year after completion of studies and work 1 year for each year that the grant was awarded. If the student fails to satisfy that requirement, the scholarship grant reverts to a loan and must be repaid with interest.

Number awarded Varies each year.

Deadline December of each year for first-time applicants; September of each year for renewal applicants.

[315]
PENS ACADEMIC EDUCATION SCHOLARSHIPS

Pediatric Endocrinology Nursing Society
Attn: President-Elect
7794 Grow Drive
Pensacola, FL 32514
(850) 484-5223   Toll Free: (877) 936-7367
Fax: (850) 484-8762   E-mail: pens@peutzamc.com
Web: www.pens.org/scholarships.html

Summary To provide financial assistance for further education to members of the Pediatric Endocrinology Nursing Society (PENS).

Eligibility This program is open to R.N.s currently employed in pediatric endocrine nursing who have been members of PENS for at least 3 years. Applicants must be working on a degree in nursing; preference is given to those working on a B.S.N. degree and to first-time applicants. Along with their application, they must submit a copy of their R.N. license card, curriculum vitae or resume, statement of fees from the college or university, transcript of grades or (if beginning course work) a letter of acceptance, a list of professional organizations to which they belong, information on PENS activities in which they have participated, a list of volunteer or community service, and documentation of financial need.

Financial Data The stipend is $1,000 per year.

Duration 1 year. Members are eligible for 2 scholarships in a 5-year period.

Number awarded Varies each year.

Deadline March or August of each year.

[316]
PETER GILI SCHOLARSHIP AWARD

ExceptionalNurse.com
Attn: Scholarship Committee
13019 Coastal Circle
Palm Beach Gardens, FL 33410
(561) 627-9872   Fax: (561) 776-9254
TDD: (561) 776-9442   E-mail: ExceptionalNurse@aol.com
Web: www.ExceptionalNurse.com/scholarship.php

Summary To provide financial assistance to nursing students who have a disability.

Eligibility This program is open to students with a documented disability or medical challenge who have applied to, or have already been admitted to, a college or university nursing program on a full-time basis. Applicants must submit an essay on how they plan to contribute to the nursing profession and how their disability will influence their practice as a nurse. Selection is based on the essay, transcripts of high school and/or college courses com-

pleted, activities and honors received, 3 letters of recommendation, and financial need.

Financial Data The stipend is $500.

Duration 1 year; nonrenewable.

Number awarded 1 each year.

Deadline May of each year.

[317]
PHILIP R. PATTON SCHOLARSHIPS

Health Occupations Students of America
6021 Morriss Road, Suite 111
Flower Mound, TX 75028
(972) 874-0062   Toll Free: (800) 321-HOSA
Fax: (972) 874-0063   E-mail: info@hosa.org
Web: www.hosa.org/member/scholar.html

Summary To provide financial assistance for college to members of the Health Occupations Students of America (HOSA).

Eligibility This program is open to high school seniors and current college students who are members of the association and planning to continue their education in the health care field (including nursing). Applicants must submit a 1-page essay describing 3 qualities they have gained through their HOSA experiences and how they plan to use them in their future college, community, and career. Selection is based on the essay (26 points), transcripts (20 points), leadership activities and recognition (30 points), community involvement (15 points), and letters of reference (9 points).

Financial Data The stipend is $1,000.

Duration 1 year.

Additional data This program, established in 2004, is sponsored by Hospital Corporation of America.

Number awarded 6 each year.

Deadline April of each year.

[318]
PHILLIPS/LAIRD SCHOLARSHIP

Minnesota Nurses Association
Attn: Minnesota Nurses Association Foundation
1625 Energy Park Drive, Suite 200
St. Paul, MN 55108
(651) 414-2822   Toll Free: (800) 536-4662, ext. 122
Fax: (651) 695-7000   E-mail: linda.owens@mnnurses.org
Web: www.mnnurses.org

Summary To provide financial assistance to members of the Minnesota Nurses Association (MNA) who are interested in working on a baccalaureate or graduate degree in nursing.

Eligibility This program is open to MNA members who have a current R.N. licensure and have been accepted into an approved program of study leading to a baccalaureate or graduate academic degree in nursing. Applicants must submit a brief description of their career goals following their graduation. Selection is based on that statement, professional activities, demonstrated leadership ability, scholarship in nursing, MNA activities, and community involvement. Preference is given to nurses who live or work in the "former" MNA District 13 (e.g., Owatonna, Waseca, Northfield, Faribault, Rice County).

Financial Data The stipend is $2,000 per year.

Duration 1 year; may be renewed.

Number awarded 1 each year.

Deadline May of each year.

[319]
PHOEBE PEMBER MEMORIAL SCHOLARSHIP

United Daughters of the Confederacy
Attn: Education Director
328 North Boulevard
Richmond, VA 23220-4057
(804) 355-1636   Fax: (804) 353-1396
E-mail: hqudc@rcn.com
Web: www.hqudc.org/scholarships/scholarships.html

Summary   To provide financial assistance for nursing education to lineal descendants of Confederate veterans.

Eligibility   Eligible to apply for these scholarships are lineal descendants of worthy Confederates or collateral descendants who are members of the Children of the Confederacy or the United Daughters of the Confederacy. Applicants must intend to study nursing and must submit a family financial report and certified proof of the Confederate record of 1 ancestor, with the company and regiment in which he served. They must have at least a 3.0 GPA in high school.

Financial Data   The amount of this scholarship depends on the availability of funds.

Duration   1 year; may be renewed for up to 3 additional years.

Additional data   Members of the same family may not hold scholarships simultaneously, and only 1 application per family will be accepted within any 1 year. All requests for applications must include a self-addressed stamped envelope.

Number awarded   1 each year.

Deadline   April of each year.

[320]
PHYSIO-CONTROL ACADEMIC SCHOLARSHIP

American Association of Occupational Health Nurses, Inc.
Attn: AAOHN Foundation
7794 Grow Drive
Pensacola, FL 32514
(850) 474-6963   Toll Free: (800) 241-8014
Fax: (850) 484-8762   E-mail: aaohn@aaohn.org
Web: www.aaohn.org/scholarships/academic-study.html

Summary   To provide financial assistance to registered nurses who are working on a bachelor's or graduate degree to prepare for a career in occupational and environmental health.

Eligibility   This program is open to registered nurses who are enrolled in a baccalaureate or graduate degree program. Applicants must demonstrate an interest in, and commitment to, occupational and environmental health. Along with their application, they must submit a 500-word narrative on their professional goals as they relate to the academic activity and the field of occupational and environmental health. Selection is based on that essay (50%), impact of education on applicant's career (20%), and 2 letters of recommendation (30%).

Financial Data   The stipend is $3,000.

Duration   1 year; may be renewed up to 2 additional years.

Additional data   Funding for this program is provided by Physio-Control, Inc.

Number awarded   1 each year.

Deadline   January of each year.

[321]
POUDRE VALLEY HEALTH SYSTEM NIGHTINGALE SCHOLARSHIP

Colorado Nurses Foundation
7400 East Arapahoe Road, Suite 211
Centennial, CO 80112
(303) 694-4728   Fax: (303) 694-4869
E-mail: mail@cnfound.org
Web: www.cnfound.org/scholarships.html

Summary   To provide financial assistance to undergraduate and graduate nursing students in Colorado who are willing to work in designated communities following graduation.

Eligibility   This program is open to Colorado residents who are enrolled in an approved nursing program in the state. Applicants may be 1) second-year students in an associate degree program; 2) junior or senior level B.S.N. undergraduate students; 3) R.N.s enrolled in a baccalaureate or higher degree program in a school of nursing; 4) R.N.s with a master's degree in nursing, currently practicing in Colorado and enrolled in a doctoral program; or 5) students in the second or third year of a Doctorate Nursing Practice (D.N.P.) program. They must be willing to work in Fort Collins, Loveland, or Estes Park, Colorado following graduation. Undergraduates must have a GPA of 3.25 or higher and graduate students must have a GPA of 3.5 or higher. Selection is based on professional philosophy and goals, dedication to the improvement of patient care in Colorado, demonstrated commitment to nursing, critical thinking skills, potential for leadership, involvement in community and professional organizations, recommendations, GPA, and financial need.

Financial Data   The stipend is $1,000.

Duration   1 year.

Number awarded   2 each year.

Deadline   October of each year.

[322]
PROMISE OF NURSING SCHOLARSHIPS

National Student Nurses' Association
Attn: Foundation
45 Main Street, Suite 606
Brooklyn, NY 11201
(718) 210-0705   Fax: (718) 797-1186
E-mail: nsna@nsna.org
Web: www.nsna.org

Summary   To provide financial assistance to nursing or pre-nursing students at schools in selected geographic locations.

Eligibility   This program is open to students currently enrolled in state-approved schools of nursing or pre-nursing associate degree, baccalaureate, diploma, generic master's, generic doctoral, R.N. to B.S.N., R.N. to M.S.N., or L.P.N./L.V.N. to R.N. programs. Graduating high school seniors are not eligible. Support for graduate education is provided only for a first degree in nursing. Applicants must be attending school in the Dallas/Fort Worth area of Texas, the Houston/Galveston area of Texas (Austin, Brazoria, Chamber, Colorado, Fort Bend, Galveston, Harris, Liberty, Matagorda, Montgomery, Walker, Waller, and Wharton counties), central Florida, southern Florida, southern California (Los Angeles, Orange, Riverside, San Bernardino, Santa Barbara, and Ventura counties), or the states of Georgia (graduate students only), Louisiana, Maryland, Massachusetts, Mississippi, New Jersey (graduate students only), Oregon, Pennsylvania, Tennessee, or Washington. Selection is based on academic achievement, financial need, and involvement in student nursing organizations and community health activities.

Financial Data   Stipends range from $1,000 to $2,500.

Duration   1 year.

Additional data   This program, offered for the first time in 2003, is supported by fundraising events sponsored by Johnson & Johnson. Applications must be accompanied by a $10 processing fee.

Number awarded   Varies each year. Recently, 57 of these scholarships were awarded: 2 in Dallas/Fort Worth, Texas; 1 in Houston/Galveston, Texas; 2 in central Florida; 9 in southern California; 9 in Maryland; 11 in Massachusetts; 4 in New Jersey; 5 in Pennsylvania; 3 in Tennessee; and 11 in Washington.

Deadline   January of each year.

[323]
REBECCA GOLDMAN FUND SCHOLARSHIP

Greater Kanawha Valley Foundation
Attn: Scholarship Coordinator
1600 Huntington Square
900 Lee Street, East
P.O. Box 3041
Charleston, WV 25331-3041
(304) 346-3620   Toll Free: (800) 467-5909
Fax: (304) 346-3640   E-mail: shoover@tgkvf.org
Web: www.tgkvf.org/scholar.htm

Summary To provide financial assistance to residents of West Virginia who are interested in studying nursing at a school in any state.

Eligibility This program is open to residents of West Virginia who are attending or planning to attend a college or university in any state. Applicants must be planning to study nursing. They must have an ACT score of 20 or higher; be able to demonstrate good moral character, academic excellence, and financial need; and have a GPA of 3.0 or higher.

Financial Data Stipends average $600 per year.

Duration 1 year; may be renewed.

Number awarded 1 or more each year.

Deadline January of each year.

[324]
REGIRER NURSING SCHOLARSHIPS

Virginia Health Care Association
Attn: Commonwealth Long Term Care Foundation, Inc.
2112 West Laburnum Avenue, Suite 206
Richmond, VA 23227
(804) 353-9101   Fax: (804) 353-3098
E-mail: Kathy.robertson@vhca.org
Web: www.vhca.org/foundation

Summary To provide financial assistance to employees of facilities of the Virginia Health Care Association (VHCA) and the Virginia Center for Assisted Living (VCIL) who are interested in working on a degree at an accredited nurse training program in any state.

Eligibility This program is open to employees of VHCA and VCIL member facilities. Applicants must be enrolled or planning to enroll in an accredited nurse training program in any state. They may be certified nursing assistants working on an L.P.N. degree or an L.P.N. working on an R.N. degree. Along with their application, they must submit a personal letter describing their reasons for wanting to become a nurse, financial need, and career goals. A personal interview is required. Selection is based on commitment to geriatrics, 3 reference letters, interviewer recommendation, and financial need.

Financial Data The stipend is $1,500.

Duration 1 year.

Additional data The Commonwealth Long Term Care Foundation is sponsored jointly by the VHCA and the VCIL. Recipients must agree to work for at least 1 year at an association member nursing or assisted living facility in Virginia following completion of their program.

Number awarded Varies each year; recently, 34 of these scholarships were awarded.

Deadline April of each year.

[325]
RICE MEMORIAL SCHOLARSHIP

Ohio Nurses Association
Attn: Ohio Nurses Foundation
4000 East Main Street
Columbus, OH 43213-2983
(614) 237-5414   Fax: (614) 237-6074
E-mail: gharsheymeade@ohnurses.org
Web: www.ohnurses.org

Summary To provide financial assistance to registered nurses in Ohio who are cancer survivors or have a relative with cancer and are working on a nursing degree at a school in the state.

Eligibility This program is open to Ohio residents who have a valid Ohio nursing license and plan to continue practicing in the state. Applicants must be a cancer survivor or have a close relative who has been diagnosed with cancer. They must have a GPA of 3.5 or higher and be planning to enroll in a nursing degree program at a school in Ohio. Along with their application, they must submit a 250-word personal statement on how the cancer experience has shaped their life and practice in Ohio. Selection is based on that statement, college academic records, school activities, and community services. Membership in the Ohio Nurses Association is considered in the selection process.

Financial Data The stipend is $500 per year.

Duration 1 year; recipients may reapply if they complete 9 credit hours during the academic year.

Number awarded 1 or more each year.

Deadline January of each year.

[326]
RN TO BSN SCHOLARSHIP

Society of Otorhinolaryngology and Head-Neck Nurses, Inc.
Attn: Ear, Nose and Throat Nursing Foundation
202 Julia Street
New Smyrna Beach, FL 32168
(386) 428-1695   Fax: (386) 423-7566
E-mail: info@sohnnurse.com
Web: www.sohnnurse.com/awards.html

Summary To provide financial assistance to members of the Society of Otorhinolaryngology and Head-Neck Nurses (SOHN) who are registered nurses interested in working on a bachelor's degree in nursing.

Eligibility This program is open to registered nurses who are SOHN members and practicing in otorhinolaryngology. Applicants must be interested in working on a B.S. degree in nursing. Along with their application, they must submit a copy of their current registration in a B.S.N. program, a copy of their latest transcript (must have at least a 3.0 GPA), a statement of current financial assistance received and required, 3 letters of recommendation, and a narrative of 750 to 1,000 words describing their past or current SOHN involvement, future SOHN goals, and desire for advancing their degree in nursing.

Financial Data Stipends range from $1,000 to $1,500.

Duration 1 year.

Number awarded 1 or more each year.

Deadline June of each year.

[327]
ROBERT BROWNING SCHOLARSHIP

Pride Foundation
Attn: Scholarship Program Director
1122 East Pike Street
PMB 1001
Seattle, WA 98122-3934
(206) 323-3318   Toll Free: (800) 735-7287
Fax: (206) 323-1017
E-mail: scholarships@pridefoundation.org
Web: www.pridefoundation.org/scholarships/scholarship-funds

Summary To provide financial assistance for undergraduate study in the health sciences to gay, lesbian, bisexual, or transgender (GLBT) students who live in the Northwest.
Eligibility This program is open to residents of Alaska, Idaho, Montana, Oregon, or Washington who are studying or planning to study the health sciences at the undergraduate level. Preference is given to students who are self-identified GLBT, members of GLBT families, or allies who have been strongly supportive of the GLBT community. Selection is based on financial need, community involvement, and commitment to civil rights for all people.
Financial Data Stipends average more than $2,100. Funds are paid directly to the recipient's school.
Duration 1 year; recipients may reapply.
Additional data The Pride Foundation was established in 1987 to strengthen the GLBT community.
Number awarded 1 or more each year. Since it began offering scholarships in 1993, the foundation has awarded $1.4 million to nearly 800 recipients.
Deadline January of each year.

[328]
ROBERTA D. THIRY ENDOWED SCHOLARSHIP

Kansas State Nurses Association
Attn: Kansas Nurses Foundation
1109 S.W. Topeka Boulevard
Topeka, KS 66612-1602
(785) 233-8638   Fax: (785) 233-5222
E-mail: ksna@ksna.net
Web: www.nursingworld.org/SNAS/KS/Knf.htm

Summary To provide financial assistance to residents of Kansas who are working on a bachelor's or higher degree in nursing.
Eligibility This program is open to R.N.s and other students in Kansas who are working on a nursing degree. Applicants must have a GPA of 3.0 or higher. Along with their application, they must submit a personal narrative describing their anticipated role in nursing in the state of Kansas. Preference is given to full-time students. First priority is given to R.N.s admitted to the B.S.N. completion program at Kansas Wesleyan University. If no applicants qualify for that first priority, second priority is given students enrolled in the third or fourth year of the B.S.N. program at Kansas Wesleyan University. If no applicants qualify for that second priority, third priority is given to students enrolled in master's or doctoral programs, especially residents of Dickinson, Ellsworth, Lincoln, Mitchell, Ottawa, and Saline counties. If no applicants qualify for that third priority, fourth priority is given to students enrolled in other Kansas B.S.N. or graduate nursing programs.
Financial Data The stipend is $500.
Duration 1 year.
Number awarded 1 each year.
Deadline June of each year.

[329]
ROBERTA PIERCE SCOFIELD BACHELOR'S SCHOLARSHIPS

Oncology Nursing Society
Attn: ONS Foundation
125 Enterprise Drive
Pittsburgh, PA 15275-1214
(412) 859-6100   Toll Free: (866) 257-4ONS
Fax: (412) 859-6163   E-mail: foundation@ons.org
Web: www.ons.org/Awards/FoundationAwards/Bachelors

Summary To provide financial assistance to nurses and other students who are interested in working on a bachelor's degree in oncology nursing.
Eligibility This program is open to students who are accepted to or currently enrolled in a bachelor's degree program at an NLN- or CCNE-accredited school of nursing. Applicants must be able to demonstrate an interest in and commitment to oncology nursing.

They may 1) already have a current license to practice as a registered nurse (R.N.); 2) currently have a postsecondary degree at some level but not be an R.N.; or 3) have only a high school diploma. Along with their application, they must submit 1) an essay of 250 words or less on their role or interest in caring for persons with cancer, and 2) a statement of their professional goals and the relationship of those goals to the advancement of oncology nursing. Non-R.N. applicants must be in the nursing component of the B.S.N. program. High school students and individuals in the liberal arts component of a B.S.N. program are not eligible. Financial need is not considered in the selection process.
Financial Data The stipend is $2,000.
Duration 1 year; nonrenewable.
Additional data These scholarships were first awarded in 1988. At the end of the year of scholarship participation, recipients must submit a summary describing their educational activities. Applications must be accompanied by a $5 fee.
Number awarded Varies each year; recently, 7 of these scholarships were awarded.
Deadline January of each year.

[330]
ROSEMARY SMITH, R.N. MEMORIAL SCHOLARSHIP

Massachusetts Nurses Association
Attn: Massachusetts Nurses Foundation
340 Turnpike Street
Canton, MA 02021
(781) 830-5745   Toll Free: (800) 882-2056, ext. 745
Fax: (781) 821-4445   E-mail: cmessia@mnarn.org
Web: www.massnurses.org/about-man/mns/scholarships

Summary To provide financial assistance to members of the Massachusetts Nurses Association (MNA) who are working on an undergraduate or graduate degree in nursing, labor studies, or public health policy.
Eligibility This program is open to MNA members who are registered nurses or other health care professionals. First preference is given to members of MNA's Unit 7. Applicants must be enrolled in a bachelor's or master's degree program in nursing, labor studies, or public health policy. Along with their application, they must submit a 500-word essay on their career goals, how education will enhance those goals, and their contribution to their profession. Selection is based on the essay, professional development activities, community work, and 2 professional references. Minorities are specifically encouraged to apply.
Financial Data A stipend is awarded (amount not specified).
Duration 1 year.
Additional data Unit 7 is a bargaining unit that represents registered nurses, public health nurses, nurse practitioners, nursing instructors, community psychiatric mental health nurses, community mental health nursing advisers, health care facility inspectors, psychologists, physical therapists, occupational therapists, and audiologists.
Number awarded 1 each year.
Deadline May of each year.

[331]
ROY ANDERSON MEMORIAL SCHOLARSHIP

Colorado Nurses Foundation
7400 East Arapahoe Road, Suite 211
Centennial, CO 80112
(303) 694-4728   Fax: (303) 694-4869
E-mail: mail@cnfound.org
Web: www.cnfound.org/scholarships.html

Summary To provide financial assistance to residents of Colorado who are working on a bachelor's or higher degree in nursing at a college or university in the state.

Eligibility This program is open to Colorado residents who have been accepted as a student in an approved nursing program in the state. Applicants must be working on a bachelor's or higher degree. Undergraduates must have a GPA of 3.25 or higher and graduate students must have a GPA of 3.5 or higher. Selection is based on professional philosophy and goals, dedication to the improvement of patient care in Colorado, demonstrated commitment to nursing, critical thinking skills, potential for leadership, involvement in community and professional organizations, recommendations, GPA, and financial need.

Financial Data The stipend is $5,000.

Duration 1 year.

Number awarded 2 each year.

Deadline October of each year.

[332]
RUTH GOODE NURSING SCHOLARSHIP

Seneca Diabetes Foundation
Attn: Lucille White
TIS Building 12837, Route 438
P.O. Box 390
Irving, NY 14081
(716) 532-4900   Fax: (716) 549-1629
E-mail: white@sni.org
Web: www.senecadiabetesfoundation.org

Summary To provide financial assistance to members of the Seneca Nation who are interested in attending college to work on a degree in nursing.

Eligibility This program is open to members of the Seneca Nation who are interested in attending college to work on a degree in nursing. Applicants must submit brief statements on 1) the professional, community, or cultural services and activities in which they have participated; 2) how this scholarship would help further their education; 3) their goals or plan for using their nursing experience to benefit the Seneca Nation and its people; and 4) the qualities about Ruth Goode's life, both personal and professional, they identify with the most. In the selection process, primary consideration is given to financial need, but involvement in community and cultural activities, personal assets, and desire to improve the quality of life for the Seneca people are also considered.

Financial Data The stipend is $5,000.

Duration 1 year.

Number awarded 1 each year.

Deadline July of each year.

[333]
RUTH LUTES BACHMANN SCHOLARSHIP

Grand Lodge of Missouri, A.F. & A.M.
Attn: Masonic Scholarship Fund of Missouri
6033 Masonic Drive, Suite B
Columbia, MO 65202-6535
(573) 474-8561
Web: www.momason.org/programs.asp

Summary To provide financial assistance to Missouri residents interested in attending college to prepare for a career as a teacher or a nurse.

Eligibility This program is open to residents of Missouri who are graduating from or have graduated from a public high school in the state. Applicants must be attending or planning to attend an accredited college or university in the United States as a full-time student with a major in education or nursing. They must have a GPA of 3.0 or higher and be able to demonstrate financial need. Along with their application, they must submit an essay of 300 to 500 words on why they are applying for this scholarship.

Financial Data The stipend is $1,000.

Duration 1 year; may be renewed if the recipient remains enrolled full time with a GPA of 3.0 or higher.

Number awarded Several each year.

Deadline March of each year.

[334]
SANDRA R. SPAULDING MEMORIAL SCHOLARSHIPS

California Nurses Association
Attn: Scholarship Fund
2000 Franklin Street, Suite 300
Oakland, CA 94612
(510) 273-2200, ext. 344   Fax: (510) 663-1625
E-mail: membershipbenefits@calnurses.org
Web: www.calnurses.org/membership

Summary To provide financial assistance to students from diverse ethnic backgrounds who are enrolled in an associate degree in nursing (A.D.N.) program in California.

Eligibility This program is open to students who have been admitted to a second-year accredited A.D.N. program in California and plan to complete the degree within 2 years. Along with their application, they must submit a 1-page essay describing their personal and professional goals. Selection is based on that essay, commitment and active participation in nursing and health-related organizations, professional vision and direction, and financial need. A goal of this scholarship program is to encourage ethnic and socioeconomic diversity in nursing.

Financial Data A stipend is awarded (amount not specified).

Duration 1 year; nonrenewable.

Additional data This program was established in 1985.

Number awarded 1 or more each year.

Deadline June of each year.

[335]
SARAH COLVIN SOCIAL JUSTICE SCHOLARSHIP

Minnesota Nurses Association
Attn: Minnesota Nurses Association Foundation
1625 Energy Park Drive, Suite 200
St. Paul, MN 55108
(651) 414-2822   Toll Free: (800) 536-4662, ext. 122
Fax: (651) 695-7000   E-mail: linda.owens@mnnurses.org
Web: www.mnnurses.org

Summary To provide financial assistance to members of the Minnesota Nurses Association (MNA) who are interested in working on a baccalaureate or graduate degree in nursing and have an interest in social justice.

Eligibility This program is open to MNA members who have a current R.N. licensure and have been accepted into an approved program of study leading to a baccalaureate or graduate academic degree in nursing. Applicants must be able to document evidence of advocating for individuals and groups harmed by inequities, environmental exploitation, discrimination, and oppression. Examples of social justice issues may include (but are not limited to) working with the mentally ill, impoverished, abused, or elderly. Selection is based on a statement of career goals, professional activities, demonstrated leadership ability, scholarship in nursing, MNA activities, and community involvement.

Financial Data The stipend is $2,000 per year.

Duration 1 year; may be renewed.

Number awarded 1 each year.

Deadline May of each year.

[336]
SCHOLARSHIP FOR RNS MAJORING IN NURSING

Ohio Nurses Association
Attn: Ohio Nurses Foundation
4000 East Main Street
Columbus, OH 43213-2983
(614) 237-5414   Fax: (614) 237-6074
E-mail: gharsheymeade@ohnurses.org
Web: www.ohnurses.org

Summary To provide financial assistance to registered nurses in Ohio who are working on a nursing degree at a school in any state.

Eligibility This program is open to Ohio residents who have a valid Ohio nursing license. Applicants must have a GPA of 2.5 or higher as an undergraduate or 3.5 or higher if working on a graduate degree. They must be planning to enroll full time in a nursing degree program at a school in any state. Along with their application, they must submit a 100-word personal statement on how they will advance the profession of nursing in Ohio. Selection is based on that statement, college academic records, school activities, and community services.

Financial Data The stipend is $1,000 per year.

Duration 1 year; recipients may reapply for 1 additional year if they maintain a cumulative GPA of 2.5 or higher.

Number awarded 1 or more each year.

Deadline January of each year.

[337]
SCHOLARSHIP FOR STUDENTS RETURNING TO SCHOOL TO MAJOR IN NURSING

Ohio Nurses Association
Attn: Ohio Nurses Foundation
4000 East Main Street
Columbus, OH 43213-2983
(614) 237-5414   Fax: (614) 237-6074
E-mail: gharsheymeade@ohnurses.org
Web: www.ohnurses.org

Summary To provide financial assistance to residents of Ohio who are interested in returning to school in any state to work on a degree in nursing.

Eligibility This program is open to Ohio residents who are not R.N.s and have been out of school for 2 or more years. Applicants must be interested in returning to school in any state to enroll full time in a nursing degree program. Along with their application, they must submit a 100-word personal statement on how they will advance the profession of nursing in Ohio. Selection is based on that statement, college academic records, school activities, and community services.

Financial Data The stipend is $1,000 per year.

Duration 1 year; recipients may reapply for 1 additional year if they maintain a cumulative GPA of 2.5 or higher.

Number awarded 1 or more each year.

Deadline January of each year.

[338]
SCHOOL NURSE ORGANIZATION OF WASHINGTON SCHOLARSHIPS

School Nurse Organization of Washington
Attn: Professional Development Chair
P.O. 141309
Spokane Valley, WA 99214-1309
Web: www.schoolnurseorganizationofwashington.org/?ID=39

Summary To provide financial assistance to members of the School Nurse Organization of Washington (SNOW) who are interested in additional training.

Eligibility This program is open to SNOW members who are interested in working on a B.S.N., master's degree, or education staff associate certification in school nursing. Applicants must

submit a 1-page essay on why they selected school nursing as a clinical specialty. Selection is based on the essay, academic achievement, professional involvement, and financial need.

Financial Data The stipend is $500.

Duration 1 year.

Additional data This program includes the Carol Hoffman Scholarship, the Martha Meyers Scholarship, and the Lifetime Members Scholarship.

Number awarded 3 each year.

Deadline February of each year.

[339]
SCOTT DOMINGUEZ-CRATERS OF THE MOON CHAPTER SCHOLARSHIP

American Society of Safety Engineers
Attn: ASSE Foundation
1800 East Oakton Street
Des Plaines, IL 60018
(847) 768-3435   Fax: (847) 768-3434
E-mail: agabanski@asse.org
Web: www.asse.org/foundation/scholarships/scholarships.php

Summary To provide financial assistance to undergraduate and graduate student members of the American Society of Safety Engineers (ASSE) from designated western states.

Eligibility This program is open to undergraduate and graduate students who are working on a degree in occupational safety, health, and environment or a closely-related field (e.g., industrial or environmental engineering, environmental science, industrial hygiene, occupational health nursing). First priority is given to residents within the service area of Craters of the Moon Chapter in Idaho; second priority is given to residents of other states in ASSE Region II (Arizona, Colorado, Montana, Nevada, New Mexico, Utah, and Wyoming). Special consideration is also given to 1) employees of a sponsoring organization or their dependents; 2) students who are serving their country through active duty in the armed forces or are honorably discharged; 3) former members of the Boy Scouts, Girl Scouts, FFA, or 4-H; 4) recipients of awards from service organizations; and 5) students who have provided volunteer service to an ASSE chapter in a leadership role. Undergraduates must have completed at least 60 semester hours with a GPA of 3.0 or higher. Graduate students must have completed at least 9 semester hours with a GPA of 3.5 or higher and have earned a GPA of 3.0 or higher as an undergraduate. Full-time students must be ASSE student members; part-time students must be ASSE general or professional members. Along with their application, they must submit 2 essays of 300 words or less: 1) why they are seeking a degree in occupational safety and health or a closely-related field, a brief description of their current activities, and how those relate to their career goals and objectives; and 2) why they should be awarded this scholarship (including career goals and financial need). U.S. citizenship is not required.

Financial Data The stipend is $1,000 per year.

Duration 1 year; recipients may reapply.

Additional data This program is sponsored by the ASSE Craters of the Moon Chapter.

Number awarded 1 each year.

Deadline November of each year.

[340]
SGNA RN ADVANCING EDUCATION SCHOLARSHIP

Society of Gastroenterology Nurses and Associates, Inc.
Attn: Awards Committee
401 North Michigan Avenue
Chicago, IL 60611-4267
(312) 321-5165   Toll Free: (800) 245-SGNA
Fax: (312) 673-6694   E-mail: sgna@smithbucklin.com
Web: www.sgna.org/Education/scholarships.cfm

Summary To provide financial assistance to registered nurses (R.N.s) working in gastroenterology who are interested in enrolling in an advanced degree program.

Eligibility This program is open to R.N.s working in gastroenterology who are members of the Society of Gastroenterology Nurses and Associates (SGNA). Applicants must be enrolled in an accredited advanced degree program working on a B.S.N., M.S.N., or Ph.D. degree with a GPA of 3.0 or higher. Along with their application, they must submit a 500-word essay on a challenging situation they see in the health care environment today and how they, as an R.N. with an advanced degree, would best address and meet that challenge. Financial need is not considered in the selection process.

Financial Data The stipend is $2,500 for full-time students or $1,000 for part-time students. Funds are issued as reimbursement after the recipient has completed the proposed course work with a GPA of 3.0 or higher.

Duration 1 year.

Number awarded 1 or more each year.

Deadline July of each year.

[341]
SGNA RN GENERAL EDUCATION SCHOLARSHIP

Society of Gastroenterology Nurses and Associates, Inc.
Attn: Awards Committee
401 North Michigan Avenue
Chicago, IL 60611-4267
(312) 321-5165   Toll Free: (800) 245-SGNA
Fax: (312) 673-6694   E-mail: sgna@smithbucklin.com
Web: www.sgna.org/Education/scholarships.cfm

Summary To provide financial assistance to full-time students working toward licensure as a registered nurse (R.N.).

Eligibility This program is open to students currently enrolled full time in an accredited nursing program with a GPA of 3.0 or higher. Applicants must be studying to become an R.N. Along with their application, they must submit a 2-page essay on a challenging situation they see in the health care environment today and how they, as an R.N., would best address and meet that challenge. Financial need is not considered in the selection process.

Financial Data The stipend is $2,500. Funds are issued as reimbursement after the recipient has completed the proposed course work with a GPA of 3.0 or higher.

Duration 1 year.

Number awarded 1 or more each year.

Deadline July of each year.

[342]
SHARON A. SMITH SCHOLARSHIP

Massachusetts Organization of Nurse Executives
Attn: Scholarship Selection Committee
101 Cambridge Street, Suite 110
Burlington, MA 01803
(781) 272-3500   Fax: (781) 272-3505
E-mail: info@massone.org
Web: www.massone.org

Summary To provide financial assistance to members of the Massachusetts Organization of Nurse Executives (MONE) and their families who are studying nursing in college or graduate school.

Eligibility This program is open to MONE members and their immediate family (spouse, children, siblings, nieces, and nephews). Applicants must be enrolled in an accredited nursing program (B.S.N., M.S.N., or advanced practice). Along with their application, they must submit a 500-word essay on why they are working on a nursing or advanced degree and what they hope to accomplish, documentation of financial need, and the names of 2 references.

Financial Data The amount of the stipend varies each year, depending on the availability of funds.

Duration 1 year.

Number awarded Varies each year.

Deadline April of each year.

[343]
SHEENA M. TAYLOR MEMORIAL SCHOLARSHIP FUND

Pittsburgh Foundation
Attn: Scholarship Coordinator
Five PPG Place, Suite 250
Pittsburgh, PA 15222-5414
(412) 394-2649   Fax: (412) 391-7259
E-mail: turnerd@pghfdn.org
Web: www.pittsburghfoundation.org

Summary To provide financial assistance to residents of western Pennsylvania and West Virginia (and of the United Kingdom) who are attending a school of nursing in those states.

Eligibility This program is open to residents of western Pennsylvania, West Virginia, or the United Kingdom who are nursing students not yet qualified to practice as registered nurses. Applicants must be enrolled in a college or hospital program in western Pennsylvania or West Virginia. They must have a GPA of 2.0 or higher and be able to demonstrate financial need.

Financial Data The stipend varies each year; recently, $1,850 was available for this program.

Duration 1 year; nonrenewable.

Number awarded 1 each year.

Deadline February of each year.

[344]
SISTER MARY FRANCES LOFTIN, D.C. FUND FOR HEALTH EDUCATION

St. Vincent's Health System
Attn: St. Vincent's Foundation
De Paul Building
2800 University Building, Suite 101
Birmingham, AL 35233
(205) 939-7296
Web: www.stvhs.com/foundations/bham/Scholarship.asp

Summary To provide scholarship/loans to nursing students interested in working at St. Vincent's Hospital in Birmingham, Alabama following certification as an R.N.

Eligibility This program is open to students working full time on an associate (A.D.N.) or bachelor's (B.S.N.) degree in nursing. Applicants must commit to working at St. Vincent's Hospital in Birmingham, Alabama following completion of their degree and certification as an R.N. Along with their application, they must submit a statement of their personal philosophy and how it relates to the mission of the Daughters of Charity and St. Vincent's Hospital. Selection is based on that statement, grades, references, school recommendation, and financial need.

Financial Data The stipend is $2,500 per year. This is a scholarship/loan program. Recipients are required to work full time at St. Vincent's for 2 years or repay all assistance received.

Duration 1 year; may be renewed 1 additional year.

Number awarded 1 each year.

Deadline April of each year.

[345]
SOCIETY OF PEDIATRIC NURSES EDUCATIONAL SCHOLARSHIP

Society of Pediatric Nurses
7794 Grow Drive
Pensacola, FL 32514
(850) 494-9467   Toll Free: (800) 723-2902
Fax: (850) 484-8762   E-mail: spn@dancyamc.com
Web: www.pedsnurses.org/awards-amp-scholarships.html

Summary To provide financial assistance to members of the Society of Pediatric Nurses (SPN) who are working on a bachelor's or graduate degree.

Eligibility This program is open to SPN members who are currently enrolled or accepted in a B.S.N. completion program or graduate program that will advance the health care of children. Students must be nominated by a current SPN member or chapter. Along with their application, they must submit a letter of recommendation from an SPN member that addresses their interest in and/or commitment to the care of children and their families, and a letter of recommendation from a faculty member who can evaluate their potential to meet professional goals.

Financial Data The stipend is $500.

Duration 1 year.

Number awarded 1 or more each year.

Deadline November of each year.

[346]
SONNE SCHOLARSHIP

Illinois Nurses Association
Attn: Sonne Scholarship Committee
105 West Adams Street, Suite 2101
Chicago, IL 60603
(312) 419-2900   Fax: (312) 419-2920
E-mail: info@illinoisnurses.com
Web: www.illinoisnurses.com

Summary To provide financial assistance to members of the Student Nurse Association of Illinois (SNAI) who are preparing for a career as a registered professional nurse.

Eligibility This program is open to SNAI members who are enrolled in a Illinois-approved nursing program that leads to eligibility to sit for licensure examination as a registered professional nurse. Applicants must have a GPA of 2.5 or higher. Along with their application, they must submit a 1-page essay on "How will membership in my state nurses association enhance my nursing career?" Financial need is also considered in the selection process.

Financial Data Stipends range from $500 to $1,500. Funds are to be used to cover tuition, fees, and other educational expenses.

Duration 1 year.

Additional data Recipients are given a year's free membership in the Illinois Nurses Association upon graduation. Although part-time students can apply, all recipients must attend school on a full-time basis.

Number awarded 2 to 4 each year.

Deadline March of each year.

[347]
SOUTH CAROLINA NURSES CARE SCHOLARSHIPS

South Carolina Nurses Foundation, Inc.
Attn: Awards Committee Chair
1821 Gadsden Street
Columbia, SC 29201
(803) 252-4781   Fax: (803) 779-3870
E-mail: brownk1@aol.com
Web: www.scnursesfoundation.org/index_files/Page316.htm

Summary To provide financial assistance to students enrolled in an undergraduate or graduate degree nursing program in South Carolina.

Eligibility This program is open to students currently enrolled in an undergraduate or graduate nursing degree program in South Carolina. Applicants must submit documentation of financial need and brief statements of their career goals, both upon graduation and in 5 years.

Financial Data The stipend is $1,500.

Duration 1 year.

Additional data This program was established in 2002 and is funded by the sale of "Nurses Care" specialty license plates.

Number awarded 4 each year: 2 to undergraduates and 2 to graduate students.

Deadline May of each year.

[348]
SOUTHWEST CHAPTER ROY KINSLOW SCHOLARSHIP

American Society of Safety Engineers
Attn: ASSE Foundation
1800 East Oakton Street
Des Plaines, IL 60018
(847) 768-3435   Fax: (847) 768-3434
E-mail: agabanski@asse.org
Web: www.asse.org/foundation/scholarships/scholarships.php

Summary To provide financial assistance to upper-division student members of the American Society of Safety Engineers (ASSE), especially those from Oklahoma and neighboring states.

Eligibility This program is open to ASSE student members who are majoring in occupational safety, health, and environment or a closely-related field (e.g., industrial or environmental engineering, environmental science, industrial hygiene, occupational health nursing). Priority is given first to students at Southeastern Oklahoma State University in Durant, Oklahoma and second to students from the ASSE Southwest Chapter area attending a school within ASSE Region III (Arkansas, Oklahoma, and Texas). Applicants must be full-time students who have completed at least 60 semester hours with a GPA of 3.0 or higher. Along with their application, they must submit 2 essays of 300 words or less: 1) why they are seeking a degree in occupational safety and health or a closely-related field, a brief description of their current activities, and how those relate to their career goals and objectives; and 2) why they should be awarded this scholarship (including career goals and financial need). U.S. citizenship is not required.

Financial Data The stipend is $1,000 per year.

Duration 1 year; recipients may reapply.

Additional data This program, established in 2006, is supported by the Southwest Chapter of ASSE.

Number awarded 1 each year.

Deadline November of each year.

[349]
ST. FRANCIS SCHOOL OF NURSING ALUMNI OF PITTSBURGH, PA SCHOLARSHIP FUND

Pittsburgh Foundation
Attn: Scholarship Coordinator
Five PPG Place, Suite 250
Pittsburgh, PA 15222-5414
(412) 394-2649   Fax: (412) 391-7259
E-mail: turnerd@pghfdn.org
Web: www.pittsburghfoundation.org

Summary To provide financial assistance to students working on an undergraduate or graduate degree in nursing.

Eligibility This program is open to 1) students working on their first academic degree or diploma that leads to professional licensure as a registered nurse, and 2) licensed registered nurses working on an advanced degree in nursing. Applicants must have a GPA of 3.0 or higher and be able to demonstrate financial need. Along with their application, they must submit brief essays on their prior work experience, prior education, financial obligations, extracurricular activities and volunteer work, past achievements related to nursing, and career goals. U.S. citizenship is required.

Financial Data A stipend is awarded (amount not specified).

Duration 1 year.

Additional data This scholarship was first awarded in 2007.

Number awarded 1 or more each year.

Deadline December of each year.

[350]
ST. VINCENT'S SCHOOL OF NURSING ALUMNI SCHOLARSHIP

St. Vincent's Health System
Attn: St. Vincent's Foundation
De Paul Building
2800 University Building, Suite 101
Birmingham, AL 35233
(205) 939-7296
Web: www.stvhs.com/foundations/bham/Scholarship.asp

Summary To provide scholarship/loans to nursing students interested in working at St. Vincent's Hospital in Birmingham, Alabama following certification as an R.N.

Eligibility This program is open to students working full time on an associate (A.D.N.) or bachelor's (B.S.N.) degree in nursing. Applicants must commit to working at St. Vincent's Hospital in Birmingham, Alabama following completion of their degree and certification as an R.N. Along with their application, they must submit a statement of their personal philosophy and how it relates to the mission of the Daughters of Charity and St. Vincent's Hospital. Selection is based on that statement, grades, references, school recommendation, and financial need.

Financial Data The stipend is $2,500 per year. This is a scholarship/loan program. Recipients are required to work full time at St. Vincent's for 2 years or repay all assistance received.

Duration 1 year; may be renewed 1 additional year.

Number awarded 1 each year.

Deadline April of each year.

[351]
STEPHANIE CARROLL SCHOLARSHIP

National Association Directors of Nursing Administration in
    Long Term Care
Attn: Education/Scholarship Committee
11353 Reed Hartman Highway, Suite 210
Cincinnati, OH 45241
(513) 791-3679   Toll Free: (800) 222-0539
Fax: (513) 791-3699   E-mail: info@nadona.org
Web: www.nadona.org/wysiwyg.php?wID=6

Summary To provide financial assistance to nursing undergraduate and graduate students who plan to practice in long-term care or geriatrics.

Eligibility This program is open to students entering or continuing in an accredited undergraduate or graduate nursing program. Applicants must indicate an intent to practice in long-term care or geriatrics for at least 2 years after graduation. Along with their application, they must submit an essay of at least 100 words on why they have chosen nursing as a career, why they are seeking this degree and how it will impact their nursing practice, and their commitment to the nursing profession, including their goals for their nursing career after graduation. Financial need is considered in the selection process.

Financial Data The stipend is $5,000.

Duration 1 year.

Number awarded At least 1 each year.

Deadline June of each year.

[352]
STRAIGHTFORWARD MEDIA NURSING SCHOLARSHIPS

StraightForward Media
508 Seventh Street, Suite 202
Rapid City, SD 57701
(605) 348-3042   Fax: (605) 348-3043
E-mail: info@straightforwardmedia.com
Web: www.straightforwardmedia.com/nursing

Summary To provide financial assistance for college to students interested in preparing for a career in nursing.

Eligibility This program is open to all students who are attending or planning to attend a school of nursing. Applicants must submit online essays (no minimum or maximum word limit) on 1) why they want to be a nurse, and 2) how this scholarship will help them meet their educational and professional goals. Financial need is not considered in the selection process.

Financial Data The stipend is $500. Funds are paid directly to the student.

Duration 1 year.

Additional data This program was established in 2004.

Number awarded 4 each year: 1 for each award cycle.

Deadline January, April, July, or October of each year.

[353]
SUSAN STEIN SCHOLARSHIP

American College of Nurse-Midwives
Attn: ACNM Foundation, Inc.
8403 Colesville Road, Suite 1550
Silver Spring, MD 20910-6374
(240) 485-1850   Fax: (240) 485-1818
Web: www.midwife.org/foundation_award.cfm

Summary To provide financial assistance for midwifery education to student members of the American College of Nurse-Midwives (ACNM) who have had a personal experience with breast cancer.

Eligibility This program is open to ACNM members who are currently enrolled in an accredited basic midwife education program and have successfully completed 1 academic or clinical semester/quarter or clinical module. Applicants must have had or currently have a personal experience with breast cancer, either their own or a family member's. Along with their application, they must submit a 300-word essay on the effect of breast cancer on their identity as a midwife. Selection is based primarily on the quality of the application, although leadership potential, financial need, academic achievement, and personal goals may also be considered.

Financial Data The stipend is $3,000.

Duration 1 year.

Additional data This program was established in 2010.

Number awarded 1 each year.

Deadline May of each year.

[354]
SYLVIA C. EDGE ENDOWMENT SCHOLARSHIP

New Jersey State Nurses Association
Attn: Institute for Nursing
1479 Pennington Road
Trenton, NJ 08618-2661
(609) 883-5335   Toll Free: (888) UR-NJSNA
Fax: (609) 883-5343   E-mail: institute@njsna.org
Web: www.njsna.org/displaycommon.cfm?an=5

Summary To provide financial assistance to New Jersey residents of African descent who are preparing for a career as a nurse.

Eligibility Applicants must be New Jersey residents of African descent currently enrolled in a diploma, associate, baccalaureate nursing program located in the state. Selection is based on financial need, GPA, and leadership potential.

Financial Data The stipend is $1,000.

Duration 1 year.

Number awarded 1 each year.

Deadline January of each year.

[355]
TENNESSEE NURSES FOUNDATION MEMORIAL EDUCATIONAL SCHOLARSHIP PROGRAM

Tennessee Nurses Association
Attn: Tennessee Nurses Foundation
545 Mainstream Drive, Suite 405
Nashville, TN 37228-1296
(615) 254-0350   Toll Free: (800) 467-1350
Fax: (615) 254-0303   E-mail: tnf@tnaonline.org
Web: www.tnaonline.org/tnf-initiatives.html

Summary To provide financial assistance to members of the Tennessee Nurses Association (TNA) who are working on a degree at a school in any state.

Eligibility This program is open to Tennessee residents who have been a continuous member of the TNA for at least 1 year. Applicants must be working on a baccalaureate, master's, or doctoral degree at an accredited institution of higher education in any state. Selection is based on available funds, financial need, leadership potential, and sustained association involvement.

Financial Data The stipend depends on the need of the recipient and the availability of funds.

Duration 1 year.

Additional data Recipients must maintain membership in the Tennessee Nurses' Association throughout the educational period.

Number awarded Varies each year.

Deadline February or August of each year.

[356]
TENNESSEE RURAL HEALTH LOAN FORGIVENESS PROGRAM

Tennessee Student Assistance Corporation
Parkway Towers
404 James Robertson Parkway, Suite 1510
Nashville, TN 37243-0820
(615) 741-1346   Toll Free: (800) 342-1663
Fax: (615) 741-6101   E-mail: TSAC.Aidinfo@tn.gov
Web: www.tn.gov/collegepays/mon_college/ruralhealth.html

Summary To provide forgivable loans to residents of Tennessee who are working on a degree at a school in the state to prepare for a career as a physician, dentist, physician assistant, or nurse practitioner and practice in an underserved area of the state.

Eligibility This program is open to students currently enrolled full time at a postsecondary educational institution in Tennessee that has a school of medicine that offers an M.D. degree, a school of osteopathic medicine that offers a D.O. degree, a school of dentistry that offers a D.D.S. or D.M.D. degree, a physician assistant program, or a master's or doctoral degree as a nurse practitioner. Applicants must have been residents of Tennessee for at least 1 year. They must agree to practice their profession in a health resource shortage area following completion of their program of study for 1 year per year of support received.

Financial Data The maximum loan is $12,000 per year or the cost of tuition, mandatory fees, books, and equipment, whichever is less. Funds are disbursed directly to the educational institution. If recipients fail to fulfill their service agreement, they must repay all funds received in cash with 9% interest.

Duration 1 year; may be renewed up to 4 additional years or until completion of the program.

Additional data This program was established in 2008.

Number awarded 50 each year.

Deadline August of each year.

[357]
TENNESSEE RURAL HEALTH NURSING SCHOLARSHIPS

Tennessee 4-H Club Foundation, Inc.
205 Morgan Hall
2621 Morgan Circle
Knoxville, TN 37996-4510
(865) 974-7436   Fax: (865) 974-1628
E-mail: mgateley@utk.edu
Web: www.utextension.utk.edu/4h/4hfoundation/index.htm

Summary To provide financial assistance to members of 4-H in Tennessee who plan to study nursing at a college in any state.

Eligibility This program is open to 4-H members in Tennessee who are graduating high school seniors or students currently enrolled in college. Applicants must be entering or attending a college, university, or technical school in any state to study nursing. Selection is based on academic record; a statement of career plans and how 4-H may have influenced their choice; school, church, and community activities; 4-H leadership roles and citizenship activities; participation in 4-H projects; and financial need.

Financial Data The stipend is $1,250.

Duration 1 year; may be renewed 1 additional year.

Additional data This program is sponsored by the Tennessee Rural Health Improvement Association.

Number awarded Up to 10 each year.

Deadline April of each year.

[358]
TEXAS 4-H TECHNICAL CERTIFICATION SCHOLARSHIP PROGRAM

Texas 4-H Youth Development Foundation
Attn: Executive Director
Texas A&M University
7606 Eastmark Drive, Suite 101
College Station, TX 77840-4027
(979) 845-1213   Fax: (979) 845-6495
E-mail: jereeves@ag.tamu.edu
Web: texas4-h.tamu.edu/youth/scholarship.html

Summary To provide financial assistance to 4-H members in Texas who plan to work on a technical certificate in selected science or social science fields at an institution in the state.

Eligibility This program is open to graduating seniors at high schools in Texas who have been actively participating in 4-H and plan to attend an institution in the state to work on a technical certificate in an approved major. Applicants must have passed all standardized tests necessary for graduation and admittance to the college or technical school of their choice. They may not have plans to continue formal education at a Texas college or university after completion of their technical program. Some scholarships require applicants to demonstrate financial need; selection for those awards is based on GPA (10%), 4-H experience (60%), financial need (20%), and a personal interview (10%). For other scholarships, selection is not based on financial need, but on GPA (10%), 4-H experience (80%), and a personal interview(10%). U.S. citizenship is required.

Financial Data Scholarships range from $1,500 to $16,000, depending on the contributions from various donors.

Duration 1 year.

Additional data The approved majors and courses of study include accounting associate, aircraft pilot training technology, applied graphic design technology, aquaculture technology, auctioneering services, automotive body/collision technology, automotive technology, aviation maintenance technology, aviation technology, biomedical equipment technology, biotechnology, business/office administration, caption reporting proficiency, carpentry, chemical laboratory technology, child development, commercial art and advertising, computer aided design and drafting, computer information systems, computer maintenance technology, computer network administration/technology, computer science technology, construction management and technology, court/realtime reporting, criminal justice, dental assistant, dental hygiene, diagnostic medical sonography, diesel and heavy equipment technology, dietary management, digital imaging technology, digital media design, drafting and design technology, echocardiology technology, e-commerce technology, educational assistant, electrical technology, electronics engineering technology, emergency medical services, environmental health and safety technology, farrier technology, fire science, food service/culinary arts, GIS/GPS technology, golf course and landscape management, HVAC technology, histology technology, horticulture technology, hotel and restaurant management, industrial maintenance and engineering technology, information management/technology, instrument and control technology, interpretation preparation program/deaf, invasive cardiovascular technology, logistics technology, machining technology, marketing, meat technology, mechanical engineering technology, media communications and information technology, medical assistant, medical data specialist, medical laboratory technology, mental health associate, mortuary science, music, nuclear medicine, nursing (associate degree and vocational), occupational therapy assistant, paralegal/legal assistant, pharmacy technology, phlebotomy, physical therapist assistant, plastics technology, process technology, radiation therapy, radiography, radio-television, ranch and feedlot operations, real estate, respiratory care, semiconductor manufacturing, surgical technology, telecommunications technology, travel/exposition/meeting management, veterinary technology, video technology, and welding technology. Students may not apply for both Texas FFA Association and Texas 4-H scholarships.

Number awarded The foundation awards approximately 225 scholarships for all of its programs each year.

Deadline Students submit their applications to their county extension office, which must forward them to the district extension office by February of each year.

[359]
TEXAS ASSOCIATION FOR ASSOCIATE DEGREE NURSING SCHOLARSHIPS

Texas Association for Associate Degree Nursing
Attn: Scholarship Committee
P.O. Box 18285
Austin, TX 78760
E-mail: contact@toadn.org
Web: www.toadn.org/scholarships.php

Summary To provide financial assistance to students working on an associate degree in nursing in Texas.

Eligibility This program is open to student who have completed at least 1 semester of nursing courses in an associate degree in nursing program in Texas. Applicants must describe their professional goals and their strengths that will contribute to their success in nursing. Selection is based on achievement as a nursing student; financial need is not considered.

Financial Data The stipend is $500.

Duration 1 year.

Number awarded 10 each year.

Deadline February of each year.

[360]
TEXAS CONFERENCE FOR WOMEN SCHOLARSHIPS

Texas Conference for Women
Attn: Scholarship Program
98 San Jacinto Boulevard, Suite 1200
Austin, TX 78701
Toll Free: (866) 375-1785   Fax: (866) 747-2857
E-mail: info@txconferenceforwomen.org
Web: www.txconferenceforwomen.org/scholarships.htm

Summary To provide financial assistance to women in Texas interested in studying nursing or other specified areas at a college in the state.

Eligibility This program is open to women who are residents of Texas and enrolled or accepted for enrollment at an institution of higher education in the state as a full- or part-time student. Applicants must be majoring or planning to major in the following 6 categories: the arts, business, education, nursing, mathematics and science, or public service. Along with their application, they must submit a 1,200-word autobiographical essay with information on their financial need, personal challenges they have experienced and how they have overcome or plan to overcome them, their plans for the future, and why they deserve this scholarship. Selection is based on that essay, academic record, volunteer community service, demonstrated leadership and participation in school and community activities, honors, work experience, and unusual personal or family circumstances and/or financial need. Top candidates may be asked to participate in a brief telephone interview.

Financial Data The stipend is $5,000.

Duration 1 year.

Additional data Recipients are expected to accept their awards at the annual Texas Conference for Women in November.

Number awarded 6 each year: 1 in each category.

Deadline June of each year.

[361]
TEXAS EXEMPTION PROGRAM FOR CLINICAL PRECEPTORS AND THEIR CHILDREN

Texas Higher Education Coordinating Board
Attn: Grants and Special Programs
1200 East Anderson Lane
P.O. Box 12788, Capitol Station
Austin, TX 78711-2788
(512) 427-6340   Toll Free: (800) 242-3062
Fax: (512) 427-6127   E-mail: grantinfo@thecb.state.tx.us
Web: www.collegeforalltexans.com

Summary To provide financial assistance for additional study at institutions in Texas 1) to residents of the state who are working as clinical preceptors in nursing programs in the state and 2) to their children.

Eligibility This program is open to residents of Texas who are either 1) registered nurses serving at least 1 day per week as a clinical preceptor for students enrolled in an undergraduate professional nursing program in the state; or 2) the children of such clinical preceptors. Applicants must be attending or planning to attend a Texas public college or university. Clinical preceptors must be taking classes related to their work. Their children may be majoring in any subject field.

Financial Data The stipend is $500 per semester or actual tuition, whichever is less.

Duration Clinical preceptors may take classes as long as they meet program requirements. Children of clinical preceptors may enroll for up to 10 semester or until they receive their bachelor's degree.

Additional data This program was established in 2005.

Number awarded Varies each year.

Deadline Deadline not specified.

[362]
TEXAS OUTSTANDING RURAL SCHOLAR RECOGNITION PROGRAM

Office of Rural Community Affairs
Attn: Rural Health Unit
1700 North Congress Street, Suite 220
P.O. Box 12877
Austin, TX 78711-2877
(512) 936-6701 Toll Free: (800) 544-2042
Fax: (512) 936-6776 E-mail: agrant@orca.state.tx.us
Web: www.orca.state.tx.us/index.php/Home/Grants

Summary To provide scholarship/loans to outstanding Texas students who are interested in preparing for a career in health care in rural areas.

Eligibility This program is open to Texas residents who are either high school seniors in the top quarter of their graduating class or college students who have earned a GPA of 3.0 or higher. Applicants must be enrolled or intend to enroll in an eligible academic institution in Texas to become a health care professional and arrange to be sponsored by an organization in 1 of the 177 rural counties in the state. Eligible health care professions include medicine (with a residency in family practice, emergency medicine, general internal medicine, general pediatrics, general surgery, or general obstetrics and gynecology), dentistry, optometry, nursing, pharmacy, chiropractic, behavioral health, and allied health (rehabilitative services, radiology technician, medical laboratory technician, health systems management, and dietary and nutritional services). Eligible sponsoring organizations include local hospitals, rural health clinics, and community organizations. Funds are awarded on a competitive basis. Selection is based on academic achievements, essay content, sponsor's financial commitment, community statement of need, and overall quality of the nominee.

Financial Data The amount of the forgivable loan award is based on the cost of attendance at the recipient's academic institution. Sponsoring communities pledge to cover half the student's educational expenses; the state covers the other half. Students must pledge to provide 1 year of work in the sponsoring community for each year of support they receive while in college.

Duration 1 year; may be renewed.

Number awarded Varies each year.

Deadline May of each year for fall semester; September of each year for spring semester; January of each year for summer semesters.

[363]
TEXAS PROFESSIONAL NURSING SCHOLARSHIPS

Texas Higher Education Coordinating Board
Attn: Grants and Special Programs
1200 East Anderson Lane
P.O. Box 12788, Capitol Station
Austin, TX 78711-2788
(512) 427-6340 Toll Free: (800) 242-3062
Fax: (512) 427-6127 E-mail: grantinfo@thecb.state.tx.us
Web: www.collegeforalltexans.com

Summary To provide financial assistance to Texas students who are interested in preparing for a career as a professional nurse.

Eligibility This program is open to undergraduate or graduate students who are residents of Texas and enrolled at least half time in a program leading to licensure as a professional nurse at a college or university in the state. Applicants must be able to demonstrate financial need.

Financial Data The stipend depends on the need of the recipient, to a maximum of $2,500.

Duration 1 academic year.

Additional data Some of these funds are targeted to students from rural communities and some to graduate students.

Number awarded Varies each year; recently, 944 of these scholarships were awarded.

Deadline Applicants should contact the financial aid director at the professional nursing school in which they plan to enroll for appropriate deadline dates.

[364]
TEXAS SAFETY FOUNDATION SCHOLARSHIP

American Society of Safety Engineers
Attn: ASSE Foundation
1800 East Oakton Street
Des Plaines, IL 60018
(847) 768-3435 Fax: (847) 768-3434
E-mail: agabanski@asse.org
Web: www.asse.org/foundation/scholarships/scholarships.php

Summary To provide financial assistance to upper-division and graduate student members of the American Society of Safety Engineers (ASSE), especially those from Texas.

Eligibility This program is open to ASSE student members who are working on an undergraduate or graduate degree in occupational safety, health, and environment or a closely-related field (e.g., industrial or environmental engineering, environmental science, industrial hygiene, occupational health nursing). Priority is given to residents of Texas or students attending a university in the state. Undergraduates must be full-time students who have completed at least 60 semester hours with a GPA of 3.0 or higher. Graduate students must also be enrolled full time, have completed at least 9 semester hours with a GPA of 3.5 or higher, and have earned a GPA of 3.0 or higher as an undergraduate. Along with their application, they must submit 2 essays of 300 words or less: 1) why they are seeking a degree in occupational safety and health or a closely-related field, a brief description of their current activities, and how those relate to their career goals and objectives; and 2) why they should be awarded this scholarship (including career goals and financial need). U.S. citizenship is not required.

Financial Data The stipend is $2,500 per year.

Duration 1 year; recipients may reapply.

Additional data This program, established in 2008, is supported by the Texas Safety Foundation.

Number awarded 1 each year.

Deadline November of each year.

[365]
TEXAS VOCATIONAL NURSING SCHOLARSHIPS

Texas Higher Education Coordinating Board
Attn: Grants and Special Programs
1200 East Anderson Lane
P.O. Box 12788, Capitol Station
Austin, TX 78711-2788
(512) 427-6340 Toll Free: (800) 242-3062, ext. 6340
Fax: (512) 427-6127 E-mail: grantinfo@thecb.state.tx.us
Web: www.collegeforalltexans.com

Summary To provide financial assistance to Texas students who are interested in preparing for a career as a vocational nurse.

Eligibility This program is open to undergraduate or graduate students who are residents of Texas and enrolled at least half time in a program leading to licensure as a vocational nurse at a college or university in the state. Applicants must be able to demonstrate financial need.

Financial Data The stipend depends on the need of the recipient, to a maximum of $1,500.

Duration 1 academic year.

Additional data Some of these funds are targeted to students from rural communities.

Number awarded Varies each year; recently, 99 of these scholarships were awarded.

Deadline Applicants should contact the financial aid director at the vocational nursing school in which they plan to enroll for appropriate deadline dates.

[366]
THE GREAT 100 SCHOLARSHIP PROGRAM

The Great 100, Inc.
P.O. Box 4875
Greensboro, NC 27404-4875
Toll Free: (800) 729-1975   E-mail: mperdue@hprhs.com
Web: www.great100.org/Scholarship/index.asp

Summary To provide financial assistance to undergraduate and graduate students in North Carolina who are interested in working on a degree in nursing.

Eligibility This program is open to students working on an associate degree in nursing, a diploma in nursing, a bachelor's degree in nursing, a master's degree in nursing, or a Ph.D. in a field related to nursing. Each year, the sponsor selects schools in North Carolina that offer nursing degrees and invites them to nominate students for these awards. The letters of nomination must indicate how the student promotes and advances the profession of nursing in a positive way in the practice setting and/or in the community, and actively seeks ways to support nurses and other health care providers; demonstrate integrity, honesty, and accountability, and functions within scope of practice; displays commitment to patients, families, and colleagues; demonstrates caring and assists others to grow and develop; and radiates energy and enthusiasm, and contributes/makes a difference to overall outcomes in the practice setting. Schools make the final selection of recipients.

Financial Data The stipend is $1,000.

Duration 1 year.

Additional data This program was established in 1989.

Number awarded Varies each year. Recently, 20 of these scholarships were awarded: 6 to A.D.N./Diploma students, 6 to B.S.N. students, 6 to M.S.N. students, and 2 to Ph.D. students.

Deadline March of each year.

[367]
THOMARA LATIMER CANCER FOUNDATION SCHOLARSHIPS

Thomara Latimer Cancer Foundation
Attn: Scholarship Committee
Franklin Plaza Center
29193 Northeastern Highway, Suite 528
Southfield, MI 48034-1006
(248) 557-2346   Fax: (248) 557-8063
E-mail: scholarships@thomlatimercares.org
Web: www.thomlatimercares.org

Summary To provide financial assistance to African American residents of Michigan, especially those who have had cancer, interested in studying a medically-related field at a college in any state.

Eligibility This program is open to African American residents of Michigan between 17 and 30 years of age. Applicants must be 1) a high school senior accepted at an accredited college or university in any state in a medically-related program (e.g., medical technician, physician assistant); 2) a student admitted to a medically-related professional program (e.g., nursing, medicine, physical or occupational therapy) at a college or university in any state. They must have a GPA of 3.0 or higher. Along with their application, they must submit a brief essay on why they should be awarded this scholarship. Financial need is not considered in the selection process. Special consideration is given to students who are cancer survivors.

Financial Data The stipend is $1,000.

Duration 1 year; may be renewed 1 additional year.

Number awarded 10 each year.

Deadline December of each year.

[368]
THOMAS M. HRICIK NURSING SCHOLARSHIPS

First Catholic Slovak Union of the United States and Canada Jednota Benevolent Foundation, Inc.
Attn: Scholarship Program
6611 Rockside Road, Suite 300
Independence, OH 44131
(216) 642-9406   Toll Free: (800) JEDNOTA
Fax: (216) 642-4310   E-mail: FCSU@aol.com
Web: www.fcsu.com

Summary To provide financial assistance to high school seniors who are interested in working on a nursing degree and are of Slovak descent and Catholic faith.

Eligibility This program is open to seniors graduating from high schools in the United States and Canada and planning to attend an approved 3- or 4-year hospital nursing program or an accredited college school of nursing. Applicants must be of Slovak descent and Catholic faith. Along with their application, they must submit 1) a transcript of grades that includes ACT or SAT scores; 2) a list of volunteer community activities in which they have participated; 3) a list of awards received for academic excellence and leadership ability; 4) a description of their career objectives; 5) an essay on why they think they should receive this scholarship; and 6) information on their financial need.

Financial Data The stipend is $500. Each winner also receives a $3,000 single premium life insurance policy upon proof of graduation from college.

Duration 1 year; nonrenewable.

Number awarded 3 each year.

Deadline September of each year.

[369]
TONY LEONE R.N. TO B.S.N. SCHOLARSHIP

American Nurses Association of California
Attn: Golden State Nursing Foundation
1121 L Street, Suite 409
Sacramento, CA 95814
(916) 447-0225   Fax: (916) 442-4394
E-mail: gsnf@goldenstatenursingfoundation.org
Web: www.goldenstatenursingfoundation.org/scholarships.html

Summary To provide financial assistance to registered nurses (R.N.s) in California who are interested in working on a bachelor's degree at a school in any state.

Eligibility This program is open to nurses registered in California who are employed in any practice field of nursing and any employment setting. Applicants must have been accepted into a baccalaureate level academic program in nursing in any state or be currently enrolled in such a program. Along with their application, they must submit a 1-page essay describing their commitment to succeed in the program and their personal vision of their nursing career following completion of the degree. Financial need is not considered in the selection process.

Financial Data The stipend is $1,000.

Duration 1 year; nonrenewable.

Number awarded Varies each year.

Deadline December of each year.

[370]
TRADITION OF CARING SCHOLARSHIPS

Newcomer Funeral Service Group
Attn: Scholarship Coordinator
520 S.W. 27th Street
Topeka, KS 66611-1228
(785) 233-6655
Web: www.newcomerfamily.com/scholarship

Summary To provide financial assistance to residents of communities served by Newcomer Funeral Homes and Crematories who are interested in attending college in any state to prepare for a career as a nurse.

Eligibility This program is open to graduating high school seniors and students already enrolled at a college or university in any state. Applicants must be permanent residents of a community served by Newcomer Funeral Homes. Along with their application, they must submit a 500-word essay on why they have chosen nursing as their field of study, why they feel nurses play an important role as care givers, and why they should be chosen to receive this scholarship. Financial need is not considered in the selection process.

Financial Data The stipend is $1,000.

Duration 1 year.

Additional data This program, established in 1999, is available from Newcomer Funeral Homes serving the following local areas: Akron, Ohio; Albany, New York; Casper, Wyoming; Columbus, Ohio; Dayton, Ohio; Denver, Colorado; Louisville, Kentucky; Orlando, Florida; Rochester, New York; Syracuse, New York; Titusville, Florida; and Toledo, Ohio. In several Kansas communities, the company does business as Penwell-Gabel Funeral Homes. To obtain contact information for each of those communities, check the company's website.

Number awarded Varies each year; recently, a total of 25 of these scholarships were awarded.

Deadline January of each year.

[371]
TYLENOL SCHOLARSHIPS

McNeil Consumer and Specialty Pharmaceuticals
c/o International Scholarship and Tuition Services, Inc.
200 Crutchfield Avenue
Nashville, TN 37210
(615) 320-3149   Toll Free: (866) 851-4275
Fax: (615) 320-3151   E-mail: contactus@applyists.com
Web: www.tylenol.com

Summary To provide financial assistance for college or graduate school to students intending to prepare for a career in nursing or another health-related field.

Eligibility This program is open to students who have completed at least 1 year of an undergraduate or graduate course of study at an accredited 2-year or 4-year college, university, or vocational/technical school. Applicants must be working on a degree in health education, medicine, nursing, pharmacy, or public health. Along with their application, they must submit 1) a 500-word essay on the experiences or persons that have contributed to their plans to prepare for a career in a health-related field, and 2) a 100-word summary of their professional plans. Selection is based on the essays, academic record, community involvement, and college GPA.

Financial Data Stipends are $10,000 or $5,000.

Duration 1 year.

Additional data This program is sponsored by McNeil Consumer and Specialty Pharmaceuticals, maker of Tylenol products, and administered by International Scholarship and Tuition Services (formerly Scholarship Program Administrators, Inc.).

Number awarded 40 each year: 10 at $10,000 and 30 at $5,000.

Deadline May of each year.

[372]
UNITED HEALTH FOUNDATION LATINO HEALTH SCHOLARS PROGRAM

Hispanic College Fund
Attn: Scholarship Processing
1301 K Street, N.W., Suite 450-A West
Washington, DC 20005
(202) 296-5400   Toll Free: (800) 644-4223
Fax: (202) 296-3774   E-mail: hcf-info@hispanicfund.org
Web: scholarships.hispanicfund.org/applications

Summary To provide financial assistance to Hispanic American undergraduate and graduate students who are interested in preparing for a career in the health field.

Eligibility This program is open to U.S. citizens and permanent residents of Hispanic background (at least 1 grandparent must be 100% Hispanic) who are high school seniors or graduates. Applicants must be enrolled or planning to enroll full time at an accredited 2- or 4-year college, university, or vocational/technical school to work on an undergraduate or graduate degree in a health-related field. They must have a GPA of 3.0 or higher, be able to demonstrate financial need, and be able to demonstrate a commitment to working in underserved communities, including community health centers. Relevant fields of study include medicine, nursing, mental health, pharmacy, public health, allied health, and health sciences.

Financial Data Stipends range from $2,500 to $5,000 per year, depending on the need of the recipient. Funds are paid directly to the student's college or university to help cover tuition and fees.

Duration 1 year; recipients may reapply.

Additional data This program is sponsored by MasterCard. All applications must be submitted online; no paper applications are available.

Number awarded Varies each year; recently, a total of $42,500 was available for this program.

Deadline March of each year.

[373]
UNITED HOSPICE FOUNDATION SCHOLARSHIP PROGRAM

United Hospice Foundation
Attn: Executive Director
1626 Jeurgens Court
Norcross, GA 30093
(678) 533-6462   Toll Free: (800) 956-5354
Fax: (678) 533-6463
E-mail: fpoole@unitedhospicefoundation.org
Web: www.unitedhospicefoundation.org/scholarships.html

Summary To provide financial assistance to residents of designated southeastern states who are working on a degree in nursing, pharmacy, or therapy to prepare for a career working in hospice or long-term care.

Eligibility This program is open to residents of Florida, Georgia, North Carolina, or South Carolina who are enrolled at an educational institution in any state. Applicants must be accepted or enrolled in 1) a nursing program and working on a diploma, associate, bachelor's, or master's degree as a registered nurse (R.N.) or licensed practical nurse (L.P.N.); 2) a school of pharmacy and working on a Pharm.D. degree; or 3) a school of rehabilitation working on a degree in physical therapy, occupational therapy, or speech therapy. They must be able to demonstrate financial need and a strong commitment to hospice nursing, long-term care, and/or pain management.

Financial Data The stipend is $1,000 per year.

Duration 1 year; recipients may reapply, provided they maintain a "B" average.

Additional data This program includes the following named awards: the Neil L. Pruitt, Sr. Scholarship, the Dorothy Shell

Scholarship, the Coy Williamson Scholarship, and the Robin W. Bryson Scholarship.

Number awarded 1 or more each year.

Deadline June of each year.

[374]
UPS FOUNDATION ACADEMIC SCHOLARSHIPS

American Association of Occupational Health Nurses, Inc.
Attn: AAOHN Foundation
7794 Grow Drive
Pensacola, FL 32514
(850) 474-6963   Toll Free: (800) 241-8014
Fax: (850) 484-8762   E-mail: aaohn@aaohn.org
Web: www.aaohn.org/scholarships/academic-study.html

Summary To provide financial assistance to registered nurses who are working on a bachelor's or graduate degree to prepare for a career in occupational and environmental health.

Eligibility This program is open to registered nurses who are enrolled in a baccalaureate or graduate degree program. Applicants must demonstrate an interest in, and commitment to, occupational and environmental health. Along with their application, they must submit a 500-word narrative on their professional goals as they relate to the academic activity and the field of occupational and environmental health. Selection is based on that essay (50%), impact of education on applicant's career (20%), and 2 letters of recommendation (30%).

Financial Data The stipend is $2,500.

Duration 1 year; may be renewed up to 2 additional years.

Additional data Funding for this program is provided by the UPS Foundation.

Number awarded 2 each year.

Deadline January of each year.

[375]
UTAH NURSES FOUNDATION GRANT-IN-AID SCHOLARSHIPS

Utah Nurses Association
Attn: Utah Nurses Foundation
4505 South Wasatch Boulevard, Suite 135
Salt Lake City, UT 84124
(801) 272-4510   Fax: (801) 272-4322
E-mail: una@xmission.com
Web: www.utahnursesassociation.com

Summary To provide scholarship/loans to Utah residents who are interested in working on a nursing degree at a school in the state.

Eligibility This program is open to Utah residents who have completed at least 1 semester of core nursing courses in an accredited registered nursing program (undergraduate or graduate) in the state. Undergraduate students must be involved in their school's chapter of the National Student Nurse Association. Registered nurses completing a baccalaureate or advanced nursing degree must be members of the Utah Nurses Association. Applicants must have a GPA of 3.0 or higher and be able to demonstration financial need. Along with their application, they must submit a narrative statement describing their anticipated role in nursing in Utah upon completion of the nursing program. Preference is given to applicants engaged in full-time study. Selection is based on the following priorities: 1) R.N.s working on a B.S.N.; 2) graduate and postgraduate nursing students; 3) students in formal nursing programs (advanced practice nurses); and 4) undergraduate nursing students. U.S. citizenship is required.

Financial Data A stipend is awarded (amount not specified). Funds may be used only for tuition and books. Recipients must agree to work for a Utah health care facility or Utah educational institution as a full-time employee for at least 1 year (2 years if part time). If they fail to complete their educational program or work requirement, they must repay all funds received.

Duration 1 year; may be renewed 1 additional year.

Additional data Recipients must agree to join the Utah Nurses Association within 6 months of graduation.

Deadline May or September of each year.

[376]
VIRGINIA "BEA" ROOT NURSING SCHOLARSHIP

Wisconsin Paralyzed Veterans of America
Attn: Scholarship Committee
2311 South 108th Street
West Allis, WI 53227-1901
(414) 328-8910   Toll Free: (800) 875-WPVA
Fax: (414) 328-8948   E-mail: info@wisconsinpva.org
Web: www.wisconsinpva.org/scholarships.html

Summary To provide financial assistance to seniors in nursing programs in Wisconsin who are interested in working in a spinal cord injury unit or rehabilitation facility after graduation.

Eligibility This program is open to students enrolled in the final year of an NLN-accredited nursing program in Wisconsin. Applicants must be willing to seek employment in a spinal cord injury unit or rehabilitation facility after graduation. They must be able to demonstrate financial need.

Financial Data The stipend is $1,000 or $500.

Duration 1 year.

Additional data Recipients are requested to seek employment in a spinal cord injury unit or rehabilitation facility for 1 year, to be completed within 3 years after graduation.

Number awarded 2 each year: 1 at $1,000 and 1 at $500.

Deadline March of each year.

[377]
VIRGINIA C. PHILLIPS UNDERGRADUATE SCHOLARSHIP AWARD

South Carolina Nurses Foundation, Inc.
Attn: Virginia C. Phillips Scholarship Fund
1821 Gadsden Street
Columbia, SC 29201
(803) 252-4781   Fax: (803) 779-3870
E-mail: brownk1@aol.com
Web: www.scnursesfoundation.org

Summary To provide financial assistance to nurses in South Carolina who are enrolled in a bachelor's degree program in public health nursing.

Eligibility This program is open to nurses who are currently employed with at least 2 years' experience in public health nursing in South Carolina. Applicants must be enrolled in a bachelor's of science in nursing program and have successfully completed 10 hours of course work. Along with their application, they must submit a 1-page narrative that describes their contributions to public/community health nursing and future career goals in public health nursing. Financial need is not considered in the selection process.

Financial Data The stipend is $1,500.

Duration 1 year.

Additional data This program, which began in 1980, is operated in partnership with the South Carolina Department of Health and Environmental Control (SCDHEC).

Number awarded 1 each year.

Deadline July of each year.

[378]
VIRGINIA ELIZABETH AND ALMA VANE TAYLOR NURSING SCHOLARSHIP

Winston-Salem Foundation
Attn: Student Aid Department
860 West Fifth Street
Winston-Salem, NC 27101-2506
(336) 725-2382   Toll Free: (866) 227-1209
Fax: (336) 727-0581   E-mail: info@wsfoundation.org
Web: www.wsfoundation.org/students

Summary   To provide financial assistance to residents of North Carolina interested in studying nursing at a school in the state.

Eligibility   This program is open to traditional and nontraditional students in North Carolina who are interested in working on an associate or baccalaureate degree in nursing at a school in the state. Applicants must have a high school or college cumulative GPA of 2.5 or higher and be able to demonstrate financial need. Preference is given to residents of Davidson, Davie, Forsyth, Stokes, Surry, and Yadkin counties. Some of the scholarships are set aside for eligible non-citizens.

Financial Data   The stipend is $1,200 per year.

Duration   1 year; may be renewed.

Additional data   There is a $20 application fee (waived if the applicant is unable to pay).

Number awarded   1 or more each year, including 5 scholarships set aside for eligible non-citizens.

Deadline   August of each year.

[379]
VIRGINIA LEGION AUXILIARY PAST PRESIDENT'S PARLEY SCHOLARSHIP

American Legion Auxiliary
Department of Virginia
Attn: Education Chair
1708 Commonwealth Avenue
Richmond, VA 23230
(804) 355-6410   Fax: (804) 353-5246

Summary   To provide financial assistance to relatives of members of the American Legion or its Auxiliary in Virginia who plan to study nursing at a college in any state.

Eligibility   This program is open to seniors graduating from high schools in Virginia and planning to attend college in any state to study nursing. Applicants must be related to a member of the American Legion or the American Legion Auxiliary.

Financial Data   The stipend is $1,000.

Duration   1 year.

Number awarded   1 each year.

Deadline   March of each year.

[380]
VIRGINIA LEYDA ROBERTS NURSING SCHOLARSHIP

Daughters of the American Revolution-Colorado State
  Society
c/o Marcy Kimminau, State Scholarship Chair
17537 West 59th Place
Golden, CO 80403-2022
E-mail: marcyk12@aol.com
Web: www.coloradodar.org/scholarships.htm

Summary   To provide financial assistance to high school seniors in Colorado who are interested in studying nursing at a school in any state.

Eligibility   Eligible to apply are graduating high school seniors in Colorado who are 1) U.S. citizens, 2) in the top third of their graduating class, and 3) accepted at an accredited school of nursing in any state. Applications must include a statement of career interest and goals (up to 500 words), 2 character references, college transcripts, a letter of sponsorship from the Daughters of the American Revolution's Colorado chapter, and a list of scholastic achievements, extracurricular activities, honors, and other significant accomplishments. Selection is based on academic excellence, commitment to field of study, and financial need.

Financial Data   The stipend is $1,000. Funds are paid directly to the student's school.

Duration   1 year; nonrenewable.

Number awarded   1 each year.

Deadline   January of each year.

[381]
VIRGINIA NURSES FOUNDATION SCHOLARSHIP

Virginia Nurses Association
Attn: Virginia Nurses Foundation
7113 Three Chopt Road, Suite 204
Richmond, VA 23226
(804) 282-1808   Toll Free: (800) 868-6877
Fax: (804) 282-4916   E-mail: admin@virginianurses.com
Web: www.virginianurses.com/displaycommon.cfm?an=9

Summary   To provide financial assistance to registered nurses in Virginia working on a bachelor's degree at a school in any state.

Eligibility   This program is open to registered nurses who are residents of Virginia. Applicants must be enrolled in an R.N. to B.S.N. program at a school in any state and have a GPA of 3.0 or higher. They must intend to practice in Virginia. Selection is based on academic achievement, commitment to nursing, and clinical and leadership abilities.

Financial Data   The stipend is $2,000.

Duration   1 year.

Number awarded   1 each year.

Deadline   September of each year.

[382]
VIRGINIA PAULSON MEMORIAL SCHOLARSHIP

Colorado Nurses Foundation
7400 East Arapahoe Road, Suite 211
Centennial, CO 80112
(303) 694-4728   Fax: (303) 694-4869
E-mail: mail@cnfound.org
Web: www.cnfound.org/scholarships.html

Summary   To provide financial assistance to undergraduate and graduate nursing students in Colorado who are members of the Colorado Nurses Association (CNA) or Colorado Student Nurses Association (CSNA).

Eligibility   This program is open to Colorado residents who have been accepted as a student in an approved nursing program in the state. Applicants may be 1) second-year students in an associate degree program; 2) junior or senior level B.S.N. undergraduate students; 3) R.N.s enrolled in a baccalaureate or higher degree program in a school of nursing; 4) R.N.s with a master's degree in nursing, currently practicing in Colorado and enrolled in a doctoral program; or 5) students in the second or third year of a Doctorate Nursing Practice (D.N.P.) program. They must be current members of CNA or CSNA. Undergraduates must have a GPA of 3.25 or higher and graduate students must have a GPA of 3.5 or higher. Selection is based on professional philosophy and goals, dedication to the improvement of patient care in Colorado, demonstrated commitment to nursing, critical thinking skills, potential for leadership, involvement in community and professional organizations, recommendations, GPA, and financial need.

Financial Data   The stipend is $1,000.

Duration   1 year.

Number awarded   1 each year.

Deadline   October of each year.

[383]
VIRGINIA TWO-YEAR COLLEGE TRANSFER GRANT PROGRAM

State Council of Higher Education for Virginia
Attn: Financial Aid Office
James Monroe Building
101 North 14th Street, Ninth Floor
Richmond, VA 23219-3659
(804) 225-2600   Toll Free: (877) 515-0138
Fax: (804) 225-2604   TDD: (804) 371-8017
E-mail: fainfo@schev.edu
Web: www.schev.edu

Summary To provide financial assistance to residents of Virginia who complete an associate degree at a 2-year public institution in the state and plan to transfer to a 4-year school to major in nursing or other fields.

Eligibility This program is open to residents of Virginia who complete an associate degree at a 2-year public institution in the state with a GPA of 3.0 or higher. Applicants must be interested in transferring to a 4-year public or private college or university in the state and work on a degree in any field except religious training or theological education. They must be able to demonstrate financial need of a federally-calculated estimated family contribution of $8,000 or less. Additional funding is available to students planning to major in science, teaching, engineering, mathematics, or nursing.

Financial Data The maximum standard award is $1,000; the additional award for students majoring in designated fields is $1,000. Funds are disbursed directly to the recipient's 4-year institution.

Duration 1 year; may be renewed up to 2 additional years, provided the recipient maintains a GPA of 3.0 or higher, satisfactory academic progress, and continued financial need.

Additional data This funding was first available to students who entered a 2-year college in fall 2007 and transferred to a 4-year institution in fall 2009.

Number awarded Varies each year.
Deadline Deadline not specified.

[384]
WALTER C. AND MARIE C. SCHMIDT SCHOLARSHIP

Oregon Student Assistance Commission
Attn: Grants and Scholarships Division
1500 Valley River Drive, Suite 100
Eugene, OR 97401-2146
(541) 687-7395   Toll Free: (800) 452-8807, ext. 7395
Fax: (541) 687-7414   TDD: (800) 735-2900
E-mail: awardinfo@osac.state.or.us
Web: www.osac.state.or.us/osac_programs.html

Summary To provide financial assistance for the study of nursing to residents of Oregon who are attending school in any state to prepare for a career in geriatric health care.

Eligibility This program is open to residents of Oregon who are enrolled at least half time in a program at a school in any state to become a registered nurse. Applicants must submit an essay on their desire to prepare for a nursing career in geriatric health care. First preference is given to students at Lane Community College; second preference is given to students at other 2-year college nursing programs.

Financial Data The stipend amount varies; recently, it was close to $1,000.

Duration 1 year.

Number awarded Varies each year; recently, 33 of these scholarships were awarded.

Deadline February of each year.

[385]
WALTER REED SMITH SCHOLARSHIP PROGRAM

United Daughters of the Confederacy
Attn: Education Director
328 North Boulevard
Richmond, VA 23220-4057
(804) 355-1636   Fax: (804) 353-1396
E-mail: hqudc@rcn.com
Web: www.hqudc.org/scholarships/scholarships.html

Summary To provide financial assistance to mature women who are lineal descendants of Confederate veterans and plan to major in nursing or other selected fields in college.

Eligibility Eligible to apply for these scholarships are women over the age of 30 who are lineal descendants of worthy Confederates or collateral descendants and members of the Children of the Confederacy or the United Daughters of the Confederacy. Applicants must intend to study business administration, computer science, home economics, nutrition, or nursing. They must submit certified proof of the Confederate record of 1 ancestor, with the company and regiment in which he served, and must have had at least a 3.0 GPA in high school.

Financial Data The amount of this scholarship depends on the availability of funds.

Duration 1 year; may be renewed.

Additional data Members of the same family may not hold scholarships simultaneously, and only 1 application per family will be accepted within any 1 year. All requests for applications must be accompanied by a self-addressed stamped envelope.

Number awarded 1 each year.
Deadline April of each year.

[386]
WARREN K. BROWN SCHOLARSHIP

American Society of Safety Engineers
Attn: ASSE Foundation
1800 East Oakton Street
Des Plaines, IL 60018
(847) 768-3435   Fax: (847) 768-3434
E-mail: agabanski@asse.org
Web: www.asse.org/foundation/scholarships/scholarships.php

Summary To provide financial assistance to upper-division student members of the American Society of Safety Engineers (ASSE), particularly those at designated universities.

Eligibility This program is open to ASSE student members who are majoring in occupational safety, health, and environment or a closely-related field (e.g., industrial or environmental engineering, environmental science, industrial hygiene, occupational health nursing). Applicants must be full-time students who have completed at least 60 semester hours with a GPA of 3.0 or higher. Along with their application, they must submit 3 essays of 300 words or less: 1) why they are seeking a degree in occupational safety and health or a closely-related field, a brief description of their current activities, and how those relate to their career goals and objectives; 2) their goals in the area of construction safety; and 3) why they should be awarded this scholarship (including career goals and financial need). U.S. citizenship is not required. Priority is given to students at Murray State University (Murray, Kentucky) and Indiana State University (Terre Haute, Indiana).

Financial Data The stipend is $1,000 per year.
Duration 1 year; recipients may reapply.
Number awarded 1 each year.
Deadline November of each year.

[387]
WASHINGTON DIVISION OF URS SAFETY SCHOLARSHIP

American Society of Safety Engineers
Attn: ASSE Foundation
1800 East Oakton Street
Des Plaines, IL 60018
(847) 768-3435   Fax: (847) 768-3434
E-mail: agabanski@asse.org
Web: www.asse.org/foundation

Summary   To provide financial assistance to upper-division student members of the American Society of Safety Engineers (ASSE) enrolled in an ASAC/ABET accredited program.

Eligibility   This program is open to ASSE student members who are majoring in occupational safety, health, and environment or a closely-related field (e.g., industrial or environmental engineering, environmental science, industrial hygiene, occupational health nursing). Applicants must be enrolled in an ASAC/ABET-accredited program. They must be full-time students who have completed at least 60 semester hours with a GPA of 3.0 or higher. Along with their application, they must submit 2 essays of 300 words or less: 1) why they are seeking a degree in occupational safety and health or a closely-related field, a brief description of their current activities, and how those relate to their career goals and objectives; and 2) why they should be awarded this scholarship (including career goals and financial need). U.S. citizenship is not required.

Financial Data   The stipend is $5,000 per year.

Duration   1 year; recipients may reapply.

Number awarded   1 each year.

Deadline   November of each year.

[388]
WASHINGTON GET READY FOR MATH AND SCIENCE CONDITIONAL SCHOLARSHIP PROGRAM

Washington Higher Education Coordinating Board
917 Lakeridge Way
P.O. Box 43430
Olympia, WA 98504-3430
(360) 753-7845   Toll Free: (888) 535-0747
Fax: (360) 753-7808   TDD: (360) 753-7809
E-mail: futureteachers@hecb.wa.gov
Web: www.hecb.wa.gov

Summary   To provide scholarship/loans to high school students in Washington who are interested in attending college to prepare for a career in a mathematics or science program (including nursing).

Eligibility   This program is open to students at high schools in Washington who participate in the Get Ready program as early as their sophomore year. Applicants must have a family income at or below 125% of the state median (currently, $97,095 or less for a family of 4) at the time of application and for the 2 preceding years. They must also 1) achieve a level 4 on the mathematics or science portion of the tenth-grade WASL, or 2) score above the 95th percentile on the mathematics section of either the SAT or ACT. Within 1 year of high school graduation, they must enroll at a college or university in Washington and major in a qualified mathematics or science program. Following graduation from college, they must work full time in Washington in a qualified mathematics or science field, including computer sciences and mathematics, engineering, physical sciences (e.g., atmospheric and space science, chemistry, environmental science, materials science, physics), life sciences (e.g., agricultural and food science, biological technology), health professions (e.g., physician, physician assistant, nursing, veterinary science), or teaching, for at least 3 years.

Financial Data   The maximum stipend is equal to resident undergraduate tuition and required state fees at the University of Washington. Students who fail to fulfill the mathematics or science service requirement must repay all funds received.

Duration   1 year; may be renewed up to 4 additional years or until completion of 180 quarter credits (or semester equivalent), whichever comes first.

Additional data   This program was first offered to high school sophomores taking the tenth-grade WASL in the 2007-2008 school year. It is administered by the College Success Foundation.

Number awarded   Varies each year.

Deadline   January of each year.

[389]
WASHINGTON STATE HEALTH PROFESSIONAL SCHOLARSHIP PROGRAM

Washington Higher Education Coordinating Board
917 Lakeridge Way
P.O. Box 43430
Olympia, WA 98504-3430
(360) 596-4817   Toll Free: (888) 535-0747
Fax: (360) 664-9273   TDD: (360) 753-7809
E-mail: health@hecb.wa.gov
Web: www.hecb.wa.gov

Summary   To provide scholarship/loans for primary care health professional education to students who agree to work in designated areas of Washington after graduation.

Eligibility   Applicants must be enrolled or accepted for enrollment in an accredited program leading to eligibility for licensure in Washington State as a physician, osteopathic physician and surgeon, pharmacist, licensed midwife or certified nurse-midwife, physician assistant, nurse practitioner, nurse faculty, dentist, dental hygienist, registered nurse, or practical nurse. They must be U.S. citizens, but Washington residency is not required. Selection is based on prior experience in a rural or shortage area, academic and humanitarian achievements, letters of recommendation, academic standing, and commitment and experience in serving the medically underserved or shortage areas. Preference is given to applicants with community sponsorship and support. The community sponsor may be a rural hospital, a rural health care facility, a community clinic, or a local health care provider that can provide training or employment opportunities. Support should be a financial commitment that may include educational and living stipends, matching funds, or employment and training opportunities.

Financial Data   The stipend is intended to cover eligible expenses: tuition, books, equipment, fees, and room and board. This is a scholarship/loan program. Recipients who fail to complete the course of study are required to repay the amount received, plus a penalty and interest. Scholars who fail to serve in a designated rural, underserved urban, or other health professional shortage areas in Washington are required to repay the scholarship, with penalty plus interest.

Duration   Up to 5 years.

Additional data   This program is jointly administered with the Washington State Department of Health.

Number awarded   Varies each year.

Deadline   April of each year.

[390]
WASHINGTON STATE NURSES FOUNDATION SCHOLARSHIPS

Washington State Nurses Association
Attn: Washington State Nurses Foundation
575 Andover Park West, Suite 101
Seattle, WA 98188-9961
(206) 575-7979   Fax: (206) 575-1908
E-mail: wsnf@wsna.org
Web: www.wsna.org/WSNF/Scholarship

Summary To provide financial assistance to students in Washington preparing for a career as a registered nurse in the state.
Eligibility This program is open to nursing students who are residents of Washington or attending a college or university in the state. Applicants must have a GPA of 3.0 or higher in a program leading to an associate, baccalaureate, or graduate degree. They must submit essays on the following topics: 1) their participation in school and volunteer activities, including offices and positions of leadership; 2) honors and awards they have received and the relevance of those to nursing; 3) special or unusual life experiences or activities that have made an impact on their nursing career or that assisted them to decide on nursing as a profession; 4) their long- and short-term goals for their nursing career; 5) what they anticipate their role in the Washington State Nurses Association (WSNA) will be, why it is important to them, and (if they are already an R.N.) their involvement in the organization and reasons for participation; and 6) their past work experience (both paid and volunteer) and why this may or may not impact their career in nursing. Undergraduate students must have completed at least 12 nursing credits in the R.N. program. Applicants who are already R.N.s must be members of the WSNA. Financial need is not considered in the selection process.
Financial Data The stipend is $1,000.
Duration 1 year.
Number awarded Varies each year; recently, 5 of these scholarships were awarded.
Deadline February of each year.

[391]
WATSON MIDWIVES OF COLOR SCHOLARSHIP
American College of Nurse-Midwives
Attn: ACNM Foundation, Inc.
8403 Colesville Road, Suite 1550
Silver Spring, MD 20910-6374
(240) 485-1850   Fax: (240) 485-1818
Web: www.midwife.org/foundation_award.cfm
Summary To provide financial assistance for midwifery education to students of color who belong to the American College of Nurse-Midwives (ACNM).
Eligibility This program is open to ACNM members of color who are currently enrolled in an accredited basic midwife education program and have successfully completed 1 academic or clinical semester/quarter or clinical module. Applicants must submit a 150-word essay on their 5-year midwifery career plans and a 100-word essay on their intended future participation in the local, regional, and/or national activities of the ACNM. Selection is based on leadership potential, financial need, academic history, and potential for future professional contribution to the organization.
Financial Data The stipend is $3,000.
Duration 1 year.
Number awarded Varies each year; recently, 3 of these scholarships were awarded.
Deadline March of each year.

[392]
WATSON PHARMA CAREER MOBILITY SCHOLARSHIP
American Nephrology Nurses' Association
Attn: ANNA National Office
200 East Holly Avenue
P.O. Box 56
Pitman, NJ 08071-0056
(856) 256-2320   Toll Free: (888) 600-2662
Fax: (856) 589-7463   E-mail: annascholarships@ajj.com
Web: www.annanurse.org
Summary To provide financial assistance to members of the American Nephrology Nurses' Association (ANNA) who are interested in working on a baccalaureate or advanced degree in nursing.
Eligibility Applicants must be current association members, have been members for at least 2 years, be actively involved in nephrology nursing related health care services, and be accepted or enrolled in a baccalaureate or higher degree program in nursing. Along with their application, they must submit a 250-word essay on their career and educational goals that includes the expected time frame for completing their degree, the application of the award to meet expected expenses, and the impact of the completion of the degree program on their nephrology nursing practice.
Financial Data The stipend is $2,500.
Duration 1 year.
Additional data This scholarship, first awarded in 2003, is sponsored by Watson Pharma, Inc.
Number awarded 1 each year.
Deadline October of each year.

[393]
WILLIAM C. RAY, CIH, CSP ARIZONA SCHOLARSHIP
American Society of Safety Engineers
Attn: ASSE Foundation
1800 East Oakton Street
Des Plaines, IL 60018
(847) 768-3435   Fax: (847) 768-3434
E-mail: agabanski@asse.org
Web: www.asse.org/foundation/scholarships/scholarships.php
Summary To provide financial assistance to upper-division and graduate student members of the American Society of Safety Engineers (ASSE).
Eligibility This program is open to ASSE student members who are working on an undergraduate or graduate degree in occupational safety, health, and environment or a closely-related field (e.g., industrial or environmental engineering, environmental science, industrial hygiene, occupational health nursing). Undergraduates must be full-time students who have completed at least 60 semester hours with a GPA of 3.0 or higher. Graduate students must also be enrolled full time, have completed at least 9 semester hours with a GPA of 3.5 or higher, and have earned a GPA of 3.0 or higher as an undergraduate. Along with their application, they must submit 2 essays of 300 words or less: 1) why they are seeking a degree in occupational safety and health or a closely-related field, a brief description of their current activities, and how those relate to their career goals and objectives; and 2) why they should be awarded this scholarship (including career goals and financial need). U.S. citizenship is not required.
Financial Data The stipend is $2,000 per year.
Duration 1 year; recipients may reapply.
Number awarded 1 each year.
Deadline November of each year.

[394]
WILLIAM R. GOLDFARB MEMORIAL SCHOLARSHIP
American Radio Relay League
Attn: ARRL Foundation
225 Main Street
Newington, CT 06111
(860) 594-0397   Fax: (860) 594-0259
E-mail: foundation@arrl.org
Web: www.arrlf.org/programs/scholarships
Summary To provide financial assistance to high school seniors who are licensed radio amateurs and interested in working on an undergraduate degree in nursing and other selected fields.
Eligibility This program is open to licensed radio amateurs of any class who are graduating high school seniors planning to attend an accredited institution of higher education. Preference is

given to students planning to major in computers, medicine, nursing, engineering, science, or a business-related field. Applicants must submit an essay on the role amateur radio has played in their lives and provide documentation of financial need.

Financial Data The stipend is at least $10,000.

Duration 1 year.

Number awarded 1 each year.

Deadline January of each year.

[395]
WISCONSIN LEGION AUXILIARY PAST PRESIDENTS PARLEY REGISTERED NURSE SCHOLARSHIPS

American Legion Auxiliary
Department of Wisconsin
Attn: Education Chair
2930 American Legion Drive
P.O. Box 140
Portage, WI 53901-0140
(608) 745-0124   Toll Free: (866) 664-3863
Fax: (608) 745-1947   E-mail: alawi@amlegionauxwi.org
Web: www.amlegionauxwi.org/Scholarships.htm

Summary To provide financial assistance to the dependents and descendants of Wisconsin veterans who are interested in studying nursing at a school in any state.

Eligibility This program is open to the wives, widows, and children of Wisconsin veterans who are enrolled or have been accepted in an accredited school of nursing in any state to prepare for a career as a registered nurse. Grandchildren and great-grandchildren of veterans are also eligible if they are American Legion Auxiliary members. Applicants must be Wisconsin residents and have a GPA of 3.5 or higher. Along with their application, they must submit a 300-word essay on "The Need for Trained Nurses Today." Financial need is considered in the selection process.

Financial Data The stipend is $1,200.

Duration 1 year.

Number awarded 3 each year.

Deadline March of each year.

[396]
WISCONSIN NURSING STUDENT LOANS

Wisconsin Higher Educational Aids Board
131 West Wilson Street, Suite 902
P.O. Box 7885
Madison, WI 53707-7885
(608) 267-2209   Fax: (608) 267-2808
E-mail: Cindy.Lehrman@wisconsin.gov
Web: heab.state.wi.us/programs.html

Summary To provide partially-forgivable loans to nursing students in Wisconsin who are interested in working in the state following licensure.

Eligibility This program is open to Wisconsin residents who are enrolled at least half time at an eligible institution in the state that prepares them to be licensed as nurses, either R.N. or L.P.N. Applicants must agree to be employed as a licensed nurse in Wisconsin following completion of their program. Financial need is considered in the selection process.

Financial Data Loans are provided up to $3,000 per year. For each of the first 2 years the recipient works as a nurse and meets the eligibility criteria, 25% of the loan is forgiven. The balance remaining after forgiveness must be repaid at an interest rate up to 5%. If the student does not practice nursing and meet the eligibility criteria, the entire loan must be repaid at an interest rate up to 5%.

Duration 1 year; may be renewed up to 4 additional years.

Additional data Eligible students should apply through their school's financial aid office.

Number awarded Varies each year.

Deadline Deadline dates vary by institution; check with your school's financial aid office.

[397]
WISCONSIN ORGANIZATION OF NURSE EXECUTIVES BACHELOR'S DEGREE EDUCATIONAL STIPEND PROGRAM

Wisconsin Organization of Nurse Executives, Inc.
c/o Kathryn Olson, Professional Development Committee
Saint Joseph's Hospital, Patient Care Services
611 St. Joseph Avenue
Marshfield, WI 54449
(715) 387-7592   Fax: (715) 387-7616
E-mail: kathryn.olson@ministryhealth.org
Web: www.w-one.org

Summary To provide financial assistance to nurses in Wisconsin who are interested in working on a bachelor's degree in nursing at a school in any state.

Eligibility This program is open to Wisconsin nurses working on a bachelor's (B.S.N.) degree in nursing. Applicants must have a GPA of 3.0 or higher. Along with their application, they must submit a letter identifying their professional goals and how they plan to attain them, the way they plan to affect nursing and patient care in Wisconsin, areas of interest, memberships in professional and community organizations and any related activities, and how they perceive their role as a nursing leader in the future.

Financial Data The stipend is $1,000.

Duration 1 year; nonrenewable.

Number awarded 1 or more each year.

Deadline July of each year.

[398]
WOCN SOCIETY ACCREDITED NURSING EDUCATION SCHOLARSHIP PROGRAM

Wound, Ostomy and Continence Nurses Society
Attn: Scholarship Committee
15000 Commerce Parkway, Suite C
Mt. Laurel, NJ 08054
Toll Free: (888) 224-WOCN   E-mail: info@wocn.org
Web: www.wocn.org/Education/Scholarships

Summary To provide financial assistance to students interested in preparing for a career in wound, ostomy, and continence nursing care.

Eligibility This program is open to students seeking education in wound, ostomy, and continence nursing care. Applicants must provide evidence of 1 of the following: 1) acceptance in a wound, ostomy, and continence education program accredited by the Wound, Ostomy and Continence Nurses (WOCN) Society; 2) current enrollment in a WOCN-accredited wound, ostomy, and continence education program; or 3) certificate of completion from a WOCN-accredited wound, ostomy, and continence education program within 3 months of completion. Selection is based on motivation to be an ET nurse and financial need.

Financial Data Stipends range from $1,000 to $3,500 per year.

Duration 1 year.

Additional data This program includes the Lee Greer Scholarship Award (for an applicant from the Pacific Coast Region) and the Beverly Hampton Award (for an applicant from the South Central Region).

Number awarded Approximately 20 each year.

Deadline April or October of each year.

[399]
WOCN SOCIETY ADVANCED EDUCATION SCHOLARSHIP PROGRAM

Wound, Ostomy and Continence Nurses Society
Attn: Scholarship Committee
15000 Commerce Parkway, Suite C
Mt. Laurel, NJ 08054
Toll Free: (888) 224-WOCN   E-mail: info@wocn.org
Web: www.wocn.org/Education/Scholarships

Summary To provide financial assistance to members of the Would, Ostomy and Continence Nurses (WOCN) Society interested in working on an undergraduate or graduate degree.

Eligibility This program is open to active members of the society who have a current, unrestricted R.N. license and are working on a baccalaureate, master's, or doctoral degree or N.P. certificate. Applicants must provide evidence of current or previous employment as a wound, ostomy, and/or continence nurse during the last 3 years, proof of WOCNCB certification, and proof of current enrollment or acceptance into an accredited nursing program or other accredited college or university program for non-nursing degrees. Selection is based on merit, compliance with the eligibility requirements, and financial need.

Financial Data The stipend is $2,000.

Duration 1 year.

Number awarded Varies each year; recently, 3 of these scholarships were awarded.

Deadline April or October of each year.

[400]
WVSNA/BERNICE L. VANCE SCHOLARSHIP

West Virginia Nurses Association
Attn: Scholarship Board of Trustees
405 Capitol Street, Suite 600
P.O. Box 1946
Charleston, WV 25327
(304) 342-1169   Toll Free: (800) 400-1226
Fax: (304) 414-3369   E-mail: centraloffice@wvnurses.org
Web: www.wvnurses.org/scholarship.html

Summary To provide financial assistance to nurses in West Virginia who are enrolled in an accredited nursing program in any state and a member of the West Virginia Nurses Association (WVNA) or the West Virginia Student Nurses Association (WVSNA).

Eligibility This program is open to native West Virginians who have been employed as a nurse in the state for at least 1 year, are enrolled in an accredited nursing program in any state, and are a member of either the WVSNA or WVNA. Applicants must submit the names of at least 2 personal references, a copy of their transcript, documentation of financial need, a self-evaluation form, an evaluation from a faculty adviser, and an evaluation from a clinical adviser.

Financial Data A stipend is awarded (amount not specified).

Duration 1 year; recipients may reapply.

Number awarded Varies each year.

Deadline June of each year.

Graduate Students

Listed alphabetically by program title are 435 fellowships, grants, awards, and other funding opportunities that support graduate study, training, research, and creative activities in the nursing field in the United States. Check here if you are looking for funding for graduate students in any area of nursing, including general practice, administration, anesthesiology, critical care, emergency, holistic health, long-term care, lung and respiratory, midwifery, nephrology, neuroscience, occupational health, oncology, operating room, ophthalmic, orthopedic, otorhinolaryngology and head-neck, pediatric, psychiatric, radiological, rehabilitative, school health, etc. All of this is free money. Not one dollar will ever need to be repaid (provided all program requirements are met)!

[401]
100 GREAT IOWA NURSES SCHOLARSHIPS

Iowa Nurses Association
Attn: Iowa Nurses Foundation
1501 42nd Street, Suite 471
West Des Moines, IA 50266
(515) 225-0495 Fax: (515) 225-2201
E-mail: info@iowanurses.org
Web: www.iowanurses.org/Default.aspx?tabid=2049

Summary To provide financial assistance to students who are working on an undergraduate or graduate nursing degree at a school in Iowa.

Eligibility This program is open to pre-licensure nursing students working on an A.D.N., practicing R.N.s working on a bachelor's degree, and graduate students working on a master's degree in nursing or doctoral degree in nursing or a related field. Pre-licensure and R.N. to B.S.N. students must have completed at least 50% of the requirements for a degree; master's and doctoral students must have completed at least 12 semester hours of graduate work. Applicants must have a career plan to work in Iowa. Along with their application, they must submit brief essays on their career goals, the areas of nursing practice where they believe they have something special to offer, their interest in that area, how their interest and goals will enhance the delivery of quality health care in Iowa, and how this assistance would impact their ability to meet their educational goals. Financial need is not considered in the selection process.

Financial Data The stipend is $500 for undergraduates or $1,500 for graduate students.

Duration 1 year.

Number awarded 4 each year: 2 to students working on an A.D.N. or R.N. to B.S.N. degree and 2 to graduate students.

Deadline February of each year.

[402]
AACN CLINICAL INQUIRY GRANTS

American Association of Critical-Care Nurses
Attn: Research Department
101 Columbia
Aliso Viejo, CA 92656-4109
(949) 362-2000, ext. 551
Toll Free: (800) 809-CARE, ext. 551
Fax: (949) 362-2020 E-mail: research@aacn.org
Web: www.aacn.org

Summary To provide small grants to investigators, including students, who wish to conduct clinical research projects that directly benefit patients and/or families.

Eligibility This program is open to investigators who are employed in a clinical setting and directly involved in patient care. Applicants must propose to conduct clinical research projects that directly benefit patients and/or families. Interdisciplinary projects are especially invited. Funding may be sought for new projects, projects in progress, or projects required for an academic degree.

Financial Data The maximum grant is $500. Funds may be used to cover direct project expenses, such as printed materials, small equipment, and supplies (including computer software). They may not be used for salaries, institutional overhead, or augmentation of funding from formal grants.

Number awarded Up to 10 each year.

Deadline September of each year.

[403]
AACN CLINICAL PRACTICE GRANT

American Association of Critical-Care Nurses
Attn: Research Department
101 Columbia
Aliso Viejo, CA 92656-4109
(949) 362-2000, ext. 551
Toll Free: (800) 809-CARE, ext. 551
Fax: (949) 362-2020 E-mail: research@aacn.org
Web: www.aacn.org

Summary To provide funding to members of the American Association of Critical-Care Nurses (AACN) who wish to conduct research directly related to the association's clinical practice research priorities.

Eligibility Registered nurses who are current members of the association may apply for these grants. They must propose to conduct research on a topic that the association has identified as a priority for critical care nursing: effective and appropriate use of technology to achieve optimal patient assessment, management, and/or outcomes; creating a healing, humane environment; processes and systems that foster the optimal contribution of critical care nurses; effective approaches to symptom management; and prevention and management of complications. Funds may be sought for research required for an academic degree.

Financial Data The grant is $6,000. Funds may be used to support direct project expenses, such as research assistants, secretarial support, equipment, supplies, and consultative assistance. They may not be used for salaries of the principle or co-investigators, travel to presentations, preparation of slides, presentation or publication of findings, or such educational expenses as tuition or books. Indirect costs are limited to 10% of direct costs.

Number awarded 1 each year.

Deadline September of each year.

[404]
AACN EVIDENCE-BASED CLINICAL PRACTICE GRANTS

American Association of Critical-Care Nurses
Attn: Research Department
101 Columbia
Aliso Viejo, CA 92656-4109
(949) 362-2000, ext. 551
Toll Free: (800) 809-CARE, ext. 551
Fax: (949) 362-2020 E-mail: research@aacn.org
Web: www.aacn.org

Summary To provide funding to investigators, including students, who wish to conduct evidence-based nursing research.

Eligibility This program is open to investigators interested in conducting research that stimulates the use of patient-focused data and/or previously generated research findings to develop, implement, and evaluate changes related to critical and acute care nursing practice. Funds may be sought for new projects, projects in progress, or projects required for an academic degree. Eligible projects may include research utilization studies, CQI projects, or outcomes evaluation projects. Interdisciplinary and collaborative projects are encouraged and may involve interdisciplinary teams, multiple nursing units, home health, subacute and transitional care, or other institutions or community agencies.

Financial Data The maximum grant is $1,000. Funds may be used to cover direct project expenses, such as printed materials, small equipment, and supplies (including computer software). They may not be used for salaries or institutional overhead.

Number awarded Up to 6 each year.

Deadline September of each year.

[405]
AACN MENTORSHIP GRANT

American Association of Critical-Care Nurses
Attn: Research Department
101 Columbia
Aliso Viejo, CA 92656-4109
(949) 362-2000, ext. 551
Toll Free: (800) 809-CARE, ext. 551
Fax: (949) 362-2020   E-mail: research@aacn.org
Web: www.aacn.org

Summary To provide funding to members of the American Association of Critical-Care Nurses (AACN) who are interested in conducting research under the direction of a mentor.

Eligibility Registered nurses who are current members of the association and have limited or no research experience may apply for these grants. They must propose to conduct research under the direction of a mentor with expertise in the area of proposed investigation. The role of the mentor must be clearly defined. The recipient may use the proposed research to meet the requirements for an academic degree, but the mentor may not. The mentor may not be a mentor on another AACN Mentorship Grant in 2 consecutive years.

Financial Data The grant is $10,000. Funds may be used to support direct project expenses, such as research assistants, secretarial support, equipment, supplies, and consultative assistance. They may not be used for salaries of the principle or co-investigators, travel to presentations, preparation of slides, presentation or publication of findings, or such educational expenses as tuition or books. Indirect costs are limited to 10% of direct costs.

Number awarded 1 each year.

Deadline September of each year.

[406]
AACN–SIGMA THETA TAU CRITICAL CARE GRANT

American Association of Critical-Care Nurses
Attn: Research Department
101 Columbia
Aliso Viejo, CA 92656-4109
(949) 362-2000, ext. 551
Toll Free: (800) 809-CARE, ext. 551
Fax: (949) 362-2020   E-mail: research@aacn.org
Web: www.aacn.org

Summary To provide funding to registered nurses who wish to conduct research directly related to the priorities of the American Association of Critical-Care Nurses (AACN).

Eligibility This program is open to registered nurses who propose to conduct research on a topic that the association has identified as a priority for critical care nursing: effective and appropriate use of technology to achieve optimal patient assessment, management, and/or outcomes; creating a healing, humane environment; processes and systems that foster the optimal contribution of critical care nurses; effective approaches to symptom management; and prevention and management of complications. The proposed research may be used to meet the requirements for an academic degree. Applicants must be a member of AACN and/or Sigma Theta Tau.

Financial Data The grant is $10,000. Funds may be used to support direct project expenses, such as research assistants, secretarial support, equipment, supplies, and consultative assistance. They may not be used for salaries of the principle or co-investigators, travel to presentations, preparation of slides, presentation or publication of findings, or such educational expenses as tuition or books. Indirect costs are limited to 10% of direct costs.

Additional data This grant is co-sponsored by AACN and Sigma Theta Tau International.

Number awarded 1 each year.

Deadline September of each year.

[407]
AAHN PRE-DOCTORAL RESEARCH AWARD

American Association for the History of Nursing
10200 West 44th Avenue, Suite 304
Wheat Ridge, CO 80033
(303) 422-2685   Fax: (303) 422-8894
E-mail: aahn@aahn.org
Web: www.aahn.org/grants.html

Summary To provide funding for graduate student research to members of the American Association for the History of Nursing (AAHN).

Eligibility This program is open to members of the association enrolled in an accredited master's or doctoral program. Applicants must be interested in conducting thesis or dissertation research on a significant question in the history of nursing. Their research adviser must be a scholar who is actively involved in the field of nursing history and who has prior experience in guiding student research. Selection is based on the scholarly merit of the proposal, the student's preparation for the study, the adviser's qualifications for guiding the study, and the project's potential for contributing to scholarship in the field of nursing history.

Financial Data The grant is $2,000.

Duration 1 year.

Additional data This program was established in 2008 as a replacement for the former American Association for the History of Nursing Competitive Student Research Award.

Number awarded 1 each year.

Deadline March of each year.

[408]
AANA FOUNDATION DOCTORAL FELLOWSHIPS

American Association of Nurse Anesthetists
Attn: AANA Foundation
222 South Prospect Avenue
Park Ridge, IL 60068-4001
(847) 655-1170   Fax: (847) 692-6968
E-mail: foundation@aana.com
Web: www.aanafoundation.com

Summary To provide financial assistance to members of the American Association of Nurse Anesthetists (AANA) who are working on a doctoral degree.

Eligibility This program is open to members of the association who are certified or recertified CRNAs working on a clinical or research doctoral degree. Applicants must be able to demonstrate a strong commitment to nurse anesthesia as a leader and to the conduct of research. Along with their application, they must submit a curriculum vitae; an abstract of their proposed research; a 250-word essay on their current involvement in nurse anesthesia education, practice, and/or research and how this funding will support them as a leader in research; 2 letters of reference; transcripts; and a copy of their program of study. transcripts; and a copy of their program of study.

Financial Data Grants are $10,000 or $5,000 per year.

Duration 1 year; grants for clinical doctorates are nonrenewable, but grants for research doctorates may be renewed 1 additional year.

Additional data This program includes 2 fellowships established in 2009: the Hershel Bradshaw Doctoral Fellowship and the New York Life Doctoral Fellowship.

Number awarded Varies each year. Recently, 8 of these grants were awarded: 3 at $10,000 and 5 at $5,000.

Deadline April of each year.

[409]
AANA STAFF SCHOLARSHIPS

American Association of Nurse Anesthetists
Attn: AANA Foundation
222 South Prospect Avenue
Park Ridge, IL 60068-4001
(847) 655-1170   Fax: (847) 692-6968
E-mail: foundation@aana.com
Web: www.aanafoundation.com

Summary To provide financial assistance to members of the American Association of Nurse Anesthetists (AANA) who are interested in obtaining further education.

Eligibility This program is open to members of the association who are currently enrolled in an accredited nurse anesthesia education program. First-year students must have completed 6 months of nurse anesthesia classes; second-year students must have completed 12 months of nurse anesthesia classes. Along with their application, they must submit a 200-word essay describing why they have chosen nurse anesthesia as a profession and their professional goals for the future. Financial need is also considered in the selection process.

Financial Data The stipend is $1,000.

Duration 1 year.

Additional data This program is supported by the staff of the AANA. The application fee is $25.

Number awarded 2 each year.

Deadline March of each year.

[410]
AANP FOUNDATION DNP CAPSTONE PROJECT GRANT

American Academy of Nurse Practitioners
Attn: AANP Foundation
P.O. Box 12924
Austin, TX 78711-2924
(512) 276-5905   Fax: (512) 442-6469
E-mail: foundation@aanp.org
Web: aanp.org

Summary To provide funding to members of the American Academy of Nurse Practitioners (AANP) who are working on their capstone/final project required for completion of a Doctor of Nursing Practice (D.N.P.) degree.

Eligibility This program is open to members of the academy who are nurse practitioners (NPs) and taking courses in an accredited doctoral program. Applicants must be interested in conducting a capstone/final project required for completion of the D.N.P. degree that relates to health care provided by NPs within the United States. They must be U.S. citizens and have a GPA of 3.75 or higher. Ed.D., D.N.Sc., and Ph.D. students are not eligible.

Financial Data The grant is $2,000. Funds may be used only for expenses related to the D.N.P. project, not for tuition.

Duration 1 year.

Additional data There is a $10 application fee.

Number awarded 1 each year.

Deadline October of each year.

[411]
AAOHN FOUNDATION ACADEMIC SCHOLARSHIP

American Association of Occupational Health Nurses, Inc.
Attn: AAOHN Foundation
7794 Grow Drive
Pensacola, FL 32514
(850) 474-6963   Toll Free: (800) 241-8014
Fax: (850) 484-8762   E-mail: aaohn@aaohn.org
Web: www.aaohn.org/scholarships/academic-study.html

Summary To provide financial assistance to registered nurses who are working on a bachelor's or graduate degree to prepare for a career in occupational and environmental health.

Eligibility This program is open to registered nurses who are enrolled in a baccalaureate or graduate degree program. Applicants must demonstrate an interest in, and commitment to, occupational and environmental health. Along with their application, they must submit a 500-word narrative on their professional goals as they relate to the academic activity and the field of occupational and environmental health. Selection is based on that essay (50%), impact of education on applicant's career (20%), and 2 letters of recommendation (30%).

Financial Data The stipend is $3,000.

Duration 1 year; may be renewed up to 2 additional years.

Number awarded 1 each year.

Deadline January of each year.

[412]
AFTERCOLLEGE/AACN NURSING SCHOLARSHIP FUND

American Association of Colleges of Nursing
One Dupont Circle, N.W., Suite 530
Washington, DC 20036
(202) 463-6930   Fax: (202) 785-8320
E-mail: scholarship@aacn.nche.edu
Web: www.aacn.nche.edu/Education/financialaid.htm

Summary To provide financial assistance to students at institutions that are members of the American Association of Colleges of Nursing (AACN).

Eligibility This program is open to students working on a baccalaureate, master's, or doctoral degree at an AACN member school. Special consideration is given to applicants who are 1) enrolled in a master's or doctoral program to prepare for a nursing faculty career; 2) completing an R.N. to baccalaureate (B.S.N.) or master's (M.S.N) program; or 3) enrolled in an accelerated baccalaureate or master's degree nursing program. Applicants must have a GPA of 3.25 or higher. Along with their application, they must submit an essay of 200 to 250 words on their goals and aspirations as related to their education, career, and future plans. They must also register and submit their resume to AfterCollege.com.

Financial Data The stipend is $2,500.

Duration 1 year.

Additional data This program, established in 2006, is sponsored by AfterCollege, an employment web site for nursing and allied health care students.

Number awarded 8 each year: 2 for each application deadline.

Deadline January, April, July, or October of each year.

[413]
AIR FORCE HEALTH PROFESSIONS SCHOLARSHIP PROGRAM

U.S. Air Force
Attn: Air Force Institute of Technology
2950 P Street, Building 642
Wright-Patterson AFB, OH 45433-7765
(937) 255-5824, ext. 3036   Toll Free: (800) 588-5260
Fax: (937) 656-7156   E-mail: afit.cimj3@afit.edu
Web: www.airforce.com/opportunities/healthcare/education

Summary To provide financial assistance for education in a medical or scientific field to future Air Force medical officers.

Eligibility This program is open to U.S. citizens who are accepted to or already enrolled in a health care professional program. They must be working on a degree that will prepare them for service in Air Force Biomedical Science Corps specialties (pharmacists, optometrists, clinical psychologists, or public health officers), Nurse Corps specialties, Medical Corps, or Dental Corps. Upon acceptance into the program, applicants are commissioned as officers in the U.S. Air Force; after completion of medical school, they must perform at least 3 years of active-duty service in the U.S. Air Force.

Financial Data This program pays full tuition at any school of medicine or osteopathy located in the United States or Puerto Rico, and it also covers the cost of fees, books, and other required equipment. In addition, recipients are awarded a stipend of $1,992 per month for 10 1/2 months of the year; for the other 1 1/2 months of each year, they perform active-duty service, usually at an Air Force medical facility, and receive the normal pay of a Second Lieutenant.

Duration 1 or 2 years for Biomedical Service Corps specialties, 2 or 3 years for Nurse Corps specialties, 3 or 4 years for Medical Corps or Dental Corps.

Additional data Following receipt of the degree, students serve an internship and residency either in an Air Force hospital (in which case they receive Air Force active-duty pay) or, if not selected for Air Force graduate medical education, in a civilian hospital (where they receive only the regular salary paid by the civilian institution). Only after completion of the residency, in either an Air Force or a civilian hospital, do the students begin the active-duty service obligation. That obligation is equal to the number of years of support received plus 1 year.

Number awarded Approximately 325 each year.

Deadline Deadline not specified.

[414]
ALABAMA NURSES FOUNDATION SCHOLARSHIPS

Alabama State Nurses Association
Attn: Alabama Nurses Foundation
360 North Hull Street
Montgomery, AL 36104-3658
(334) 262-8321   Fax: (334) 262-8578
E-mail: alabamasna@mindspring.com
Web: www.alabamanurses.org

Summary To provide financial assistance to residents of Alabama enrolled in an undergraduate or graduate program in nursing at a school in any state.

Eligibility This program is open to residents of Alabama who are enrolled in an accredited associate, baccalaureate (either initial or R.N. to B.S.N.), master's, or doctoral program in nursing. Applicants may be attending school in any state, but they should be planning to remain employed in Alabama for at least 2 years after graduation. Along with their application, they must submit a 100-word statement on their career goals. Financial need is not considered in the selection process. Priority is given to graduate students interested in teaching at a school of nursing.

Financial Data The stipend is $1,000 for undergraduates or $2,500 for graduate students.

Duration 1 year.

Number awarded 1 or more each year.

Deadline June of each year.

[415]
ALANA SCHOLARSHIP

American Association of Nurse Anesthetists
Attn: AANA Foundation
222 South Prospect Avenue
Park Ridge, IL 60068-4001
(847) 655-1170   Fax: (847) 692-6968
E-mail: foundation@aana.com
Web: www.aanafoundation.com

Summary To provide financial assistance to members of the American Association of Nurse Anesthetists (AANA) from Alabama who are interested in obtaining further education.

Eligibility This program is open to members of the association from Alabama who are currently enrolled in an accredited nurse anesthesia education program. Applicants must be second-year students who have completed 12 months of nurse anesthesia classes. They must have a GPA of 3.4 or higher. Preference is given to applicants who can demonstrate extracurricular or politi-

cal involvement. Along with their application, they must submit a 200-word essay describing why they have chosen nurse anesthesia as a profession and their professional career goals for the future. Financial need is also considered in the selection process.

Financial Data The stipend is $1,000.

Duration 1 year.

Additional data Funds for this scholarship, first awarded in 2002, are provided by the Alabama Association of Nurse Anesthetists (ALANA). The application fee is $25.

Number awarded 1 each year.

Deadline March of each year.

[416]
ALCAVIS INTERNATIONAL CAREER MOBILITY SCHOLARSHIP

American Nephrology Nurses' Association
Attn: ANNA National Office
200 East Holly Avenue
P.O. Box 56
Pitman, NJ 08071-0056
(856) 256-2320   Toll Free: (888) 600-2662
Fax: (856) 589-7463   E-mail: annascholarships@ajj.com
Web: www.annanurse.org

Summary To provide financial assistance to members of the American Nephrology Nurses' Association (ANNA) who are interested in working on a baccalaureate or advanced degree in nursing.

Eligibility Applicants must be current association members, have been members for at least 2 years, be actively involved in nephrology nursing-related health care services, and be accepted or enrolled in a baccalaureate or higher degree program in nursing. Along with their application, they must submit a 250-word essay on their career and educational goals that includes the expected time frame for completing their degree, the application of the award to meet expected expenses, and the impact of the completion of the degree program on their nephrology nursing practice.

Financial Data The stipend is $2,500.

Duration 1 year.

Additional data Funds for this scholarship, first awarded in 2006, are supplied by Alcavis International, Inc.

Number awarded 1 each year.

Deadline October of each year.

[417]
ALICE FISHER SOCIETY HISTORICAL SCHOLARSHIP

University of Pennsylvania
School of Nursing
Attn: Barbara Bates Center for the Study of the History of Nursing
307 Nursing Education Building
Philadelphia, PA 19104-6906
(215) 898-4502   Fax: (215) 573-2168
E-mail: dantonio@nursing.upenn.edu
Web: www.nursing.upenn.edu/history/research.htm

Summary To provide funding to graduate students interested in conducting research at the Barbara Bates Center for the Study of the History of Nursing in Philadelphia, Pennsylvania.

Eligibility This program is open to nurses working on a master's or doctoral degree on the history of nursing. Proposals should cover aims, background significance, previous work, methods, facilities needed, other research support needed, budget, and professional accomplishments. Selection is based on evidence of interest in and aptitude for historical research related to nursing.

Financial Data The grant is $2,500.

Duration 2 weeks.

Additional data Scholars must be in residence at the Barbara Bates Center for the Study of the History of Nursing for the duration of the program. They are expected to participate in Center activities and present their research at a Center seminar.
Number awarded 1 each year.
Deadline December of each year.

[418]
ALICE WISE MEMORIAL FUND SCHOLARSHIP

PeriAnesthesia Nurses Association of California
P.O. Box 10841
Westminster, CA 92685-0841
Toll Free: (866) 321-3582   E-mail: treasurer@panac.org
Web: www.panac.org/scholarships.html

Summary To provide financial assistance to members of the American Society of PeriAnesthesia Nurses (ASPAN) and the PeriAnesthesia Nurses Association of California (PANAC) who are interested in working on a nursing degree.
Eligibility This program is open to students working on a B.S.N. or M.S.N. degree who have been ASPAN/PANAC members for at least the past 2 consecutive years. Applicants must have compiled at least 10 points from the PANAC activity list (for the complete list of acceptable activities, contact PANAC). Selection is based on merit as indicated by involvement with PANAC on the district and state level.
Financial Data The stipend is $500.
Duration 1 year; members may not receive more than 1 scholarship or other grant in any 2-year period.
Number awarded 1 or more each year.
Deadline December of each year.

[419]
ALPHARMA PAIN MANAGEMENT AWARDS

Nurse Practitioner Healthcare Foundation
Attn: Scholarship Selection Committee
2647 134th Avenue N.E.
Bellevue, WA 98005-1813
(425) 861-0911   Fax: (425) 861-0907
Web: www.nphealthcarefoundation.org

Summary To provide funding to nurse practitioners and graduate nurse practitioner students interested in conducting a research or educational project related to pain management.
Eligibility This program is open to professional nurse practitioners and students currently enrolled in a nationally-accredited graduate nurse practitioner program. Applicants must be interested in conducting a research or educational project related to pain management. Priority is given to projects that target pain relief while avoiding misuse, abuse, or diversion. U.S. citizenship or permanent resident status is required.
Financial Data The initial grant is $3,500, paid at the time of the award. Upon completion of the project, an additional $1,500 is awarded to support project dissemination (e.g., travel expenses for presenting at a national meeting, editing a paper for publication, preparing a poster).
Duration The project must be completed within 2 years.
Additional data This program is sponsored by Alpharma Pharmaceuticals, LLC.
Number awarded 4 each year.
Deadline January of each year.

[420]
ALUMNI PRN GRANT

Alpha Tau Delta
Attn: Lynn Zeman, Scholarship Chair
1904 Poinsettia Avenue
Manhattan Beach, CA 90266
E-mail: bilynzeman@yahoo.com
Web: www.atdnursing.org/awards.htm

Summary To provide financial assistance for graduate education in nursing to members of Alpha Tau Delta (the national fraternity for professional nurses).
Eligibility This program is open to members in good standing who have been accepted into a graduate or doctoral program in a course of study to "enhance and further nursing service." Selection is based on involvement in the organization, community involvement, professional accomplishments, and financial need.
Financial Data Stipends range from $100 to $1,000.
Duration 1 year.
Number awarded 1 each year.
Deadline May of each year.

[421]
AMERICAN ACADEMY OF NURSE PRACTITIONERS FOUNDATION DOCTORAL STUDENT NP SCHOLARSHIPS

American Academy of Nurse Practitioners
Attn: AANP Foundation
P.O. Box 12924
Austin, TX 78711-2924
(512) 276-5905   Fax: (512) 442-6469
E-mail: foundation@aanp.org
Web: aanp.org

Summary To provide financial assistance to members of the American Academy of Nurse Practitioners (AANP) who are working on a doctoral degree.
Eligibility This program is open to members of the academy who are working on a doctoral degree (e.g., D.N.P., D.N.Sc., Ed.D., Ph.D.) and have a GPA of 3.75 or higher. Applicants must be currently licensed practicing nurse practitioners (NPs) in the United States. They must have completed at least 1 course for their doctoral program requirements but not be finishing their degree during the current year. U.S. citizenship is required.
Financial Data The stipend is $2,000. Funds may be used only for educational expenses (tuition, books, equipment, etc.), not for expenses related to dissertation and/or general research projects.
Duration 1 year.
Additional data This program includes the Julia Smith Memorial NP Doctoral Student Scholarship and the Reckitt Benckiser NP Doctoral Student Scholarships. There is a $10 application fee.
Number awarded Varies each year; recently, 11 of these scholarships were awarded.
Deadline October of each year.

[422]
AMERICAN ACADEMY OF NURSE PRACTITIONERS FOUNDATION MSN-NP STUDENT SCHOLARSHIPS

American Academy of Nurse Practitioners
Attn: AANP Foundation
P.O. Box 12924
Austin, TX 78711-2924
(512) 276-5905   Fax: (512) 442-6469
E-mail: foundation@aanp.org
Web: aanp.org

Summary To provide financial assistance to members of the American Academy of Nurse Practitioners (AANP) who are working on a master's degree.

Eligibility This program is open to members of the academy who are enrolled in an M.S.N. degree program with a nurse practitioner (NP) specialty. Applicants must have a GPA of 3.5 or higher. They must have completed at least 1 course for their master's program requirements but not be finishing their degree during the current year. U.S. citizenship is required.

Financial Data The stipend is $1,000. Funds may be used only for educational expenses (tuition, books, equipment, etc.), not for expenses related to master's thesis and/or general research projects.

Duration 1 year.

Additional data Recent corporate sponsors included Advanced Practice Education Associates (APEA), Endo Pharmaceuticals, Home Diagnostics, Inc., King Pharmaceuticals, the National Heartburn Alliance, Pfizer Inc., Pharmavite LLC, Redi-Clinic, Take Care Health Systems, UCB, Inc., and the United Soybean Board. There is a $10 application fee.

Number awarded Varies each year; recently, 13 of these scholarships were awarded.

Deadline October of each year.

[423]
AMERICAN ACADEMY OF NURSE PRACTITIONERS FOUNDATION POST-MS NP STUDENT SCHOLARSHIP

American Academy of Nurse Practitioners
Attn: AANP Foundation
P.O. Box 12924
Austin, TX 78711-2924
(512) 276-5905   Fax: (512) 442-6469
E-mail: foundation@aanp.org
Web: aanp.org

Summary To provide financial assistance to members of the American Academy of Nurse Practitioners (AANP) who are pursuing post-master's degree study.

Eligibility This program is open to members of the academy who have a master's degree in nursing and are pursuing nurse practitioner (NP) education in an accredited post-M.S. program. Applicants must have at least a 3.5 GPA in their post-master's program. They must have completed at least 1 course for their post-M.S. program requirements but not be finishing their degree during the current year. U.S. citizenship is required.

Financial Data The stipend is $1,500. Funds may be used only for educational expenses (tuition, books, equipment, etc.), not for expenses related to thesis and/or general research projects.

Duration 1 year.

Additional data There is a $10 application fee.

Number awarded 1 each year.

Deadline October of each year.

[424]
AMERICAN ASSEMBLY FOR MEN IN NURSING ESSAY CONTEST

American Assembly for Men in Nursing
Education Committee
6700 Oporto-Madrid Boulevard
P.O. Box 130220
Birmingham, AL 35213
(205) 956-0146   Fax: (205) 956-0149
E-mail: aamn@aamn.org
Web: www.aamn.org/awards.html

Summary To recognize and reward nursing students who prepare outstanding creative works dealing with men's health or men's place in the nursing profession.

Eligibility This program is open to undergraduate and graduate nursing students who submit creative work in fiction, fine arts, photography, essay, or research. Applicants may be either male or female, but the submission must relate to how nursing can

become more involved in men's health initiatives in order to improve the health and well-being of men and their families. They must be members of either the American Assembly for Men in Nursing or the National Student Nurses' Association.

Financial Data The award is $500. Funds may be spent at the student's discretion.

Duration The award is presented annually.

Number awarded 1 each year.

Deadline April of each year.

[425]
AMERICAN ASSOCIATION OF CRITICAL-CARE NURSES PROFESSIONAL ADVANCEMENT SCHOLARSHIPS

American Association of Critical-Care Nurses
Attn: Scholarships
101 Columbia
Aliso Viejo, CA 92656-4109
(949) 362-2000, ext. 507
Toll Free: (800) 809-CARE, ext. 507
Fax: (949) 362-2020   E-mail: scholarships@aacn.org
Web: www.aacn.org

Summary To provide financial assistance to members of the American Association of Critical-Care Nurses (AACN) who are interested in participating in professional development activities.

Eligibility This program is open to members of the association who are interested in participating in a career enrichment program. Applicants must show a direct link between the content of the learning activity they are proposing and what they need to learn in order to overcome the gaps in their knowledge and skills. Eligible programs demonstrate a relationship to nursing practice and include those that focus on communication, collaboration, mediation, leadership and governance, organizational effectiveness, informatics, political processes, safety, and quality. Students working on an academic degree may apply for funding of specific courses, but not an entire degree program over more than a year's time. They should focus on the content of a specific course and show how that content fills an individual learning gap. All applicants must submit 300-word essays that 1) describe the gaps in their knowledge and skills; 2) describe their learning plan, their goals for addressing the gaps in their knowledge and skills, and how the learning activity they are proposing will help them achieve their professional goals; and 3) list professional activities related to the proposed learning activity. Selection is based on the applicant's ability to 1) assess and articulate gaps in their own knowledge and skills; 2) set professional learning goals on the basis of identified gaps; and 3) identify and evaluate learning opportunities that will move them toward achieving their goals.

Financial Data A maximum of $3,000 per person per year is available.

Duration 1 year; recipients may reapply.

Number awarded Varies each year.

Deadline Applications may be submitted at any time, but they must be received at least 4 to 6 months prior to the beginning of the proposed activity.

[426]
AMERICAN COLLEGE OF NURSE PRACTITIONERS STUDENT SCHOLARSHIP AWARD

American College of Nurse Practitioners
Attn: Student Scholarship Committee
1501 Wilson Boulevard, Suite 509
Arlington, VA 22209
(703) 740-2529   Fax: (703) 740-2533
E-mail: acnp@acnpweb.org
Web: www.acnpweb.org/i4a/pages/index.cfm?pageid=3310

Summary To provide financial assistance to members of the American College of Nurse Practitioners (ACNP) who are working on an advanced degree.
Eligibility This program is open to student members of ACNP who have a current GPA of 3.4 or higher. Applicants must be enrolled in an accredited nurse practitioner program. Along with their application, they must submit a current curriculum vitae; 2 letters of recommendation from professional colleagues that indicate their leadership roles and involvement in public, student, or organizational policy development; and a 200-word statement on their personal goals as related to the ACNP mission statement.
Financial Data The stipend is $1,000. The award also includes 1-year's membership in ACNP, complimentary registration for the ACNP annual national clinical symposium where the award is presented, and up to $750 to pay travel and lodging expenses.
Duration 1 year.
Additional data Only the first 20 applications received are considered.
Number awarded 1 each year.
Deadline July of each year.

[427]
AMERICAN COLLEGE OF NURSE-MIDWIVES FOUNDATION FELLOWSHIP FOR GRADUATE EDUCATION

American College of Nurse-Midwives
Attn: ACNM Foundation, Inc.
8403 Colesville Road, Suite 1550
Silver Spring, MD 20910-6374
(240) 485-1850   Fax: (240) 485-1818
Web: www.midwife.org/foundation_award.cfm

Summary To provide financial assistance for midwifery education to graduate student members of the American College of Nurse-Midwives (ACNM).
Eligibility This program is open to ACNM members who are currently enrolled in a doctoral or postdoctoral midwife education program. Applicants must be a certified nurse midwife (CNM) or a certified midwife (CM). Along with their application, they must submit a curriculum vitae; a sample of up to 30 pages of scholarly work; and brief essays on their 5-year academic career plans, intended use of the fellowship money, and intended future participation in the local, regional, and/or national activities of ACNM or other activities that contribute to midwifery research, education, or practice.
Financial Data A stipend is awarded (amount not specified).
Duration 1 year.
Additional data This program was established in 1997.
Number awarded 1 each year.
Deadline March of each year.

[428]
AMERICAN NURSES ASSOCIATION PRESIDENTIAL SCHOLAR AWARD

American Nurses Foundation
Attn: Nursing Research Grants Program
8515 Georgia Avenue, Suite 400
Silver Spring, MD 20910-3492
(301) 628-5227   Fax: (301) 628-5354
E-mail: anf@ana.org
Web: www.anfonline.org

Summary To provide funding to nurses interested in conducting research.
Eligibility This program is open to registered nurses who have earned a baccalaureate or higher degree. Applicants must be beginning researchers who have had no more than 3 research-based publications in refereed journals and have received, as a principal investigator, no more than $15,000 in extramural funding in any 1 research area. The topic of the research changes peri-odically; recently, it was health disparities. Proposed research may be for a master's thesis or doctoral dissertation, if the project has been approved by the principal investigator's thesis or dissertation committee.
Financial Data The grant is $3,500. Funds may not be used as a salary for the principal investigator.
Duration 1 year.
Additional data This program was established in 1993. There is a $100 application fee.
Number awarded Up to 3 each year.
Deadline April of each year.

[429]
AMERICAN PSYCHIATRIC NURSES FOUNDATION RESEARCH GRANTS

American Psychiatric Nurses Association
Attn: APN Foundation
1555 Wilson Boulevard, Suite 530
Arlington, VA 22209
(703) 243-2443   Toll Free: (866) 243-2443
Fax: (703) 243-3390   E-mail: info@apna.org
Web: www.apna.org/i4a/pages/index.cfm?pageid=3741

Summary To provide funding for research to nurses who are members of the American Psychiatric Nurses Association (APNA).
Eligibility This program is open to licensed registered nurses in psychiatric mental health nursing who are APNA members. Applicants must be interested in conducting a research project; if it is for a master's thesis or doctoral dissertation, it must have the approval of their thesis or dissertation committee. Selection is based on the project's scientific merit, potential for knowledge development, and relevance to the advancement of knowledge and the practice of psychiatric and mental health nursing. Preference is given to investigators in the early stages of their research careers.
Financial Data The stipend is $5,000.
Duration 1 year; recipients may reapply after 2 years.
Number awarded 5 each year.
Deadline February of each year.

[430]
ANAC STUDENT DIVERSITY MENTORSHIP SCHOLARSHIP

Association of Nurses in AIDS Care
Attn: Awards Committee
3538 Ridgewood Road
Akron, OH 44333-3122
(330) 670-0101   Toll Free: (800) 260-6780
Fax: (330) 670-0109   E-mail: anac@anacnet.org
Web: www.anacnet.org/i4a/pages/index.cfm?pageid=3321

Summary To provide financial assistance to student nurses from minority groups who are interested in HIV/AIDS nursing and in attending the national conference of the Association of Nurses in AIDS Care (ANAC).
Eligibility This program is open to student nurses from a diverse racial or ethnic background, defined to include African Americans, Hispanics/Latinos, Asians/Pacific Islanders, and American Indians/Alaskan Natives. Candidates must have a genuine interest in HIV/AIDS nursing, be interested in attending the ANAC national conference, and desire to develop a mentorship relationship with a member of the ANAC Diversity Specialty Committee. They must be currently enrolled in an accredited nursing program at any level (e.g., L.P.N., A.D.N., diploma, B.S.N., or graduate nursing). Nominees may be recommended by themselves, nursing faculty members, or ANAC members, but their nomination must be supported by an ANAC member. Along with their nomination form, they must submit a 500-word personal

statement describing their interest or experience in HIV/AIDS care and why they want to attend the ANAC conference.

Financial Data Recipients are awarded a $1,000 scholarship (paid directly to the school), up to $599 in reimbursement of travel expenses to attend the ANAC annual conference, free conference registration, an award plaque, a free ticket to the awards ceremony at the conference, and a 1-year ANAC membership.

Duration 1 year.

Additional data The mentor will be assigned at the conference and will maintain contact during the period of study.

Number awarded 1 each year.

Deadline June of each year.

[431]
ANDREW CMELKO CRNA MEMORIAL SCHOLARSHIPS

American Association of Nurse Anesthetists
Attn: AANA Foundation
222 South Prospect Avenue
Park Ridge, IL 60068-4001
(847) 655-1170   Fax: (847) 692-6968
E-mail: foundation@aana.com
Web: www.aanafoundation.com

Summary To provide financial assistance to members of the American Association of Nurse Anesthetists (AANA), especially married males with children, who are interested in obtaining further education.

Eligibility This program is open to members of the association who are currently enrolled in an accredited nurse anesthesia education program. Preference is given to married male nurse anesthesia students who have children. First-year students must have completed 6 months of nurse anesthesia classes; second-year students must have completed 12 months of nurse anesthesia classes. Along with their application, they must submit a 200-word essay describing why they have chosen nurse anesthesia as a profession and their professional goals for the future. Financial need is also considered in the selection process.

Financial Data The stipend is $1,000.

Duration 1 year.

Additional data This scholarship was first awarded in 2006. The application processing fee is $25.

Number awarded 5 each year.

Deadline March of each year.

[432]
ANN OLSON MEMORIAL DOCTORAL SCHOLARSHIP

Oncology Nursing Society
Attn: ONS Foundation
125 Enterprise Drive
Pittsburgh, PA 15275-1214
(412) 859-6100   Toll Free: (866) 257-4ONS
Fax: (412) 859-6163   E-mail: foundation@ons.org
Web: www.ons.org/Awards/FoundationAwards/Doctoral

Summary To provide financial assistance to registered nurses interested in working on a doctoral degree in oncology nursing.

Eligibility This program is open to registered nurses who have an interest in and commitment to oncology nursing. Applicants must be enrolled in or applying to a doctoral nursing degree program or related program. If they do not have a master's degree, they must have completed the first 2 years of a doctoral program. Along with their application, they must submit brief essays on their role in caring for persons with cancer; their research area of interest and plans for a dissertation; their professional goals and how those goals relate to the advancement of oncology nursing; and how the doctoral program will assist them in achieving their goals.

Financial Data The stipend is $3,000.

Duration 1 year; nonrenewable.

Additional data This program, established in 1991, is currently sponsored by Pfizer Oncology. At the end of each year of scholarship participation, recipients must submit a summary of their educational activities. Applications must be accompanied by a $5 fee.

Number awarded 1 each year.

Deadline January of each year.

[433]
ANNA/ABBOTT-PAMELA BALZER CAREER MOBILITY SCHOLARSHIP

American Nephrology Nurses' Association
Attn: ANNA National Office
200 East Holly Avenue
P.O. Box 56
Pitman, NJ 08071-0056
(856) 256-2320   Toll Free: (888) 600-2662
Fax: (856) 589-7463   E-mail: annascholarships@ajj.com
Web: www.annanurse.org

Summary To provide financial assistance to members of the American Nephrology Nurses' Association (ANNA) who are interested in working on a baccalaureate or advanced degree in nursing.

Eligibility Applicants must be current association members, have been members for at least 2 years, be actively involved in nephrology nursing-related health care services, and be accepted or enrolled in a baccalaureate or higher degree program in nursing. Along with their application, they must submit a 250-word essay on their career and educational goals that includes the expected time frame for completing their degree, the application of the award to meet expected expenses, and the impact of the completion of the degree program on their nephrology nursing practice.

Financial Data The stipend is $2,500.

Duration 1 year.

Additional data Funds for this program, established in 2002, are supplied by Abbott Renal Care Group.

Number awarded 1 each year.

Deadline October of each year.

[434]
ANNA MAY ROLANDO SCHOLARSHIP AWARD

ExceptionalNurse.com
Attn: Scholarship Committee
13019 Coastal Circle
Palm Beach Gardens, FL 33410
(561) 627-9872   Fax: (561) 776-9254
TDD: (561) 776-9442   E-mail: ExceptionalNurse@aol.com
Web: www.ExceptionalNurse.com/scholarship.php

Summary To provide financial assistance to nursing students who have a disability.

Eligibility This program is open to students with a documented disability who have applied to, or have already been admitted to, a college or university nursing program on a full-time basis. Preference is given to graduate students who have demonstrated a commitment to working with people with disabilities. Applicants must submit an essay on how they plan to contribute to the nursing profession and how their disability will influence their practice as a nurse. Selection is based on the essay, transcripts of high school and/or college courses completed, activities and honors received, 3 letters of recommendation, and financial need.

Financial Data The stipend is $500.

Duration 1 year; nonrenewable.

Number awarded 1 each year.

Deadline May of each year.

[435]
ANNE ZIMMERMAN AMERICAN NURSES FOUNDATION SCHOLAR AWARD

American Nurses Foundation
Attn: Nursing Research Grants Program
8515 Georgia Avenue, Suite 400
Silver Spring, MD 20910-3492
(301) 628-5227   Fax: (301) 628-5354
E-mail: anf@ana.org
Web: www.anfonline.org

Summary To provide funding to nurses interested in conducting research related to nursing practice or social policy issues that will advance the profession.

Eligibility This program is open to registered nurses who have earned a baccalaureate or higher degree. Applicants may be either beginning or experienced researchers. They must be planning to conduct research that is intended to advance the profession of nursing by strengthening clinical nursing practice, supporting pertinent social policies, and underpinning the economic and general welfare of both nurses and nursing. Proposed research may be for a master's thesis or doctoral dissertation, if the project has been approved by the principal investigator's thesis or dissertation committee.

Financial Data The grant is $5,000. Funds may not be used as a salary for the principal investigator.

Duration 1 year.

Additional data This program was established in 1995. There is a $100 application fee. A publication, preferably a monograph, is expected at the conclusion of the award term.

Number awarded 1 each year.

Deadline April of each year.

[436]
AORN DEGREE COMPLETION RESEARCH GRANT PROGRAM

Association of periOperative Registered Nurses
Attn: Research and Nursing Resources Department
2170 South Parker Road, Suite 400
Denver, CO 80231-5711
(303) 755-6300, ext. 244 Toll Free: (800) 755-2676, ext. 244
Fax: (303) 750-2927   E-mail: rchard@aorn.org
Web: www.aorn.org

Summary To provide funding for research to student members of the Association of periOperative Registered Nurses (AORN).

Eligibility This program is open to student members of the association who are enrolled in an accredited baccalaureate, master's, or doctoral program. Applicants must be interested in conducting a research project that is related to perioperative nursing practice and consistent with AORN's research priorities, which emphasize patient outcomes and workforce issues. Except for generic baccalaureate nursing students, applicants must be a registered nurse with a current and valid license.

Financial Data The maximum grant is $15,000.

Duration These are 1-time grants.

Number awarded Varies each year.

Deadline March or October of each year.

[437]
AORN FOUNDATION DOCTORAL DEGREE SCHOLARSHIP

Association of periOperative Registered Nurses
Attn: AORN Foundation
2170 South Parker Road, Suite 400
Denver, CO 80231-5711
(303) 755-6300, ext. 230 Toll Free: (800) 755-2676, ext. 230
Fax: (303) 755-4219   E-mail: foundation@aorn.org
Web: www.aorn.org/AORNFoundation/Scholarships

Summary To provide financial assistance to students who wish to work on a doctoral degree in a field of interest to the Association of periOperative Registered Nurses (AORN).

Eligibility This program is open to registered nurses who are committed to perioperative nursing and are currently enrolled in a doctoral program at an accredited university. Along with their application, they must submit 4 essays: 1) their role as a perioperative nurse, their professional goals, and what AORN does to support their professional goals; 2) why they chose this doctoral program; 3) how this program will assist them in achieving their professional goals and advancing perioperative nursing; and 4) their research area of interest and their plan for a dissertation. Financial need is not considered in the selection process. Membership in AORN is not required, but applicants are encouraged to become members.

Financial Data A stipend is awarded (amount not specified); funds are intended to be used for payment of tuition, related fees, and books.

Duration 1 year.

Additional data This program was established in 1991.

Number awarded Varies each year; recently, 3 of these scholarships were awarded.

Deadline June each year.

[438]
AORN FOUNDATION MASTER'S DEGREE SCHOLARSHIP

Association of periOperative Registered Nurses
Attn: AORN Foundation
2170 South Parker Road, Suite 400
Denver, CO 80231-5711
(303) 755-6300, ext. 230 Toll Free: (800) 755-2676, ext. 230
Fax: (303) 755-4219   E-mail: foundation@aorn.org
Web: www.aorn.org/AORNFoundation/Scholarships

Summary To provide financial assistance to students who wish to work on a master's degree in a field of interest to the Association of periOperative Registered Nurses (AORN).

Eligibility This program is open to registered nurses who are committed to perioperative nursing and are currently enrolled in an accredited master's degree program. Along with their application, they must submit 4 essays: 1) their role as a perioperative nurse, their professional goals, and what AORN does to support their professional goals; 2) why they chose this master's program and how it will assist them in achieving their goals; 3) the perioperative nursing role this program prepares them for; and 4) the courses and clinical learning activities that are related to perioperative nursing. Financial need is not considered in the selection process. Membership in AORN is not required, but applicants are encouraged to become members.

Financial Data A stipend is awarded (amount not specified); funds are intended to be used for payment of tuition, related fees, and books.

Duration 1 year.

Additional data This program was established in 1991.

Number awarded Varies each year; recently, 24 of these scholarships were awarded.

Deadline June of each year.

[439]
AORN FOUNDATION NURSING STUDENT SCHOLARSHIPS

Association of periOperative Registered Nurses
Attn: AORN Foundation
2170 South Parker Road, Suite 400
Denver, CO 80231-5711
(303) 755-6300, ext. 230 Toll Free: (800) 755-2676, ext. 230
Fax: (303) 755-4219   E-mail: foundation@aorn.org
Web: www.aorn.org/AORNFoundation/Scholarships

Summary To provide financial assistance to students interested in preparing for a career in nursing, especially perioperative nursing.
Eligibility This program is open to students currently enrolled in an accredited nursing program leading to initial licensure as an R.N. The program may be for a diploma or an A.D.N., B.S.N., master's entry, or accelerated second B.S.N. degree. Applicants must submit 3 essays: 1) why they have chosen to prepare for a career in nursing and their career goals; 2) their academic and/or clinical experience or exposure to the operating room/surgical field; and 3) how they believe the Association of periOperative Registered Nurses (AORN) promotes the specialty of perioperative nursing. Financial need is not considered in the selection process. Membership in AORN is not required, but applicants are encouraged to become members.
Financial Data A stipend is awarded (amount not specified); funds are intended to be used for payment of tuition, related fees, and books.
Duration 1 year.
Additional data This program was established in 2001.
Number awarded Varies each year; recently, 12 of these scholarships were awarded.
Deadline June of each year.

[440]
ARIZONA ASSOCIATION OF NURSE ANESTHETISTS STUDENT SCHOLARSHIP

American Association of Nurse Anesthetists
Attn: AANA Foundation
222 South Prospect Avenue
Park Ridge, IL 60068-4001
(847) 655-1170　　　　　Fax: (847) 692-6968
E-mail: foundation@aana.com
Web: www.aanafoundation.com

Summary To provide financial assistance to members of the American Association of Nurse Anesthetists (AANA), especially residents of Arizona, who are interested in obtaining further education.
Eligibility This program is open to members of the association who are currently enrolled in an accredited nurse anesthesia education program. Preference is given to residents of Arizona. First-year students must have completed 6 months of nurse anesthesia classes; second-year students must have completed 12 months of nurse anesthesia classes. Along with their application, they must submit a 200-word essay describing why they have chosen nurse anesthesia as a profession and their professional goals for the future. Financial need is also considered in the selection process.
Financial Data The stipend is $3,000.
Duration 1 year.
Additional data This scholarship, first awarded in 2009, is supported by the Arizona Association of Nurse Anesthetists. The application processing fee is $25.
Number awarded 1 each year.
Deadline March of each year.

[441]
ARIZONA NURSES FOUNDATION ACADEMIC SCHOLARSHIP PROGRAM

Arizona Nurses Association
Attn: Arizona Nurses Foundation
1850 East Southern Avenue, Suite 1
Tempe, AZ 85282-5832
(480) 831-0404　　　　　Fax: (480) 839-4780
E-mail: info@aznurse.org
Web: www.aznurse.org/foundation/index.html

Summary To provide financial assistance to undergraduate and graduate students from any state enrolled in or accepted to nursing programs in Arizona.
Eligibility This program is open to undergraduate and graduate students from any state enrolled in, or accepted for enrollment in, an academic nursing education program in Arizona. Selection is based on potential for leadership in nursing, commitment to professional nursing in Arizona, and financial need. For graduate students, priority is given to applicants planning to teach nursing.
Financial Data Stipends are $500 per semester for associate degree students, $1,000 per semester for R.N. to B.S.N. students, $1,000 per semester for direct entry B.S.N. students, $1,000 per semester for master's degree students, and $2,500 per semester for doctoral students.
Duration 1 semester; recipients may reapply.
Number awarded 18 each semester: 4 for associate degree students, 4 for R.N. to B.S.N. students, 4 for direct entry B.S.N. students, 4 for master's degree students, and 2 for doctoral students.
Deadline February or October of each year.

[442]
ARKANSAS NURSES FOUNDATION SCHOLARSHIPS

Arkansas Nurses Association
Attn: Arkansas Nurses Foundation
1123 South University, Suite 1015
Little Rock, AR 72204
(501) 244-2363　　　　　Fax: (501) 244-9903
E-mail: arna@arna.org
Web: www.arna.org/snas/ar/fdtn/info.htm

Summary To provide financial assistance to residents of Arkansas interested in working on a graduate degree in nursing at a school in any state.
Eligibility This program is open to residents of Arkansas who have a current nursing license and have graduated from a regionally-accredited program (i.e., L.P.N., R.N., B.S.N., M.S.N., or A.P.N.). Applicants must be interested in working on an advanced degree in an accredited program in any state. Along with their application, they must submit a cover letter describing their desire for the scholarship and intended use of funds, a statement regarding institutional financial assistance, a current resume, 2 letters of recommendation, official transcripts, a letter of acceptance into an advanced degree program accredited by NLNAC or CCNE (except doctoral programs), and a list of extracurricular activities.
Financial Data A stipend is awarded (amount not specified).
Duration 1 year.
Number awarded 1 or more each year.
Deadline May of each year.

[443]
ARMY FUNDED NURSE EDUCATION PROGRAM (FNEP)

U.S. Army
Attn: Recruiting Command, RCHS-SVD-FNEP
1307 Third Avenue
Fort Knox, KY 40121-2726
(502) 626-0364　　　Toll Free: (800) 223-3735, ext. 60364
Fax: (502) 626-0952　　　E-mail: fnep@usarec.army.mil
Web: www.usarec.army.mil/AECP

Summary To provide financial assistance to Army officers who are interested in completing a bachelor's or master's degree in nursing and continuing to serve in the Army Nurse Corps.
Eligibility This program is open to active component Army officers who are currently in grade O-3 and have completed at least 38 months but no more than 7 years of active federal service. Applicants must be interested in enrolling full time at an accred-

ited school of nursing to work on a bachelor's or entry-level master's degree. They must agree to serve an additional 2 years for each year of support received for a bachelor's degree or an additional 3 years for the first year of support for a master's degree plus 1 year for each additional 6 months of support. U.S. citizenship is required.

Financial Data The stipend is $12,000 per year, including $11,000 for tuition and fees and $1,000 for books. Participants are not allowed to pay tuition in excess of $11,000 per year from other sources. If the university's tuition is more than $11,000, it must either waive the additional amount or direct the participant to another school. Army officers continue to draw their regular pay and allowances while attending nursing school.

Duration Participants must be able to complete all degree requirements in 24 consecutive months or less. They must remain enrolled full time and maintain a GPA of 2.5 or higher.

Number awarded Up to 25 each year.

Deadline February of each year.

[444]
ARMY HEALTH PROFESSIONS SCHOLARSHIP PROGRAM

U.S. Army
Human Resources Command, Health Services Division
Attn: AHRC-OPH-AN
200 Stovall Street, Room 9N47
Alexandria, VA 22332-0417
(703) 325-2330   Toll Free: (800) USA-ARMY
Fax: (703) 325-2358
Web: www.goarmy.com/amedd/hpsp.jsp

Summary To provide financial assistance to future Army officers who are interested in preparing for a career in psychiatric nursing or other medically-related fields.

Eligibility This program is open to U.S. citizens under 35 years of age. Applicants must be enrolled in or accepted as a full-time student at an accredited professional school located in the United States or Puerto Rico in 1 of the following areas: allopathic or osteopathic medicine, dentistry, clinical or counseling psychology, optometry, veterinary science, or psychiatric nurse practitioner. Upon acceptance into the program, applicants are commissioned as officers in the U.S. Army Reserve; after completion of school, they must perform active-duty service in the U.S. Army Medical Corps, Dental Corps, Medical Service Corps (for clinical psychology and optometry), Nurse Corps, or Veterinary Corps.

Financial Data This program pays full tuition at any school or college granting a doctoral or other relevant professional degree located in the United States or Puerto Rico and covers the cost of fees, books, and other required equipment. Recipients are also awarded a stipend of $1,992 per month for 10 1/2 months of the year. During the other 1 1/2 months of each year, they perform active-duty service, usually at an Army medical facility, and receive the normal pay of a Second Lieutenant.

Duration 1 to 4 years for the medical program; 1 to 4 years for the dental program; 2 or 3 years for the clinical or counseling psychology program; 2 to 4 years for the optometry program; and 1 to 3 years for the veterinary program.

Additional data Participants incur an active-duty obligation based on existing Department of Defense and Army Directives in effect at the time they sign their contract accepting support through this program. Recently, the obligation has been 1 year for each year of support and a minimum of 2 years for the medical program or 3 years for the dental, clinical or counseling psychology, optometry, or veterinary programs.

Number awarded Varies each year.

Deadline Applications may be submitted at any time.

[445]
ARMY MEDICAL AND DENTAL SCHOOL STIPEND PROGRAM (MDSSP)

U.S. Army
Human Resources Command, Health Services Division
Attn: AHRC-OPH-AN
200 Stovall Street, Room 9N47
Alexandria, VA 22332-0417
(703) 325-2330   Toll Free: (800) USA-ARMY
Fax: (703) 325-2358
Web: www.goarmy.com/amedd/graduate.jsp

Summary To provide financial assistance to students in designated medically-related fields (including psychiatric nursing) who are interested in serving in the U.S. Army Reserve after graduation.

Eligibility This program is open to U.S. citizens under 35 years of age. Applicants must be enrolled in or accepted as a full-time student at an accredited professional school located in the United States or Puerto Rico in 1 of the following areas: allopathic or osteopathic medicine, dentistry, psychology (doctoral level only), optometry, or psychiatric nurse practitioner. Upon acceptance into the program, applicants are commissioned as officers in the U.S. Army Reserve; after completion of school, they must train as part of an Army Reserve unit and serve when needed.

Financial Data This program pays a stipend of $1,992 per month.

Duration Until completion of a degree.

Additional data Participants incur an obligation to serve 1 year in the Selected Reserve for each 6 months of support received, including 12 days of annual training or active duty for training.

Number awarded Varies each year.

Deadline Applications may be submitted at any time.

[446]
ARMY NURSE CORPS ASSOCIATION SCHOLARSHIPS

Army Nurse Corps Association
Attn: Education Committee
P.O. Box 39235
San Antonio, TX 78218-1235
(210) 650-3534   Fax: (210) 650-3494
E-mail: education@e-anca.org
Web: e-anca.org/ANCAEduc.htm

Summary To provide financial assistance to students who have a connection to the Army and are interested in working on an undergraduate or graduate degree in nursing.

Eligibility This program is open to students attending colleges or universities that have accredited programs offering associate, bachelor's, master's, or doctoral degrees in nursing. Applicants must be 1) nursing students who plan to enter the active Army, Army National Guard, or Army Reserve and are not participating in a program funded by the active Army, Army National Guard, or Army Reserve; 2) nursing students who have previously served in the active Army, Army National Guard, or Army Reserve; 3) Army Nurse Corps officers enrolled in an undergraduate or graduate nursing program not funded by the active Army, Army National Guard, or Army Reserve; 4) enlisted soldiers in the active Army, Army National Guard, or Army Reserve who are working on a baccalaureate degree in nursing not funded by the active Army, Army National Guard, or Army Reserve; or 5) nursing students whose parent(s) or spouse are serving or have served in the active Army, Army National Guard, or Army Reserve. Along with their application, they must submit a personal statement on their professional career objectives, reasons for applying for this scholarship, financial need, special considerations, personal and academic interests, and why they are preparing for a nursing career.

Financial Data The stipend is $3,000. Funds are sent directly to the recipient's school.

Duration 1 year.

Additional data Although the sponsoring organization is made up of current, retired, and honorably discharged officers of the Army Nurse Corps, it does not have an official affiliation with the Army. Therefore, students who receive these scholarships do not incur any military service obligation.

Number awarded 1 or more each year.

Deadline March of each year.

[447]
ARMY SPECIALIZED TRAINING ASSISTANCE PROGRAM (STRAP)

U.S. Army
Human Resources Command, Health Services Division
Attn: AHRC-OPH-AN
200 Stovall Street, Room 9N47
Alexandria, VA 22332-0417
(703) 325-2330   Toll Free: (800) USA-ARMY
Fax: (703) 325-2358
Web: www.goarmy.com/amedd/postgrad.jsp

Summary To provide funding for service to members of the United States Army Reserve (USAR) or Army National Guard (ARNG) who are engaged in additional training in designated health care fields (including nursing) that are considered critical for war time medical needs.

Eligibility This program is open to members of the USAR or ARNG who are currently 1) medical residents (in orthopedic surgery, family practice, emergency medicine, general surgery, obstetrics/gynecology, or internal medicine); 2) dental residents (in oral surgery, prosthodontics, or comprehensive dentistry); 3) nursing students working on a master's degree in critical care or nurse anesthesia; or 4) associate degree or diploma nurses working on a bachelor's degree. Applicants must agree to a service obligation of 1 year for every 6 months of support received.

Financial Data This program pays a stipend of $1,992 per month.

Additional data During their obligated period of service, participants must attend Extended Combat Training (ECT) at least 12 days each year and complete the Officer Basic Leadership Course (OBLC) within the first year.

Number awarded Varies each year.

Deadline Applications may be submitted at any time.

[448]
ARNA/DOROTHY BUDNEK MEMORIAL SCHOLARSHIP

Association for Radiologic & Imaging Nursing
7794 Grow Drive
Pensacola, FL 32514
(850) 474-7292   Toll Free: (866) 486-2762
Fax: (850) 484-8762   E-mail: arin@dancyamc.com
Web: www.arinursing.org/awards-amp-scholarships.html

Summary To provide financial assistance to members of the Association for Radiologic & Imaging Nursing (ARIN) who are interested in working on a higher degree in a health-related field.

Eligibility This program is open to association members (must have been members for at least 3 years) who have a current nursing license and have returned to school to advance their nursing education. Applicants must have a GPA of 2.5 or higher at their current educational institution. Along with their application, they must submit a statement of purpose on how these funds would be utilized to further or enhance their educational goal, 2 letters of recommendation, a transcript, a statement of financial support throughout their postsecondary education, and a copy of their current nursing license.

Financial Data The stipend is $600.

Duration 1 year.

Additional data The ARIN was formerly named the American Radiological Nurses Association.

Number awarded 1 or more each year.

Deadline October of each year.

[449]
ARTHUR L. DAVIS PUBLISHING AGENCY SCHOLARSHIP OF MASSACHUSETTS

Massachusetts Association of Registered Nurses
P.O. Box 285
Milton, MA 02186
(617) 990-2856   Toll Free: (866) MARN-ANA
E-mail: info@marnonline.org
Web: www.marnonline.org

Summary To provide financial assistance to members of the Massachusetts Association of Registered Nurses (MARN) who are working on an additional degree and their children and significant others who are entering a nursing program.

Eligibility This program is open to 1) registered nurses who have been members of MARN for at least 1 year and are enrolled in a baccalaureate, master's, or doctoral degree program in nursing, and 2) children and significant others of MARN members who have been accepted into a nursing education program. Applicants must be enrolled or planning to enroll at an accredited school of nursing in any state. They must be nominated by themselves or by a colleague. Along with their application, they must submit a 2-page essay describing their career goals and how this scholarship would assist them in achieving their goals. Financial need is not considered in the selection process.

Financial Data The stipend is $1,000. Funds are paid jointly to the student and to the college or university and may be used for tuition and fees only.

Duration 1 year; nonrenewable.

Additional data This program is supported by the Arthur L. Davis Publishing Agency.

Number awarded 1 each year.

Deadline March of each year.

[450]
ARTHUR M. MILLER FUND SCHOLARSHIPS

Arthur M. Miller Fund
c/o Bank of America, N.A.
P.O. Box 1122
Wichita, KS 67201
(316) 261-4609

Summary To provide financial assistance to students working on a nursing or medical degree in Kansas.

Eligibility This program is open to students working on a nursing or medical degree in any area except osteopathy, podiatry, chiropractic, or optometry. They must be enrolled full time at a school in Kansas. Applicants working on a degree for a registered nurse must have been accepted into the professional phase of the program. Selection is based on financial need, general character, and career choice.

Financial Data The stipend is $2,000. Funds are to be used for tuition only and cannot be spent on textbooks, living expenses, or other fees.

Duration 1 year.

Number awarded Several each year.

Deadline March of each year.

[451]
ASPAN DEGREE SCHOLARSHIPS

American Society of PeriAnesthesia Nurses
Attn: Scholarship Program
90 Frontage Road
Cherry Hill, NJ 08034-1424
(856) 616-9600   Toll Free: (877) 737-9696, ext. 13
Fax: (856) 616-9601   E-mail: aspan@aspan.org
Web: www.aspan.org

Summary To provide financial assistance for additional education to members of the American Society of PeriAnesthesia Nurses (ASPAN).

Eligibility This program is open to registered nurses who have been members of the society for at least 2 years and have been employed for at least 2 years in any phase of the perianesthesia setting (preanesthesia, postanesthesia, ambulatory surgery, management, research, or education). Applicants must be interested in working on a bachelor of science in nursing, a master of science in nursing, or a doctorate in nursing. Along with their application, they must submit a statement of financial need; 2 letters of recommendation; and a narrative statement describing their level of activity or involvement in a phase of perianesthesia nursing, ASPAN and/or a component, or their community. Their statement should explain how they see their perianesthesia practice changing and benefiting as a result of their degree and how receiving this scholarship will help them obtain their professional goals and contribute to the perianesthesia community.

Financial Data The stipend is $1,000 per year; funds are sent directly to the recipient's university.

Duration 1 year; recipients may not reapply for additional funding until 3 years have elapsed.

Number awarded At least 2 each year.

Deadline June of each year.

[452]
ASSOCIATES IN BEHAVIORAL HEALTH SCHOLARSHIP

Pride Foundation
Attn: Scholarship Program Director
1122 East Pike Street
PMB 1001
Seattle, WA 98122-3934
(206) 323-3318   Toll Free: (800) 735-7287
Fax: (206) 323-1017
E-mail: scholarships@pridefoundation.org
Web: www.pridefoundation.org/scholarships/scholarship-funds

Summary To provide financial assistance to gay, lesbian, bisexual, or transgender (GLBT) graduate students who live in the Northwest and are working on a degree related to behavioral health (including psychiatric nursing).

Eligibility This program is open to GLBT residents of Alaska, Idaho, Montana, Oregon, or Washington who are enrolled or planning to enroll in graduate school in any state. Applicants must be planning to work on a degree in psychology, psychiatry, social work, or psychiatric nursing. Preference is given to students who are already enrolled in graduate school and can demonstrate financial need. Selection is based on financial need, community involvement, and commitment to civil rights for all people.

Financial Data Stipends average more than $2,100. Funds are paid directly to the recipient's school.

Duration 1 year; recipients may reapply.

Additional data The Pride Foundation was established in 1987 to strengthen the lesbian, gay, bisexual, and transgender community.

Number awarded 1 or more each year. Since it began offering scholarships in 1993, the foundation has awarded $1.4 million to nearly 800 recipients.

Deadline January of each year.

[453]
ASSOCIATION OF BRETHREN CARING MINISTRIES NURSING SCHOLARSHIPS

Church of the Brethren
Attn: Caring Ministries
1451 Dundee Avenue
Elgin, IL 60120-1694
(847) 742-5100, ext. 300   Toll Free: (800) 323-8039
Fax: (847) 742-6103
Web: www.brethren.org

Summary To provide financial assistance to members of the Church of the Brethren working on an undergraduate or graduate degree in nursing.

Eligibility This program is open to students who are members of the Church of the Brethren or employed in a Church of the Brethren agency. Applicants must be enrolled in a L.P.N., R.N., or graduate program in nursing. Along with their application, they must submit 1) a statement describing their reasons for wanting to enter nursing or continue their nursing education, including something of their aspirations for service in the profession; and 2) a description of how the scholarship will assist them in reaching their educational and career goals.

Financial Data The stipend is $2,000 for R.N. and graduate nurse candidates or $1,000 for L.P.N. candidates.

Duration 1 year. Recipients are eligible for only 1 scholarship per degree.

Number awarded Varies each year.

Deadline March of each year.

[454]
ASSOCIATION OF CALIFORNIA NURSE LEADERS RESEARCH SCHOLARSHIPS

Association of California Nurse Leaders
3835 North Freeway Boulevard, Suite 120
Sacramento, CA 95834
(916) 779-6949   Fax: (916) 779-6945
E-mail: info@acnl.org
Web: www.acnl.org

Summary To provide funding for research to graduate nursing students, especially members of the Association of California Nurse Leaders (ACNL).

Eligibility This program is open students working on a graduate degree in nursing and conducting a research project as part of their degree requirements. Preference is given to members of ACNL. The project must show promise of having relevance to nursing practice, education, or research. Applicants must be available to present a summary of their work at the ACNL annual conference the year following the award. Along with their application, they must submit an academic transcript and a 750-word essay on their specific long- and short-term career goals, how a graduate degree will help them to accomplish those goals, their leadership contributions to the profession of nursing and/or their community, and their recent work experience and work-related achievements.

Financial Data Grants range from $500 to $2,500. Funds must be used for research expenses; support is not provided for compensation of the investigator, travel to meetings, preparation of manuscripts or slides, or educational expenses.

Duration 1 year.

Number awarded Varies each year.

Deadline October of each year.

[455]
ASSOCIATION OF CALIFORNIA NURSE LEADERS SCHOLARSHIPS

Association of California Nurse Leaders
3835 North Freeway Boulevard, Suite 120
Sacramento, CA 95834
(916) 779-6949   Fax: (916) 779-6945
E-mail: info@acnl.org
Web: www.acnl.org

Summary To provide financial assistance to members of the Association of California Nurse Leaders (ACNL) who are working on a graduate degree in nursing or a field related to health care leadership.

Eligibility This program is open to ACNL members enrolled or accepted in a graduate degree program in nursing or another field related to health care leadership (e.g., M.N., M.S.N., M.B.A., M.P.H., D.N.Sc., D.N.P., Ph.D.). Applicants must submit an academic transcript and a 750-word essay on their specific long- and short-term career goals, how a graduate degree will help them to accomplish those goals, their leadership contributions to the profession of nursing and/or their community, and their recent work experience and work-related achievements.

Financial Data Stipends range from $500 to $10,000.

Duration 1 year.

Additional data This program includes the Barbara Brantley Nursing Education Scholarship (established by Catalyst Systems, LLC), the Claire V. Cunningham Masonic Fund for Supporting Leadership in Nursing (established by the California Masonic Foundation), and the Victor E. Schimmel Memorial Nursing Scholarships (established by The Camden Group).

Number awarded Varies each year; recently, 9 of these scholarships were awarded.

Deadline October of each year.

[456]
ASSOCIATION OF UNITED NURSES SCHOLARSHIPS

Scholarship Administrative Services, Inc.
Attn: AUN Program
457 Ives Terrace
Sunnyvale, CA 94087

Summary To provide financial assistance to undergraduate and graduate students working on a degree in nursing.

Eligibility This program is open to full-time students working on or planning to work on an undergraduate or graduate degree in nursing. Applicants must have a GPA of 3.0 or higher and be able to demonstrate a record of involvement in extracurricular and work activities related to nursing. Along with their application, they must submit a 1,000-word essay on their educational and career goals, why they believe nursing is essential to America, and why they have decided to prepare for a career in nursing. Financial need is not considered in the selection process.

Financial Data The stipend is $5,000 per year.

Duration 1 year; may be renewed 1 additional year if the recipient maintains full-time enrollment and a GPA of 3.0 or higher.

Additional data This program is sponsored by the Association of United Nurses (AUN) and administered by Scholarship Administrative Services, Inc. AUN was established in 2005 to encourage more American students to consider a career as a nurse. Requests for applications should be accompanied by a self-addressed stamped envelope, the student's e-mail address, and the source where they found the scholarship information.

Number awarded Up to 20 each year.

Deadline April of each year.

[457]
ASTRAZENECA DIVERSITY SCHOLARSHIP PROGRAM

Nurse Practitioner Healthcare Foundation
Attn: Scholarship Selection Committee
2647 134th Avenue N.E.
Bellevue, WA 98005-1813
(425) 861-0911   Fax: (425) 861-0907
Web: www.nphealthcarefoundation.org

Summary To provide financial assistance to members of minority groups enrolled in a graduate nurse practitioner program.

Eligibility This program is open to members of minority ethnic and racial groups, currently defined to include African Americans, Hispanics/Latinos, Asians/Pacific Islanders, Native Americans/Alaska Natives, and Middle Easterners. Applicants must be enrolled in a graduate nurse practitioner program at the master's, post-master's, or doctoral level. They must have a GPA of 3.0 or higher. Along with their application, they must submit a 350-word personal statement on their commitment to serving vulnerable populations and eliminating health disparities. U.S. citizenship or permanent resident status is required.

Financial Data The stipend is $4,000.

Additional data This program is sponsored by AstraZeneca Pharmaceuticals.

Number awarded 6 each year.

Deadline January of each year.

[458]
ATI EDUCATIONAL ASSESSMENT NURSING RESEARCH GRANT

Sigma Theta Tau International
Attn: Research Services
550 West North Street
Indianapolis, IN 46202-3191
(317) 634-8171   Toll Free: (888) 634-7575
Fax: (317) 634-8188   E-mail: research@stti.iupui.edu
Web: www.nursingsociety.org

Summary To provide funding to nurses interested in conducting research on the use of standardized assessments in nursing programs.

Eligibility This program is open to registered nurses who have a master's or doctoral degree or are enrolled in a doctoral program. Applicants must be interested in conducting a research project on the appropriate use of standardized assessments at the end of a nursing program, including (but not limited to) 1) use of diagnostic data to inform group or individual remediation; 2) use of group data to guide curricular evaluation and revision; and 3) identification of key markets of students at risk for NCLEX failure.

Financial Data The maximum grant is $6,000.

Duration 1 year.

Additional data Funding for this program is provided by Assessment Technologies Institute (ATI).

Number awarded 1 each year.

Deadline June of each year.

[459]
BANNER HEALTH SYSTEM NORTH COLORADO MEDICAL CENTER NIGHTINGALE SCHOLARSHIP

Colorado Nurses Foundation
7400 East Arapahoe Road, Suite 211
Centennial, CO 80112
(303) 694-4728   Fax: (303) 694-4869
E-mail: mail@cnfound.org
Web: www.cnfound.org/scholarships.html

Summary To provide financial assistance to undergraduate and graduate nursing students in Colorado who are willing to work at a designated facility following graduation.

Eligibility This program is open to Colorado residents who are enrolled in an approved nursing program in the state. Applicants may be 1) second-year students in an associate degree program; 2) junior or senior level B.S.N. undergraduate students; 3) R.N.s enrolled in a baccalaureate or higher degree program in a school of nursing; 4) R.N.s with a master's degree in nursing, currently practicing in Colorado and enrolled in a doctoral program; or 5) students in the second or third year of a Doctorate Nursing Practice (D.N.P.) program. They must be willing to work for a Banner Health Facility following graduation. Undergraduates must have a GPA of 3.25 or higher and graduate students must have a GPA of 3.5 or higher. Selection is based on professional philosophy and goals, dedication to the improvement of patient care in Colorado, demonstrated commitment to nursing, critical thinking skills, potential for leadership, involvement in community and professional organizations, recommendations, GPA, and financial need.

Financial Data The stipend is $1,000.

Duration 1 year.

Number awarded 1 each year.

Deadline October of each year.

[460]
BARBARA F. PROWANT NURSING RESEARCH GRANT

American Nephrology Nurses' Association
Attn: ANNA National Office
200 East Holly Avenue
P.O. Box 56
Pitman, NJ 08071-0056
(609) 256-2320   Toll Free: (888) 600-2662
Fax: (856) 589-7463   E-mail: annascholarships@ajj.com
Web: www.annanurse.org

Summary To provide funding to members of the American Nephrology Nurses' Association (ANNA) who are interested in conducting pilot, thesis, or dissertation research.

Eligibility This program is open to ANNA members who are currently certified by the Nephrology Nursing Certification Commission (NNCC). Applicants must be interested in conducting research for a pilot study, master's thesis, or doctoral dissertation. They must be enrolled in a graduate program at the master's, doctoral, or postdoctoral level. Preference is given to graduate students, but if funding is available the grant may be awarded to members who already have a master's degree. The proposed project may be a new endeavor or already in process. The proposals must demonstrate the following: significance and applicability of the project to nephrology, transplantation, or related therapies; sound methodology in accordance with recognized nursing research guidelines; approval by the appropriate internal review board; feasibility and likelihood of successful completion; and support from the institution where the project will be implemented.

Financial Data The grant is $5,000.

Duration 1 year.

Additional data Funds for this program, established in 2009, are supplied by the NNCC.

Number awarded 1 each year.

Deadline November of each year.

[461]
BARBARA PALO FOSTER MEMORIAL SCHOLARSHIP

Ulman Cancer Fund for Young Adults
Attn: Scholarship Program Coordinator
10440 Little Patuxent Parkway, Suite 1G
Columbia, MD 21044
(410) 964-0202, ext. 106   Toll Free: (888) 393-FUND
E-mail: scholarship@ulmanfund.org
Web: www.ulmanfund.org/Services/tabid/53/Default.aspx

Summary To provide financial assistance to undergraduate and graduate nursing students who have a parent with cancer.

Eligibility This program is open to nursing students who have or have lost a parent to cancer. Applicants must be younger than 35 years of age and enrolled in, or planning to enroll in, an undergraduate or graduate program in nursing. They must demonstrate an interest in furthering patient education, focusing on persons from medically underserved communities and/or women's health issues. Along with their application, they must submit an essay of at least 1,000 words on the ways in which their experiences as a member of a marginalized group within the cancer community (i.e., young adults affected by cancer) have taught them lessons that inspire them to be of service to other socially, politically, and or economically marginalized people in the healthcare system. Selection is based on demonstrated dedication to community service, commitment to educational and professional goals, use of their cancer experience to impact the lives of other young adults affected by cancer, medical hardship, and financial need.

Financial Data The stipend is $2,500. Funds are paid directly to the educational institution.

Duration 1 year; nonrenewable.

Additional data Recipients must agree to complete 50 hours of community service.

Number awarded 1 each year.

Deadline April of each year.

[462]
BASIC MIDWIFERY STUDENT SCHOLARSHIPS

American College of Nurse-Midwives
Attn: ACNM Foundation, Inc.
8403 Colesville Road, Suite 1550
Silver Spring, MD 20910-6374
(240) 485-1850   Fax: (240) 485-1818
Web: www.midwife.org/foundation_award.cfm

Summary To provide financial assistance for midwifery education to student members of the American College of Nurse-Midwives (ACNM).

Eligibility This program is open to ACNM members who are currently enrolled in an accredited basic midwife education program and have successfully completed 1 academic or clinical semester/quarter or clinical module. Applicants must submit a 150-word essay on their midwifery career plans and a 100-word essay on their intended future participation in the local, regional, and/or national activities of the ACNM. Selection is based on leadership potential, financial need, academic history, and potential for future professional contribution to the organization.

Financial Data The stipend is $3,000.

Duration 1 year.

Additional data This program includes the following named scholarships: the A.C.N.M. Foundation Memorial Scholarship, the TUMS Calcium for Life Scholarship (presented by GlaxoSmithKline), the Edith B. Wonnell CNM Scholarship, and the Margaret Edmundson Scholarship.

Number awarded Varies each year; recently, 4 of these scholarships were awarded.

Deadline March of each year.

[463]
BCSP MICHAEL ORN SCHOLARSHIP

American Society of Safety Engineers
Attn: ASSE Foundation
1800 East Oakton Street
Des Plaines, IL 60018
(847) 768-3435   Fax: (847) 768-3434
E-mail: agabanski@asse.org
Web: www.asse.org/foundation/scholarships/scholarships.php

Summary   To provide financial assistance to upper-division and graduate student members of the American Society of Safety Engineers (ASSE).
Eligibility   This program is open to ASSE student members who are working on an undergraduate or graduate degree in occupational safety, health, and environment or a closely-related field (e.g., industrial or environmental engineering, environmental science, industrial hygiene, occupational health nursing). Undergraduates must be full-time students who have completed at least 60 semester hours with a GPA of 3.0 or higher. Graduate students must also be enrolled full time, have completed at least 9 semester hours with a GPA of 3.5 or higher, and have earned a GPA of 3.0 or higher as an undergraduate. Along with their application, they must submit 2 essays of 300 words or less: 1) why they are seeking a degree in occupational safety and health or a closely-related field, a brief description of their current activities, and how those relate to their career goals and objectives; and 2) why they should be awarded this scholarship (including career goals and financial need). U.S. citizenship is not required.
Financial Data   The stipend is $1,000 per year.
Duration   1 year; recipients may reapply.
Additional data   This program is supported by the Board of Certified Safety Professionals (BCSP).
Number awarded   1 each year.
Deadline   November of each year.

[464]
BOSTONWORKS NURSING FACULTY SCHOLARSHIP

Massachusetts Hospital Association
Attn: Human Resources Manager
5 New England Executive Park
Burlington, MA 01803-5096
(781) 262-6000   E-mail: workforce@mhalink.org
Web: www.mhalink.org/public/education/scholarship.cfm
Summary   To provide financial assistance to registered nurses interested in working on a graduate degree to prepare for a career as a faculty member.
Eligibility   This program is open to registered nurses who are enrolled or accepted for enrollment in a graduate nursing program (M.S.N. or Ph.D.) on at least a half-time basis. Applicants must be able to document a commitment to nursing faculty role preparation and plans to serve as academic faculty after graduation. Selection is based on academic excellence. U.S. citizenship is required.
Financial Data   The stipend is $15,000.
Duration   1 year.
Additional data   This program was established in 2006 with a donation from BostonWorks.
Number awarded   1 each year.
Deadline   April of each year.

[465]
BRAINTRACK NURSING SCHOLARSHIP

BrainTrack
c/o FutureMeld, LLC
221 Boston Post Road East
Marlborough, MA 01772
(978) 451-0471   E-mail: info@braintrack.com
Web: www.braintrack.com/about-braintrack-scholarships.htm
Summary   To provide financial assistance to students and nurses working on an undergraduate or graduate degree in nursing.
Eligibility   This program is open to students preparing for a career in nursing as an L.P.N. or R.N. and to nurses advancing their education by working on an associate, bachelor's, master's, or doctoral degree. Applicants must have completed at least 1 semester of study as a full- or part-time student in an on-campus

and/or online program. They must be a U.S. citizen, have permanent resident status, or have an appropriate student visa. Along with their application, they must submit essays between 200 and 800 words each on 1) what led them to choose nursing as a career path; 2) what they have enjoyed most and least during their nursing degree program so far; 3) what they wish they had known about selecting and entering their nursing school that would be helpful to others going into nursing. Selection is based entirely on the creativity, focus, overall thoughtfulness, accuracy, and practical value of their essays.
Financial Data   Stipends are $1,000 or $500.
Duration   1 year.
Number awarded   4 each year: 2 at $1,000 and 2 at $500.
Deadline   October or February of each year.

[466]
BREAKTHROUGH TO NURSING SCHOLARSHIPS

National Student Nurses' Association
Attn: Foundation
45 Main Street, Suite 606
Brooklyn, NY 11201
(718) 210-0705   Fax: (718) 797-1186
E-mail: nsna@nsna.org
Web: www.nsna.org
Summary   To provide financial assistance to minority undergraduate and graduate students who wish to prepare for careers in nursing.
Eligibility   This program is open to students currently enrolled in state-approved schools of nursing or pre-nursing associate degree, baccalaureate, diploma, generic master's, generic doctoral, R.N. to B.S.N., R.N. to M.S.N., or L.P.N./L.V.N. to R.N. programs. Graduating high school seniors are not eligible. Support for graduate education is provided only for a first degree in nursing. Applicants must be members of a racial or ethnic minority underrepresented among registered nurses (American Indian or Alaska Native, Hispanic or Latino, Native Hawaiian or other Pacific Islander, Black or African American, or Asian). They must be committed to providing quality health care services to underserved populations. Along with their application, they must submit a 200-word description of their professional and educational goals and how this scholarship will help them achieve those goals. Selection is based on academic achievement, financial need, and involvement in student nursing organizations and community health activities. U.S. citizenship or permanent resident status is required.
Financial Data   Stipends range from $1,000 to $2,500. A total of approximately $155,000 is awarded each year by the foundation for all its scholarship programs.
Duration   1 year.
Additional data   Applications must be accompanied by a $10 processing fee.
Number awarded   Varies each year. Recently, 5 of these scholarships were awarded: 2 sponsored by the American Association of Critical-Care Nurses and 3 sponsored by the Mayo Clinic.
Deadline   January of each year.

[467]
BROTHER FRANCES SMITH SCHOLARSHIP

Connecticut Nurses' Association
Attn: Connecticut Nurses' Foundation
377 Research Parkway, Suite 2D
Meriden, CT 06450-7155
(203) 238-1207   Fax: (203) 238-3437
E-mail: info@ctnurses.org
Web: www.ctnurses.org/displaycommon.cfm?an=12
Summary   To provide financial assistance to Connecticut residents interested in preparing for a career as a licensed practical

nurse (L.P.N.) or working on a degree in nursing at a school in any state.

Eligibility This program is open to residents of Connecticut who are entering or enrolled at an accredited practical nurse education program in any state to earn a license as an L.P.N. or work on an associate, bachelor's, master's, or doctoral degree. Selection is based on employment experience; professional, community, and student activities; a statement of educational and practice goals; and financial need.

Financial Data The stipend depends on the qualifications of the recipient and the availability of funds.

Duration 1 year.

Number awarded 1 or more each year.

Deadline June of each year.

[468]
BUILDING ACADEMIC GERIATRIC NURSING CAPACITY PROGRAM PREDOCTORAL SCHOLARSHIP PROGRAM

American Academy of Nursing
Attn: Building Academic Geriatric Nursing Capacity Program
888 17th Street, N.W., Suite 800
Washington, DC 20006
(202) 777-1170   Fax: (202) 777-0107
E-mail: bagnc@aannet.org
Web: www.geriatricnursing.org

Summary To provide funding to nurses interested in working on a doctoral degree in gerontological nursing.

Eligibility This program is open to registered nurses who hold a degree in nursing and have been admitted to a doctoral program as a full-time student. Applicants must plan an academic career in geriatric nursing. They must identify a mentor/adviser with whom they will work and whose program of research in geriatric nursing is a good match with their own research interest area. Selection is based on potential for substantial long-term contributions to the knowledge base in geriatric nursing; leadership potential; evidence of commitment to a career in academic geriatric nursing; and evidence of involvement in educational, research, and professional activities. Members of underrepresented minority groups (American Indians, Alaska Natives, Asians, Blacks or African Americans, Hispanics or Latinos/Latinas, Native Hawaiians or other Pacific Islanders) are especially encouraged to apply. U.S. citizenship or permanent resident status is required.

Financial Data The stipend is $50,000 per year. An additional stipend of $5,000 is available to fellows whose research includes the study of pain in the elderly.

Duration 2 years.

Additional data This program began in 2001 with funding from the John A. Hartford Foundation. In 2004, the Mayday Fund added support to scholars who focus on the study of pain in the elderly.

Number awarded Varies each year; recently, 12 of these scholarships were awarded.

Deadline January of each year.

[469]
CATHERINE J. DODD HEALTH POLICY SCHOLARSHIP

American Nurses Association of California
Attn: Golden State Nursing Foundation
1121 L Street, Suite 409
Sacramento, CA 95814
(916) 447-0225   Fax: (916) 442-4394
E-mail: gsnf@goldenstatenursingfoundation.org
Web: www.goldenstatenursingfoundation.org/scholarships.html

Summary To provide financial assistance to registered nurses (R.N.s) in California who have some experience in health policy

issues and are interested in working on a graduate degree at a school in any state.

Eligibility This program is open to nurses registered in California employed in any practice field of nursing and any employment setting. Applicants must have been accepted into a graduate level academic program in nursing in any state or be currently enrolled in such a program. They must be able to demonstrate evidence of prior government relations or health policy activities and an intent to remain active in health policy issues. Along with their application, they must submit a 1-page essay describing their personal vision of their future involvement in government relations or health policy issues.

Financial Data The stipend is $1,000.

Duration 1 year; nonrenewable.

Number awarded Varies each year.

Deadline December of each year.

[470]
CENTENNIAL SCHOLARSHIP

New Jersey State Nurses Association
Attn: Institute for Nursing
1479 Pennington Road
Trenton, NJ 08618-2661
(609) 883-5335   Toll Free: (888) UR-NJSNA
Fax: (609) 883-5343   E-mail: institute@njsna.org
Web: www.njsna.org/displaycommon.cfm?an=5

Summary To provide financial assistance to New Jersey residents who are preparing for a career as a nurse at a school in the state.

Eligibility Applicants must be New Jersey residents currently enrolled in a diploma, associate, baccalaureate, or master's nursing program located in the state. Registered nurses in an R.N.-B.S.N. program are also eligible if they are members of the New Jersey State Nurses Association. Selection is based on financial need, GPA, and leadership potential.

Financial Data The stipend is $1,000.

Duration 1 year.

Number awarded 1 each year.

Deadline January of each year.

[471]
CENTRAL INDIANA ASSE SCHOLARSHIP

American Society of Safety Engineers
Attn: ASSE Foundation
1800 East Oakton Street
Des Plaines, IL 60018
(847) 768-3435   Fax: (847) 768-3434
E-mail: agabanski@asse.org
Web: www.asse.org/foundation/scholarships/scholarships.php

Summary To provide financial assistance to upper-division and graduate student members of the American Society of Safety Engineers (ASSE) from Indiana.

Eligibility This program is open to ASSE student members who are working on an undergraduate or graduate degree in occupational safety, health, and environment or a closely-related field (e.g., industrial or environmental engineering, environmental science, industrial hygiene, occupational health nursing). Priority is given to residents of Indiana attending school in the state or anywhere in the United States and to nonresidents attending school in Indiana. Undergraduates must be full-time students who have completed at least 60 semester hours with a GPA of 3.0 or higher. Graduate students must also be enrolled full time, have completed at least 9 semester hours with a GPA of 3.5 or higher, and have earned a GPA of 3.0 or higher as an undergraduate. Along with their application, they must submit 2 essays of 300 words or less: 1) why they are seeking a degree in occupational safety and health or a closely-related field, a brief description of their current activities, and how those relate to their career goals and objectives; and 2) why they should be awarded this scholarship (including career goals and financial need). U.S. citizenship is not required.

Financial Data   The stipend is $1,500 per year.

Duration   1 year; recipients may reapply.

Additional data   This program is supported by the Central Indiana Chapter of ASSE.

Number awarded   1 each year.

Deadline   November of each year.

[472]
CHARLOTTE LIDDELL SCHOLARSHIP

Florida Nurses Association
Attn: Florida Nurses Foundation
1235 East Concord Street
P.O. Box 536985
Orlando, FL 32853-6985
(407) 896-3261   Fax: (407) 896-9042
E-mail: foundation@floridanurse.org
Web: www.floridanurse.org/foundationGrants/index.asp

Summary   To provide financial assistance to Florida residents who are interested in working on an undergraduate or graduate degree in nursing.

Eligibility   Applicants must have been Florida residents for at least 1 year and have completed at least 1 semester at an accredited nursing program in the state. They may be working on an associate, baccalaureate, master's, or doctoral degree. Undergraduates must have a GPA of 2.5 or higher and graduate students 3.0 or higher. Preference is given to students focusing on psychiatric nursing and attending school in south Florida. Along with their application, they must submit 1-page essays on 1) why it is necessary for them to receive this scholarship; and 2) their goals and their assessment of their potential for making a contribution to nursing and society.

Financial Data   A stipend is awarded (amount not specified).

Duration   1 semester or year.

Number awarded   1 or more each year.

Deadline   May of each year.

[473]
CHIMSS SCHOLARSHIP

Healthcare Information and Management Systems Society-
Colorado Chapter
c/o Bob Barrett, Treasurer
4375 Golden Glow View, Number 102
Colorado Springs, CO 80922
E-mail: academic@chimss.org
Web: www.chimss.org/scholarship/scholarship.html

Summary   To provide financial assistance to residents of Colorado working on an undergraduate or graduate degree in health care informatics at a school in any state.

Eligibility   This program is open to Colorado residents currently enrolled in an undergraduate, master's, or Ph.D. program in any state in health care informatics or a sub-specialty, such as nursing informatics or healthcare information management. Applicants must submit a 500-word essay on how they will impact the field of health care informatics and 2 letters of recommendation.

Financial Data   The stipend is $2,500. The winner also receives a 1-year complimentary membership in the Colorado Healthcare Information and Management Systems Society (CHIMSS).

Duration   1 year.

Number awarded   2 each year.

Deadline   April of each year.

[474]
CLAIRE MARTIN MEMORIAL SCHOLARSHIPS

New Hampshire Nurse Practitioner Association
Attn: Executive Director
P.O. Box 820
New London, NH 03257-0820
(603) 848-4341   Fax: (603) 526-7841
E-mail: lkcarpenter@tds.net
Web: www.npweb.org

Summary   To provide financial assistance to residents of New Hampshire who are interested in working on an undergraduate or graduate degree in nursing at a school in any state.

Eligibility   This program is open to residents of New Hampshire who are enrolled or planning to enroll at a college or university in any state to work on an undergraduate or graduate degree in nursing. Applicants must submit a 250-word essay on why they chose nursing as a career and the qualities they possess that will help them succeed. Financial need is not considered in the selection process.

Financial Data   The stipend is $500.

Duration   1 year.

Number awarded   4 each year.

Deadline   August of each year.

[475]
CLARE SULLIVAN MEMORIAL NURSE LEADER SCHOLARSHIP

Nursing Foundation of Rhode Island
Attn: Scholarship Committee
P.O. Box 41702
Providence, RI 02940
(401) 223-9680   E-mail: nfri@rinursingfoundation.org
Web: www.rinursingfoundation.org/scholarships.htm

Summary   To provide financial assistance to registered nurses working on a postbaccalaureate degree at an institution in Rhode Island.

Eligibility   This program is open to registered nurses enrolled in a nursing program in Rhode Island to work on a postbaccalaureate degree. Applicants must submit a 1-page essay that demonstrates their commitment to nursing and outlines their short-term goals related to nursing, a long-term goal related to nursing, and how they plan to use their leadership skills as an outcome of their nursing program. Preference is given to Rhode Island residents.

Financial Data   The stipend ranges from $500 to $1,000. Checks are written jointly to the recipient and the recipient's school.

Duration   1 year.

Additional data   This program was established in 1999.

Number awarded   1 each year.

Deadline   March of each year.

[476]
CLARK-PHELPS SCHOLARSHIP

Oregon Student Assistance Commission
Attn: Grants and Scholarships Division
1500 Valley River Drive, Suite 100
Eugene, OR 97401-2146
(541) 687-7395   Toll Free: (800) 452-8807, ext. 7395
Fax: (541) 687-7414   TDD: (800) 735-2900
E-mail: awardinfo@osac.state.or.us
Web: www.osac.state.or.us/osac_programs.html

Summary   To provide financial assistance to residents of Oregon and Alaska who are interested in studying nursing, dentistry, or medicine at schools in Oregon.

Eligibility   This program is open to residents of Oregon and Alaska who are currently enrolled or planning to enroll at a public college or university in Oregon. Applicants must be interested in working on a 4-year or graduate degree in nursing, a doctoral degree in dentistry, or a doctoral degree in medicine. Preference is given to applicants who are interested in studying at Oregon Health and Science University, including the nursing programs at Eastern Oregon University, Southern Oregon University, and Oregon Institute of Technology.

Financial Data A stipend is awarded (amount not specified).

Duration 1 year; recipients may reapply.

Additional data This program is administered by the Oregon Student Assistance Commission (OSAC) with funds provided by the Oregon Community Foundation, 1221 S.W. Yamhill, Suite 100, Portland, OR 97205, (503) 227-6846, Fax: (503) 274-7771.

Number awarded Varies each year.

Deadline February of each year.

[477]
CLIFFORD JORDAN SCHOLARSHIP

Florida Council of periOperative Registered Nurses
c/o Carol Morris, Scholarship Chair
223 S.E. Ninth Terrace
Cape Coral, FL 33990
(239) 458-8539   E-mail: Christmascat721@aol.com
Web: community.aorn.org:8080

Summary To provide financial assistance to nursing students and registered nurses in Florida who are working on a degree to advance their career as a perioperative nurse.

Eligibility This program is open to residents of Florida who are 1) students in the final year of an accredited nursing program, or 2) perioperative nurses. Students must have a GPA of 3.0 or higher and be planning to work in a perioperative setting after graduation. Current perioperative nurses must be interested in working on a diploma to A.D.N., diploma/A.D.N., A.D.N. to M.S.N., B.S.N. to M.S.N., degree in hospital administration or health care administration, or Ph.D. in nursing. Applicants must submit information on their educational history, professional activities, civic and school activities, work experience, personal philosophy of perioperative nursing, and reasons for applying. Financial need is not considered.

Financial Data A stipend is awarded (amount not specified).

Duration 1 year.

Number awarded 1 or more each year.

Deadline June of each year.

[478]
CLINICAL PRACTICE PROJECTS IN MEMORY OF LINDA KNAUFF

Minnesota Nurses Association
Attn: Minnesota Nurses Association Foundation
1625 Energy Park Drive, Suite 200
St. Paul, MN 55108
(651) 414-2822   Toll Free: (800) 536-4662, ext. 122
Fax: (651) 695-7000   E-mail: linda.owens@mnnurses.org
Web: www.mnnurses.org

Summary To provide funding to members of the Minnesota Nurses Association (MNA) and the Minnesota Student Nurses Association (MSNA) who are interested in conducting a clinical practice project.

Eligibility This program is open to Registered Nurses who are MNA or MSNA members and to nursing students who are MSNA members. Applicants must be interested in conducting a staff nurse project designed to improve patient care. They must provide a budget, literature review, description of the purpose and goals of the project, and an assessment of the potential contribution to the quality of patient care. Preference is given to first-time applicants.

Financial Data The maximum grant is $2,000.

Duration The project must be completed within 2 years.

Number awarded Varies each year.

Deadline March, May, September, or December of each year.

[479]
CNA FOUNDATION SCHOLARSHIPS

American Society of Safety Engineers
Attn: ASSE Foundation
1800 East Oakton Street
Des Plaines, IL 60018
(847) 768-3435   Fax: (847) 768-3434
E-mail: agabanski@asse.org
Web: www.asse.org/foundation/scholarships/scholarships.php

Summary To provide financial assistance to upper-division and graduate student members of the American Society of Safety Engineers (ASSE).

Eligibility This program is open to ASSE student members who are working on an undergraduate or graduate degree in occupational safety, health, and environment or a closely-related field (e.g., industrial or environmental engineering, environmental science, industrial hygiene, occupational health nursing). Undergraduates must be full-time students who have completed at least 60 semester hours with a GPA of 3.0 or higher. Graduate students must also be enrolled full time, have completed at least 9 semester hours with a GPA of 3.5 or higher, and have earned a GPA of 3.0 or higher as an undergraduate. Along with their application, they must submit 2 essays of 300 words or less: 1) why they are seeking a degree in occupational safety and health or a closely-related field, a brief description of their current activities, and how those relate to their career goals and objectives; and 2) why they should be awarded this scholarship (including career goals and financial need). U.S. citizenship is not required.

Financial Data The stipend is $4,650 per year.

Duration 1 year; recipients may reapply.

Additional data This program, established in 2006, is supported by the CNA Foundation.

Number awarded 2 each year.

Deadline November of each year.

[480]
COLLEGE NETWORK MOLN MEMBER SCHOLARSHIPS

Minnesota Organization of Leaders in Nursing
1821 University Avenue West, Suite S256
St. Paul, MN 55104
(651) 999-5344   Fax: (651) 917-1835
E-mail: office@moln.org
Web: www.moln.org/sections/scholarships.php

Summary To provide financial assistance to members of the Minnesota Organization of Leaders in Nursing (MOLN) who are interested in returning to school to earn an additional degree in nursing.

Eligibility This program is open to MOLN members (must have been voting members for at least 12 months) who are currently enrolled or have been admitted to a relevant bachelor's, master's, or doctoral degree program. Applicants must have a GPA of 3.0 or higher in their current academic work. Along with their application, they must submit a 2-page essay on their goals in returning to school to complete a degree, how attainment of this degree will facilitate their professional development as a leader in nursing, and how their educational and career goals relate to the goals of MOLN. Selection is based on the essay, a letter of recommendation, and transcripts. Financial need is not considered.

Financial Data A total of $3,000 is available to MOLN members who attend a partnership university in The College Network and an additional $1,000 is available to MOLN members who attend a college or university of their choice.

Duration 1 year.

Additional data This program is sponsored by The College Network.

Number awarded Varies each year.

Deadline June of each year.

[481]
COLORADO NURSES ASSOCIATION NIGHTINGALE SCHOLARSHIP

Colorado Nurses Foundation
7400 East Arapahoe Road, Suite 211
Centennial, CO 80112
(303) 694-4728   Fax: (303) 694-4869
E-mail: mail@cnfound.org
Web: www.cnfound.org/scholarships.html

Summary To provide financial assistance to undergraduate and graduate nursing students in Colorado who are members of the Colorado Nurses Association (CNA) or Colorado Student Nurses Association (CSNA).

Eligibility This program is open to Colorado residents who have been accepted as a student in an approved nursing program in the state. Applicants may be 1) second-year students in an associate degree program; 2) junior or senior level B.S.N. undergraduate students; 3) R.N.s enrolled in a baccalaureate or higher degree program in a school of nursing; 4) R.N.s with a master's degree in nursing, currently practicing in Colorado and enrolled in a doctoral program; or 5) students in the second or third year of a Doctorate Nursing Practice (D.N.P.) program. They must be current members of CNA or CSNA. Undergraduates must have a GPA of 3.25 or higher and graduate students must have a GPA of 3.5 or higher. Selection is based on professional philosophy and goals, dedication to the improvement of patient care in Colorado, demonstrated commitment to nursing, critical thinking skills, potential for leadership, involvement in community and professional organizations, recommendations, GPA, and financial need.

Financial Data The stipend is $1,000.

Duration 1 year.

Number awarded 1 each year.

Deadline October of each year.

[482]
COLORADO NURSES FOUNDATION SCHOLARSHIPS

Colorado Nurses Foundation
7400 East Arapahoe Road, Suite 211
Centennial, CO 80112
(303) 694-4728   Fax: (303) 694-4869
E-mail: mail@cnfound.org
Web: www.cnfound.org/scholarships.html

Summary To provide financial assistance to undergraduate and graduate nursing students in Colorado.

Eligibility This program is open to Colorado residents who have been accepted as a student in an approved nursing program in the state. Applicants may be 1) second-year students in an associate degree program; 2) junior or senior level B.S.N. undergraduate students; 3) R.N.s enrolled in a baccalaureate or higher degree program in a school of nursing; 4) R.N.s with a master's degree in nursing, currently practicing in Colorado and enrolled in a doctoral program; or 5) students in the second or third year of a Doctorate Nursing Practice (D.N.P.) program. They must be committed to practicing nursing in Colorado. Undergraduates must have a GPA of 3.25 or higher and graduate students must have a GPA of 3.5 or higher. Selection is based on professional philosophy and goals, dedication to the improvement of patient care in Colorado, demonstrated commitment to nursing, critical thinking skills, potential for leadership, involvement in community and professional organizations, recommendations, GPA, and financial need.

Financial Data The stipend is $1,000.

Duration 1 year.

Additional data The program includes the following named scholarships: the Johnson and Johnson Nightingale Scholarship, the Donor Alliance Nightingale Scholarship, the National Jewish Health Nightingale Scholarship, the Colorado Trust Nightingale Scholarship, the Colorado Nurses Association District 3 Scholarship, the Colorado Nurses Association District 16 Scholarship in Honor of Eleanor Bent, the University of Colorado Denver College of Nursing Scholarship (limited to students in the nursing program at the University of Colorado at Denver), the Denver Metro Regional Nightingale Scholarship, the Exempla Lutheran Medical Center Nightingale Scholarship, the Medical Center of Aurora Nightingale Scholarship, the Rose Medical Center Nightingale Scholarship, the St. Anthony's Hospitals Nightingale Scholarship, the Nightingale Scholarships, the Arthur L. Davis Publishing Agency Scholarship, the Colorado Organization of Nurse Leaders Scholarship in Memory of Dorothy Babcock, the LaFawn Biddle Nightingale Scholarship, and the Patty Walter Memorial Scholarship (limited to graduate students in urology or oncology at the University of Northern Colorado).

Number awarded Varies each year; recently, 15 of these scholarships were awarded.

Deadline October of each year.

[483]
COLORADO SOCIETY OF ADVANCED PRACTICE NURSES EDUCATOR SCHOLARSHIP

Colorado Society of Advanced Practice Nurses
Attn: Colorado Nurses Association, DNA 30
P.O. Box 100158
Denver, CO 80250-0158
(303) 757-7483   Toll Free: (800) 757-7310
Fax: (303) 757-8833   E-mail: CSAPN@msn.com
Web: www.enpnetwork.com

Summary To provide financial assistance to members of the Colorado Society of Advanced Practice Nurses (CSAPN) who are working on an advanced degree in order to prepare for a career as a nursing educator.

Eligibility This program is open to CSAPN members working on an advanced degree in nursing at a Colorado college or university to prepare for a career as a nursing educator. Applicants must submit brief statements on why they should be the recipient of this scholarship, their goals after they finish school, in the nursing activities and organizations in which they are involved, the community service activities in which they have been involved, and how they would use this scholarship.

Financial Data The stipend is $750.

Duration 1 year.

Additional data The CSAPN serves as DNA 30 of the Colorado Nurses Association.

Number awarded 1 each year.

Deadline May of each year.

[484]
COMMISSION ON GRADUATES OF FOREIGN NURSING SCHOOLS/AMERICAN NURSES FOUNDATION SCHOLAR AWARD

American Nurses Foundation
Attn: Nursing Research Grants Program
8515 Georgia Avenue, Suite 400
Silver Spring, MD 20910-3492
(301) 628-5227   Fax: (301) 628-5354
E-mail: anf@ana.org
Web: www.anfonline.org

Summary To provide funding to nurses interested in conducting research on international aspects.

Eligibility This program is open to registered nurses who have earned a baccalaureate or higher degree. Applicants may be either beginning or experienced researchers. They must be interested in conducting research on international nursing issues or issues related to internationally educated nurses in the U.S. workforce. Proposed research may be for a master's thesis or doctoral dissertation if the project has been approved by the principal investigator's thesis or dissertation committee.

Financial Data The grant is $5,000. Funds may not be used as a salary for the principal investigator.

Duration 1 year.

Additional data Funding for this program is provided by the Commission on Graduates of Foreign Nursing Schools. There is a $100 application fee.

Number awarded 1 each year.

Deadline April of each year.

[485]
CONNECTICUT CHAPTER HFMA SCHOLARSHIPS

Healthcare Financial Management Association-Connecticut Chapter
c/o Cassandra L. Mitchell, Scholarship Committee Chair
UConn Health Center/John Dempsey Hospital
263 Farmington Avenue
Farmington, CT 06030-5355
(860) 679-2916   Fax: (860) 679-3071
E-mail: mitchellc@uche.edu
Web: www.cthfma.org/site/epage/18079_473.htm

Summary To recognize and reward, with scholarships, undergraduate and graduate students in fields related to health care financial management (including nursing) at colleges and universities in Connecticut who submit outstanding essays on topics in the field.

Eligibility This competition is open to undergraduate and graduate students at colleges and universities in Connecticut, children of members of the Connecticut chapter of the Healthcare Financial Management Association (HFMA) attending a school outside of Connecticut, residents of Connecticut commuting to a college or university in a state that borders the state, and Connecticut health care industry employees who are currently attending college. Applicants must be enrolled in a business, finance, accounting, or information systems program and have an interest in health care or be enrolled in a nursing or allied health program. They must submit an essay, up to 5 pages, on a topic that changes annually but relates to financing of health care. Finalists may be interviewed.

Financial Data The first-place winner (undergraduate or graduate) receives a $4,000 award and the second-place winner (undergraduate or graduate) receives a $1,000 award. Both winners also receive membership in the Connecticut chapter of HFMA, a 1-year subscription to *Healthcare Financial Management,* and waiver of chapter program fees for 1 year.

Duration 1 year.

Number awarded 2 each year: 1 for an undergraduate and 1 for a graduate student.

Deadline March of each year.

[486]
CONNECTICUT NURSES' FOUNDATION NURSING RESEARCH AWARD

Connecticut Nurses' Association
Attn: Connecticut Nurses' Foundation
377 Research Parkway, Suite 2D
Meriden, CT 06450-7155
(203) 238-1207   Fax: (203) 238-3437
E-mail: info@ctnurses.org
Web: www.ctnurses.org/displaycommon.cfm?an=12

Summary To provide funding to residents of Connecticut interested in conducting research relevant to nursing.

Eligibility This program is open to residents of Connecticut at all academic levels. Applicants must be interested in conducting research investigating problems applicable to nursing. They must submit information on the purpose of the research study, review of

the literature, research questions, research design, timetable, budget, and their curriculum vitae or resume.

Financial Data The grant is $1,000.

Duration 1 year.

Number awarded 1 or more each year.

Deadline June of each year.

[487]
CONNECTICUT NURSES' FOUNDATION SCHOLARSHIPS

Connecticut Nurses' Association
Attn: Connecticut Nurses' Foundation
377 Research Parkway, Suite 2D
Meriden, CT 06450-7155
(203) 238-1207   Fax: (203) 238-3437
E-mail: info@ctnurses.org
Web: www.ctnurses.org/displaycommon.cfm?an=12

Summary To provide financial assistance to Connecticut residents interested in preparing for a career as a registered nurse (R.N.) or working on a degree in nursing at a school in any state.

Eligibility This program is open to residents of Connecticut who are entering or enrolled at an accredited school of nursing in any state to earn an R.N. certificate or work on an associate, bachelor's, master's, or doctoral degree. Selection is based on employment experience; professional, community, and student activities; a statement of educational and practice goals; and financial need.

Financial Data The stipend depends on the qualifications of the recipient and the availability of funds.

Duration 1 year.

Additional data This program includes the following named scholarships: the Dominion Enterprises Scholarship, the Frank Chant Memorial Scholarship, and the Polly Barey Scholarship.

Number awarded 1 or more each year.

Deadline June of each year.

[488]
CONNIE SCHEFFER PUBLIC HEALTH NURSE ENDOWED SCHOLARSHIP

Kansas State Nurses Association
Attn: Kansas Nurses Foundation
1109 S.W. Topeka Boulevard
Topeka, KS 66612-1602
(785) 233-8638   Fax: (785) 233-5222
E-mail: ksna@ksna.net
Web: www.nursingworld.org/SNAS/KS/Knf.htm

Summary To provide financial assistance to residents of Kansas who are working on a degree in public health nursing at the undergraduate, master's, or doctoral level at a school in the state.

Eligibility This program is open to students who are working on a nursing degree on the undergraduate or graduate level at a school in Kansas. Applicants must have a GPA of 3.0 or higher. Along with their application, they must submit a personal narrative describing their anticipated role in nursing in the state of Kansas. Preference is given to full-time students. The following priority is used in awarding scholarships: 1) R.N.s working on B.S.N.s and employed in public health settings; and 2) graduate and postgraduate nursing students in public health nursing or public health (e.g., M.P.H. degree).

Financial Data The stipend is $500.

Duration 1 year.

Number awarded 1 each year.

Deadline June of each year.

[489]
COUNCIL FOR THE ADVANCEMENT OF NURSING SCIENCE/SOUTHERN NURSING RESEARCH SOCIETY NURSING SCIENCE ADVANCEMENT DISSERTATION GRANT AWARD

Southern Nursing Research Society
10200 West 44th Avenue, Suite 304
Wheat Ridge, CO 80033
Toll Free: (877) 314-SNRS
E-mail: snrs@resourcecenter.com
Web: snrs.org/research/dissertationgrants.html

Summary To provide dissertation research funding to doctoral candidates who are members of both the Southern Nursing Research Society (SNRS) and the Council for the Advancement of Nursing Science (CANS).

Eligibility This program is open to students currently enrolled in doctoral study at a school or college of nursing in the southern states. Applicants must be members of both the SNRS and the CANS. Their dissertation topic must have been approved; they must submit evidence that their proposed research topic meets the requirements for the dissertation and that it can be supported at the proposed institution or facility. Selection is based on significance to nursing, scientific merit, innovation, appropriateness of methodology to the research question, qualifications of the applicant to conduct the study, adequacy of human subjects and/or animal protection, and appropriateness of the environment, budget, and time frame.

Financial Data The grant is $3,000.

Duration 1 year.

Additional data The application fee is $25.

Number awarded 1 each year.

Deadline August of each year.

[490]
CWG SCHOLARSHIP FUND

Maine Community Foundation
Attn: Program Director
245 Main Street
Ellsworth, ME 04605
(207) 667-9735   Toll Free: (877) 700-6800
Fax: (207) 667-0447   E-mail: info@mainecf.org
Web: www.mainecf.org/GraduateScholars.aspx

Summary To provide financial assistance to Maine residents who are registered nurses or college graduates interested in graduate training in mental health services.

Eligibility This program is open to 2 categories of Maine residents: 1) college graduates employed by providers of mental health service in the state who are interested in continuing their professional education by obtaining an M.S.W. or other degree related to work in the mental health field; and 2) registered nurses working for hospitals or outpatient providers of social and mental health services who are interested in obtaining specialized, post-R.N. training in order to work more effectively with patients who have mental health problems. Special consideration is given to applicants whose career goals include work with adolescents and adults and who wish to continue to work in Maine. Financial need is considered in the selection process.

Financial Data A stipend is paid (amount not specified).

Duration 1 year.

Additional data This program was established in 1999.

Number awarded 1 or more each year.

Deadline April of each year.

[491]
CYNTHIA HUNT-LINES SCHOLARSHIP

Minnesota Nurses Association
Attn: Minnesota Nurses Association Foundation
1625 Energy Park Drive, Suite 200
St. Paul, MN 55108
(651) 414-2822   Toll Free: (800) 536-4662, ext. 122
Fax: (651) 695-7000   E-mail: linda.owens@mnnurses.org
Web: www.mnnurses.org

Summary To provide financial assistance to members of the Minnesota Nurses Association (MNA) and the Minnesota Student Nurses Association (MSNA) who are single parents and interested in working on a baccalaureate or master's degree in nursing.

Eligibility This program is open to MNA and MSNA members who are enrolled or entering a baccalaureate or master's program in nursing in Minnesota or North Dakota. Applicants must be single parents, at least 21 years of age, with at least 1 dependent. Along with their application, they must submit: a current transcript; a short essay describing their interest in nursing, their long-range career goals, and how their continuing education will have an impact on the profession of nursing in Minnesota; a description of their financial need; and 2 letters of support.

Financial Data The stipend is $2,000 per year.

Duration 1 year; may be renewed.

Number awarded 1 each year.

Deadline May of each year.

[492]
CYNTHIA MCNERNEY SCHOLARSHIP

American Association of Nurse Anesthetists
Attn: AANA Foundation
222 South Prospect Avenue
Park Ridge, IL 60068-4001
(847) 655-1170   Fax: (847) 692-6968
E-mail: foundation@aana.com
Web: www.aanafoundation.com

Summary To provide financial assistance to members of the American Association of Nurse Anesthetists (AANA) who are interested in obtaining further education, especially at programs in North Carolina.

Eligibility This program is open to members of the association who are currently enrolled in an accredited nurse anesthesia education program. Preference is given to students attending a program in North Carolina. First-year students must have completed 6 months of nurse anesthesia classes; second-year students must have completed 12 months of nurse anesthesia classes. Along with their application, they must submit a 200-word essay describing why they have chosen nurse anesthesia as a profession and their professional goals for the future. Financial need is also considered in the selection process.

Financial Data The stipend is $1,000.

Duration 1 year.

Additional data This scholarship was first awarded in 2002. The application processing fee is $25.

Number awarded 1 each year.

Deadline March of each year.

[493]
DAVIS SCHOLARSHIP FOR FUTURE NURSE EDUCATORS

Illinois Nurses Association
Attn: Illinois Nurses Foundation
105 West Adams Street, Suite 2101
Chicago, IL 60603
(312) 419-2900   Fax: (312) 419-2920
E-mail: info@illinoisnurses.com
Web: www.illinoisnurses.com

Summary To provide financial assistance to graduate nursing students interested in becoming a faculty member at a school of nursing in Illinois.

Eligibility This program is open to students enrolled in an accredited graduate program in nursing with an emphasis on nursing education. Applicants must have a GPA of 3.5 or higher. They must 1) demonstrate recognition for modeling a pattern of excellence; 2) evidence leadership in the profession of nursing; 3) contribute to 1 or more professional organizations; 4) reflect skills of strong communications and interactions with colleagues, students, and clients; and 5) intend to serve on the faculty of a school of nursing in Illinois for 1 academic year.

Financial Data The stipend is $1,000.

Duration 1 year.

Number awarded 1 or more each year.

Deadline March of each year.

[494]
DEAN AND FRED HAYDEN MEMORIAL NATIONAL SCHOLARSHIP

American Association of Nurse Anesthetists
Attn: AANA Foundation
222 South Prospect Avenue
Park Ridge, IL 60068-4001
(847) 655-1170   Fax: (847) 692-6968
E-mail: foundation@aana.com
Web: www.aanafoundation.com

Summary To provide financial assistance to members of the American Association of Nurse Anesthetists (AANA) who are interested in obtaining further education.

Eligibility This program is open to members of the association who are currently enrolled in an accredited nurse anesthesia education program. Applicants must be second-year students who have completed 12 months of nurse anesthesia classes. Along with their application, they must submit a 200-word essay describing why they have chosen nurse anesthesia as a profession and their professional goals for the future. Financial need is also considered in the selection process.

Financial Data The stipend is $3,000.

Duration 1 year.

Additional data This scholarship was first awarded in 1999. The application processing fee is $25.

Number awarded 1 each year.

Deadline March of each year.

[495]
DEAN HAYDEN STUDENT RESEARCH SCHOLARSHIP

American Association of Nurse Anesthetists
Attn: AANA Foundation
222 South Prospect Avenue
Park Ridge, IL 60068-4001
(847) 655-1170   Fax: (847) 692-6968
E-mail: foundation@aana.com
Web: www.aanafoundation.com

Summary To provide funding to student members of the American Association of Nurse Anesthetists who are interested in conducting research.

Eligibility This program is open to nurse anesthesia students in good academic standing who are members of the association. Applicants must be proposing a research project related to their field. Along with their application, they must submit a 300-word abstract of their proposed research and a 50-word statement on how their research impacts nurse anesthesia practice and/or education. Selection is based on the anticipated value of the research finding for nurse anesthetists.

Financial Data Grants are currently limited to $5,000.

Duration 1 year.

Number awarded 1 each year.

Deadline April of each year.

[496]
DEAN M. COX MEMORIAL SCHOLARSHIPS

American Association of Nurse Anesthetists
Attn: AANA Foundation
222 South Prospect Avenue
Park Ridge, IL 60068-4001
(847) 655-1170   Fax: (847) 692-6968
E-mail: foundation@aana.com
Web: www.aanafoundation.com

Summary To provide financial assistance to members of the American Association of Nurse Anesthetists (AANA) who are interested in obtaining further education.

Eligibility This program is open to members of the association who are currently enrolled in an accredited nurse anesthesia education program. Applicants must have a record of promoting education in the CRNA profession. First-year students must have completed 6 months of nurse anesthesia classes; second-year students must have completed 12 months of nurse anesthesia classes. Along with their application, they must submit a 200-word essay describing why they have chosen nurse anesthesia as a profession and their professional goals for the future. Financial need is also considered in the selection process.

Financial Data The stipend is $3,000.

Duration 1 year.

Additional data This scholarship was first awarded in 2006. The application processing fee is $25.

Number awarded 3 each year.

Deadline March of each year.

[497]
DEBORAH HAGUE MEMORIAL SCHOLARSHIP

Ohio Nurses Association
Attn: Ohio Nurses Foundation
4000 East Main Street
Columbus, OH 43213-2983
(614) 237-5414   Fax: (614) 237-6074
E-mail: gharsheymeade@ohnurses.org
Web: www.ohnurses.org

Summary To provide financial assistance to registered nurses in Ohio who are interested in working on a graduate nursing degree at a school in the state.

Eligibility This program is open to Ohio residents who have a valid Ohio nursing license and plan to continue practicing in the state. Applicants must be able to demonstrate a willingness and ability to become a dynamic nursing leader. They must have a GPA of 3.0 or higher and be planning to enroll in a nursing degree program at a school in Ohio. Along with their application, they must submit a 250-word personal statement about the leader they envision becoming and how this education will assist them. Selection is based on that statement, college academic records, school activities, and community services. Membership in the Ohio Nurses Association is considered in the selection process.

Financial Data The stipend is $500 per year.

Duration 1 year; recipients may reapply if they complete 9 credit hours during the academic year.

Number awarded 1 or more each year.

Deadline January of each year.

[498]
DEMPSTER NP DOCTORAL DISSERTATION RESEARCH GRANT

American Academy of Nurse Practitioners
Attn: AANP Foundation
P.O. Box 12924
Austin, TX 78711-2924
(512) 276-5905   Fax: (512) 442-6469
E-mail: foundation@aanp.org
Web: aanp.org

Summary To provide funding to members of the American Academy of Nurse Practitioners (AANP) who wish to conduct research for a doctoral degree project.

Eligibility This program is open to current student and full members of the academy who are working on a doctoral degree and their dissertation research. Applicants must be a currently licensed, practicing nurse practitioner (NP) in the United States and the principal investigator on a research project that is to be used for their degree program. Their GPA in their doctoral program must be 3.75 or higher. U.S. citizenship is required. The research must have an evidence-based and/or outcomes-based primary care focus relevant to health care provided by NPs within the United States.

Financial Data The grant is $2,000. Funds must be used for the proposed research, not tuition expenses.

Duration 1 year.

Additional data There is a $10 application fee.

Number awarded 1 each year.

Deadline October of each year.

[499]
DERMATOLOGY NURSES' ASSOCIATION CAREER MOBILITY SCHOLARSHIPS

Dermatology Nurses' Association
Attn: Recognition Program
15000 Commerce Parkway, Suite C
Mt. Laurel, NJ 08055
Toll Free: (800) 454-4DNA   Fax: (856) 439-0525
E-mail: dna@dnanurse.org
Web: www.dnanurse.org

Summary To provide financial assistance to members of the Dermatology Nurses' Association (DNA) who are working on an undergraduate or graduate degree.

Eligibility Applicants for these scholarships must 1) have been members of the association for at least 2 years, 2) be employed in the specialty of dermatology, and 3) be working on a degree or advanced degree in nursing. Selection is based on a letter in which applicants describe their professional goals, proposed course of study, time frame for completion of study, funds necessary to meet their educational needs, and financial need.

Financial Data The stipend is $2,500.

Duration 1 year.

Number awarded 1 or more each year.

Deadline September of each year.

[500]
DISTRICT 6 GENERIC SCHOLARSHIPS FOR FLORIDA

Florida Nurses Association
Attn: Florida Nurses Foundation
1235 East Concord Street
P.O. Box 536985
Orlando, FL 32853-6985
(407) 896-3261   Fax: (407) 896-9042
E-mail: foundation@floridanurse.org
Web: www.floridanurse.org/foundationGrants/index.asp

Summary To provide financial assistance to residents of Florida who are interested in working on an undergraduate or graduate degree in nursing.

Eligibility Applicants must have been residents of Florida for at least 1 year and have completed at least 1 semester at an accredited nursing program in the state. They may be working on an associate, baccalaureate, master's, or doctoral degree. Undergraduates must have a GPA of 2.5 or higher and graduate students a GPA of 3.0 or higher. Along with their application, they must submit 1-page essays on 1) why it is necessary for them to receive this scholarship; and 2) their goals and their assessment of their potential for making a contribution to nursing and society.

Financial Data A stipend is awarded (amount not specified).

Duration 1 semester or year.

Number awarded 4 each year.

Deadline May of each year.

[501]
DIVERSITY COMMITTEE SCHOLARSHIP

American Society of Safety Engineers
Attn: ASSE Foundation
1800 East Oakton Street
Des Plaines, IL 60018
(847) 768-3435   Fax: (847) 768-3434
E-mail: agabanski@asse.org
Web: www.asse.org/foundation/scholarships/scholarships.php

Summary To provide financial assistance to upper-division and graduate student members of the American Society of Safety Engineers (ASSE) who come from diverse groups.

Eligibility This program is open to ASSE student members who are majoring in occupational safety, health, and environment or a closely-related field (e.g., industrial or environmental engineering, environmental science, industrial hygiene, occupational health nursing). Undergraduates must be full-time students who have completed at least 60 semester hours with a GPA of 3.0 or higher. Graduate students must also be enrolled full time, have completed at least 9 semester hours with a GPA of 3.5 or higher, and have earned a GPA of 3.0 or higher as an undergraduate. Along with their application, they must submit 2 essays of 300 words or less: 1) why they are seeking a degree in occupational safety and health or a closely-related field, a brief description of their current activities, and how those relate to their career goals and objectives; and 2) why they should be awarded this scholarship (including career goals and financial need). A goal of this program is to support individuals regardless of race, ethnicity, gender, religion, personal beliefs, age, sexual orientation, physical challenges, geographic location, university, or specific area of study. U.S. citizenship is not required.

Financial Data The stipend is $1,000 per year.

Duration 1 year; recipients may reapply.

Number awarded 1 each year.

Deadline November of each year.

[502]
DNA 30 STUDENT SCHOLARSHIP

Colorado Society of Advanced Practice Nurses
Attn: Colorado Nurses Association, DNA 30
P.O. Box 100158
Denver, CO 80250-0158
(303) 757-7483   Toll Free: (800) 757-7310
Fax: (303) 757-8833   E-mail: CSAPN@msn.com
Web: www.enpnetwork.com

Summary To provide financial assistance to registered nurses in Colorado who are interested in working on a degree in advanced practice.

Eligibility This program is open to Colorado residents who are R.N.s preparing to become advanced practice nurses and advanced practice nurses working on an advanced degree in nursing (M.S. or higher). Applicants must submit brief statements on why they should be the recipient of this scholarship, their goals after they finish school, in the nursing activities and organizations in which they are involved, the community service activities in which they have been involved, and how they would use this scholarship. Membership in the Colorado Society of Advanced Practice Nurses (DNA 30 of the Colorado Nurses Association) is not required, but members received preference.

Financial Data The stipend is $750.

Duration 1 year; recipients may reapply.

Number awarded 2 each year.

Deadline May of each year.

[503]
DOCTORAL DEGREE SCHOLARSHIPS IN CANCER NURSING

American Cancer Society
Attn: Research Department
250 Williams Street, N.W.
Atlanta, GA 30303-1002
(404) 329-7558   Toll Free: (800) ACS-2345
Fax: (404) 417-5974   TDD: (866) 228-4327
E-mail: grants@cancer.org
Web: www.cancer.org

Summary To provide financial assistance to graduate students working on a doctoral degree in cancer nursing.

Eligibility This program is open to registered nurses with a current license to practice who are enrolled in or applying to a doctoral degree program in cancer nursing at an academic institution within the United States. The institution must offer an organized multidisciplinary program in cancer control or cancer care that allows a student the flexibility to develop educational and research activities related to cancer nursing. Applicants must be U.S. citizens or permanent residents; be committed to preparing for a career full time; have had experience in professional nursing (as well as cancer nursing); be involved in professional organizations; be involved in the American Cancer Society and other volunteer organizations; have published or contributed to publications and creative works; have received professional and personal awards and honors; have clear, explicit, and realistic professional goals; have considered geographic location and financial needs as well as program components in selecting a doctoral program; have conducted or plan to conduct research that is meritorious, methodologically sound, and relevant to cancer nursing; have identified a faculty sponsor who is experienced in their area of study and will provide guidance in academic and research activities; have selected a doctoral program that will support their professional goals and research; and have made a career commitment to cancer nursing. They must be preparing to work in the following fields of cancer nursing: research, education, administration, or clinical practice.

Financial Data The stipend is $15,000 per year. Payments are made to the institution at the beginning of each semester.

Duration 2 years; may be renewed for an additional 2-year period.

Number awarded Varies each year.

Deadline October of each year.

[504]
DORIS BLOCH RESEARCH AWARD

Sigma Theta Tau International
Attn: Research Services
550 West North Street
Indianapolis, IN 46202-3191
(317) 634-8171   Toll Free: (888) 634-7575
Fax: (317) 634-8188   E-mail: research@stti.iupui.edu
Web: www.nursingsociety.org

Summary To provide funding to nurses, especially members of Sigma Theta Tau International, interested in conducting research.

Eligibility This program is open to registered nurses who have a current license. Applicants must have a master's or doctoral degree in nursing or be enrolled in a doctoral program. Novice researchers who have received no other national research funds are especially encouraged to apply. Preference is given to members of Sigma Theta Tau International. Selection is based on the quality of the proposed research, future promise of the applicant, and the research budget.

Financial Data The maximum grant is $5,000.

Duration 1 year.

Number awarded 1 each year.

Deadline November of each year.

[505]
DOROTHEA FUNK SCHOLARSHIP

Arkansas Nurses Association
Attn: Arkansas Nurses Foundation
1123 South University, Suite 1015
Little Rock, AR 72204
(501) 244-2363   Fax: (501) 244-9903
E-mail: arna@arna.org
Web: www.arna.org/snas/ar/fdtn/info.htm

Summary To provide financial assistance to residents of Arkansas interested in working on a graduate degree in community health nursing at a school in any state.

Eligibility This program is open to residents of Arkansas who have a current nursing license and have graduated from a regionally-accredited program (i.e., L.P.N., R.N., B.S.N., M.S.N., or A.P.N.). Applicants must be interested in working on an advanced degree in community health nursing at a school in any state. Along with their application, they must submit a cover letter describing their desire for the scholarship and intended use of funds, a statement regarding institutional financial assistance, a current resume, 2 letters of recommendation, official transcripts, a letter of acceptance into an advanced degree program accredited by NLNAC or CCNE (except doctoral programs), and a list of extracurricular activities.

Financial Data A stipend is awarded (amount not specified).

Duration 1 year.

Number awarded 1 each year.

Deadline May of each year.

[506]
DOROTHY CORNELIUS AMERICAN NURSES FOUNDATION SCHOLAR AWARD

American Nurses Foundation
Attn: Nursing Research Grants Program
8515 Georgia Avenue, Suite 400
Silver Spring, MD 20910-3492
(301) 628-5227   Fax: (301) 628-5354
E-mail: anf@ana.org
Web: www.anfonline.org

Summary To provide funding to nurses interested in conducting research.

Eligibility This program is open to registered nurses who have earned a baccalaureate or higher degree. Applicants must be beginning researchers who have had no more than 3 research-based publications in refereed journals and have received, as a principal investigator, no more than $15,000 in extramural funding in any 1 research area. Proposed research may be for a master's thesis or doctoral dissertation, if the project has been approved by the principal investigator's thesis or dissertation committee. There are no restrictions on the research topic.

Financial Data The grant is $5,000. Funds may not be used as a salary for the principal investigator.

Duration 1 year.

Additional data　There is a $100 application fee.
Number awarded　1 each year.
Deadline　April of each year.

[507]
DOROTHY E. GENERAL SCHOLARSHIP

Seattle Foundation
Attn: African American Scholarship Program
1200 Fifth Avenue, Suite 1300
Seattle, WA 98101-3151
(206) 622-2294　　　　　　　　Fax: (206) 622-7673
E-mail: scholarships@seattlefoundation.org
Web: www.seattlefoundation.org/page32313.cfm

Summary　To provide financial assistance to African Americans from any state working on an undergraduate or graduate degree in a field related to health care.

Eligibility　This program is open to African American undergraduate and graduate students who are preparing for a career in a health care profession, including public health, medicine, nursing, or dentistry; pre-professional school students are also eligible. Applicants must be able to demonstrate financial need, academic competence, and leadership of African American students. They may be residents of any state attending school in any state. Along with their application, they must submit a 2-page essay describing their future aspirations, including their career goals and how their study of health care will help them achieve those goals and contribute to the African American community.

Financial Data　The stipend is $1,000 per year. Payments are made directly to the recipient's educational institution.

Duration　1 year; may be renewed.

Number awarded　1 or more each year.

Deadline　February of each year.

[508]
DOROTHY E. REILLY AMERICAN NURSES FOUNDATION SCHOLAR AWARD

American Nurses Foundation
Attn: Nursing Research Grants Program
8515 Georgia Avenue, Suite 400
Silver Spring, MD 20910-3492
(301) 628-5227　　　　　　　　Fax: (301) 628-5354
E-mail: anf@ana.org
Web: www.anfonline.org

Summary　To provide funding to nurses interested in conducting research on pediatric or life-span immunization issues.

Eligibility　This program is open to registered nurses who have earned a baccalaureate or higher degree. Applicants may be either beginning or experienced researchers. They must be interested in conducting research on nursing education or curriculum development. Proposed research may be for a master's thesis or doctoral dissertation, if the project has been approved by the principal investigator's thesis or dissertation committee.

Financial Data　The grant is $5,000. Funds may not be used as a salary for the principal investigator.

Duration　1 year.

Additional data　This program was established in 2005. There is a $100 application fee. Recipients are expected to make the results of their research available to nurses either through publication (monograph, abstract, or journal article) or conference presentation.

Number awarded　1 each year.

Deadline　April of each year.

[509]
DR. LORRAINE G. SPRANZO MEMORIAL SCHOLARSHIP

Community Foundation of Greater New Britain
Attn: Scholarship Manager
74A Vine Street
New Britain, CT 06052-1431
(860) 229-6018, ext. 305　　　　Fax: (860) 225-2666
E-mail: cfarmer@cfgnb.org
Web: www.cfgnb.org

Summary　To provide financial assistance to Connecticut residents or students who are working on a graduate degree in nursing at a school in the state.

Eligibility　This program is open to Connecticut residents or students at accredited schools of nursing in the state. Applicants must be registered nurses seeking an advanced degree in nursing (beyond the 4-year degree nursing level) who have been accepted at an NLN-accredited graduate program leading to an advanced degree in nursing. They must have a GPA of 3.0 or higher, a record of distinguished professional service, and the intent to prepare for a career in community health nursing or nursing informatics.

Financial Data　A stipend is awarded (amount not specified).

Duration　1 year.

Number awarded　1 each year.

Deadline　October of each year.

[510]
DR. SANDRA J. TUNAJEK SCHOLARSHIP FOR NURSE ANESTHESIA EDUCATION

American Association of Nurse Anesthetists
Attn: AANA Foundation
222 South Prospect Avenue
Park Ridge, IL 60068-4001
(847) 655-1170　　　　　　　　Fax: (847) 692-6968
E-mail: foundation@aana.com
Web: www.aanafoundation.com

Summary　To provide financial assistance to members of the American Association of Nurse Anesthetists (AANA) who are residents of Kentucky pursuing further education at a program in any state.

Eligibility　This program is open to members of the association who are residents of Kentucky attending a nurse anesthesia program in any state. Applicants may be working on an entry-level or advanced degree. They must intend to practice in Kentucky after graduation. Along with their application, they must submit a 200-word essay describing why they have chosen nurse anesthesia as a profession and their professional goals for the future. Financial need is also considered in the selection process.

Financial Data　The stipend is $1,500.

Duration　1 year.

Additional data　This program, which began in 2008, is sponsored by the Kentucky Association of Nurse Anesthetists. The application processing fee is $25.

Number awarded　1 each year.

Deadline　March of each year.

[511]
DR. SHEILA PACKARD MEMORIAL SCHOLARSHIP

Connecticut Nurses' Association
Attn: Connecticut Nurses' Foundation
377 Research Parkway, Suite 2D
Meriden, CT 06450-7155
(203) 238-1207　　　　　　　　Fax: (203) 238-3437
E-mail: info@ctnurses.org
Web: www.ctnurses.org/displaycommon.cfm?an=12

Summary To provide funding to students, faculty, and alumni of designated nursing schools who are interested in conducting research on nursing as a healing art.
Eligibility This program is open to students, faculty members, and alumni of the schools of nursing of Boston College, the University of Connecticut, or Yale University. Applicants must be interested in conducting a research project on nursing as a healing art.
Financial Data The grant is $1,500.
Duration 1 year.
Number awarded 2 each year.
Deadline June of each year.

[512]
EASTERN NURSING RESEARCH SOCIETY/ AMERICAN NURSES FOUNDATION SCHOLAR AWARD

American Nurses Foundation
Attn: Nursing Research Grants Program
8515 Georgia Avenue, Suite 400
Silver Spring, MD 20910-3492
(301) 628-5227   Fax: (301) 628-5354
E-mail: anf@ana.org
Web: www.anfonline.org

Summary To provide funding to members of the Eastern Nursing Research Society (ENRS) who are interested in conducting research.
Eligibility This program is open to registered nurses who have earned a baccalaureate or higher degree. Applicants may be either beginning or experienced researchers. Proposed research may be for a master's thesis or doctoral dissertation if the project has been approved by the principal investigator's thesis or dissertation committee. There are no restrictions on the research topic, but applicants must be current ENRS members.
Financial Data The grant is $3,500. Funds may not be used as a salary for the principal investigator.
Duration 1 year.
Additional data Funding for this program is provided by the ENRS. There is a $100 application fee.
Number awarded 1 each year.
Deadline April of each year.

[513]
EASTERN NURSING RESEARCH SOCIETY/ COUNCIL FOR THE ADVANCEMENT OF NURSING SCIENCE DISSERTATION AWARD

Eastern Nursing Research Society
Attn: Associate Director
100 North 20th Street, Fourth Floor
Philadelphia, PA 19103
(215) 599-6700   Fax: (215) 564-2175
E-mail: info@enrs-go.org
Web: www.enrs-go.org

Summary To provide dissertation research funding to doctoral candidates who are members of both the Eastern Nursing Research Society (ENRS) and the Council for the Advancement of Nursing Science (CANS).
Eligibility This program is open to doctoral candidates in nursing at schools or colleges of nursing that award a research doctoral degree requiring a dissertation. Applicants must be members of both ENRS and CANS. They must submit a research proposal conforming to the standard NIH format. Selection is based on significance of the research study to nursing science, innovativeness of proposed methods, likelihood that the study will lead to an important program of research, qualification and scholarly activity of the applicant, and clarity and preciseness of the proposal.
Financial Data Grants range up to $4,000.

Duration 1 year.
Number awarded 1 or more each year.
Deadline January of each year.

[514]
ECLIPSYS CLINICAL INFORMATICS SCHOLARSHIP

Healthcare Information and Management Systems Society
Attn: HIMSS Foundation
230 East Ohio Street, Suite 500
Chicago, IL 60611-3270
(312) 915-9277   Fax: (312) 664-6143
E-mail: foundation@himss.org
Web: www.himss.org/foundation/schlr_Eclipsys.asp

Summary To provide financial assistance to student members of the Healthcare Information and Management Systems Society (HIMSS) who are working on an undergraduate or graduate degree in health care information management.
Eligibility This program is open to upper-division and graduate students working full time on a degree in a health care information management systems field. Applicants must be members of HIMSS. They may be studying in any relevant field, but preference is given to students enrolled in a nursing, medical, or health informatics program. Along with their application, they must submit a personal statement that includes their career goals, past achievements, and future goals. Selection is based on that statement, academic achievement, and financial need.
Financial Data The stipend is $5,000. The award includes an all-expense paid trip to the annual conference and exhibition of HIMSS.
Duration 1 year; nonrenewable.
Additional data This scholarship, first offered in 2008, is sponsored by Eclipsys Corporation.
Number awarded 1 each year.
Deadline October of each year.

[515]
EDWARD HYLAND, CRNA SCHOLARSHIP

American Association of Nurse Anesthetists
Attn: AANA Foundation
222 South Prospect Avenue
Park Ridge, IL 60068-4001
(847) 655-1170   Fax: (847) 692-6968
E-mail: foundation@aana.com
Web: www.aanafoundation.com

Summary To provide financial assistance to members of the American Association of Nurse Anesthetists (AANA) from Delaware who are interested in obtaining further education.
Eligibility This program is open to members of the association who are currently enrolled in an accredited nurse anesthesia education program. Applicants must have completed 1 year in a program whose primary clinical site is a hospital in Delaware. Preference is given to residents of Delaware. Along with their application, they must submit a 200-word essay describing why they have chosen nurse anesthesia as a profession and their professional goals for the future. Financial need is also considered in the selection process.
Financial Data The stipend is $1,000.
Duration 1 year.
Additional data This scholarship was first awarded in 2003. The application processing fee is $25.
Number awarded 1 each year.
Deadline March of each year.

[516]
EDWARD J. AND VIRGINIA M. ROUTHIER NURSING SCHOLARSHIP

Rhode Island Foundation
Attn: Funds Administrator
One Union Station
Providence, RI 02903
(401) 427-4017   Fax: (401) 331-8085
E-mail: lmonahan@rifoundation.org
Web: www.rifoundation.org

Summary To provide financial assistance to undergraduate and graduate students enrolled in nursing programs in Rhode Island.

Eligibility This program is open to students enrolled or accepted at an accredited nursing program in Rhode Island. Applicants must be 1) registered nurses (R.N.s) enrolled in a nursing baccalaureate degree program; 2) students enrolled in a baccalaureate nursing program; or 3) R.N.s working on a graduate degree (master's or Ph.D.). They must be able to demonstrate financial need and a commitment to practice in Rhode Island. Along with their application, they must submit an essay, up to 300 words, on their career goals, particularly as they relate to practicing in or advancing the field of nursing in Rhode Island.

Financial Data The stipend ranges from $500 to $3,000 per year.

Duration 1 year; may be renewed.

Number awarded Varies each year. Recently, 11 of these scholarships were awarded: 6 new awards and 5 renewals.

Deadline April of each year.

[517]
EIGHT AND FORTY LUNG AND RESPIRATORY DISEASE NURSING SCHOLARSHIP

American Legion
Attn: Americanism and Children & Youth Division
700 North Pennsylvania Street
P.O. Box 1055
Indianapolis, IN 46206-1055
(317) 630-1323   Fax: (317) 630-1223
E-mail: acy@legion.org
Web: www.legion.org/programs/resources/scholarships

Summary To provide financial assistance to registered nurses who wish to prepare for advanced positions in lung and respiratory disease nursing supervision, administration, or teaching.

Eligibility This program is open to registered nurses who are graduates of an accredited school of nursing and who wish to continue their studies in the field of lung and respiratory disease nursing on either a full-time or part-time basis. Awards are based on personal and academic qualifications, especially past experience and future employment prospects as they relate to lung and respiratory disease nursing. U.S. citizenship is required.

Financial Data The stipend is $3,000 per year.

Duration 1 year.

Additional data The Eight and Forty was organized by members of the American Legion Auxiliary in 1922; it began awarding these scholarships in 1957.

Number awarded Varies each year.

Deadline May of each year.

[518]
ELEANOR BINDRUM SCHOLARSHIP

Florida Nurses Association
Attn: Florida Nurses Foundation
1235 East Concord Street
P.O. Box 536985
Orlando, FL 32853-6985
(407) 896-3261   Fax: (407) 896-9042
E-mail: foundation@floridanurse.org
Web: www.floridanurse.org/foundationGrants/index.asp

Summary To provide financial assistance to Florida residents who are interested in working on an undergraduate or graduate degree in nursing.

Eligibility Applicants must have been Florida residents for at least 1 year and have completed at least 1 semester at an accredited nursing program in the state. They may be working on an associate, baccalaureate, master's, or doctoral degree. Preference is given to perioperative nurses returning to school in south Florida. Undergraduates must have a GPA of 2.5 or higher and graduate students a GPA of 3.0 or higher. Along with their application, they must submit 1-page essays on 1) why it is necessary for them to receive this scholarship; and 2) their goals and their assessment of their potential for making a contribution to nursing and society.

Financial Data A stipend is awarded (amount not specified).

Duration 1 semester or year.

Number awarded 1 or more each year.

Deadline May of each year.

[519]
ELEANOR LAMBERTSON AMERICAN NURSES FOUNDATION SCHOLAR AWARD

American Nurses Foundation
Attn: Nursing Research Grants Program
8515 Georgia Avenue, Suite 400
Silver Spring, MD 20910-3492
(301) 628-5227   Fax: (301) 628-5354
E-mail: anf@ana.org
Web: www.anfonline.org

Summary To provide funding to nurses interested in conducting research.

Eligibility This program is open to registered nurses who have earned a baccalaureate or higher degree. Applicants must be beginning researchers who have had no more than 3 research-based publications in refereed journals and have received, as a principal investigator, no more than $15,000 in extramural funding in any 1 research area. Proposed research may be for a master's thesis or doctoral dissertation, if the project has been approved by the principal investigator's thesis or dissertation committee. There are no restrictions on the research topic.

Financial Data The grant is $3,500. Funds may not be used as a salary for the principal investigator.

Duration 1 year.

Additional data There is a $100 application fee.

Number awarded 1 each year.

Deadline April of each year.

[520]
ELIZABETH GARDE NATIONAL SCHOLARSHIP

Danish Sisterhood of America
Attn: Donna Hansen, Scholarship Chair
1605 South 58th Street
Lincoln, NE 68506
(402) 488-5820   E-mail: djhansen@windstream.net
Web: www.danishsisterhood.org/dssScholGrant.asp

Summary To provide financial assistance for nursing or medical education to members or relatives of members of the Danish Sisterhood of America.

Eligibility This program is open to members or the family of members of the sisterhood who have been members for at least 1 year. Applicants must be working on an undergraduate or graduate degree in the nursing or medical profession. They must have a GPA of 3.0 or higher.

Financial Data The stipend is $850.

Duration 1 year; nonrenewable.

Number awarded 1 each year.

Deadline February of each year.

[521]
ENA FOUNDATION DOCTORAL SCHOLARSHIPS

Emergency Nurses Association
Attn: ENA Foundation
915 Lee Street
Des Plaines, IL 60016-6569
(847) 460-4100   Toll Free: (800) 900-9659, ext. 4100
Fax: (847) 460-4004   E-mail: foundation@ena.org
Web: www.ena.org

Summary To provide financial assistance for doctoral study to nurses who are members of the Emergency Nurses Association (ENA).

Eligibility This program is open to nurses (R.N.) who are working on a doctoral degree (Ph.D. or D.N.P.) to prepare for a career as a faculty member at a college of nursing. Applicants must have been members of the association for at least 12 months and have a GPA of 3.0 or higher. Along with their application, they must submit 1) a 100-word statement on their professional and educational goals and how this scholarship will help them attain those goals; and 2) a 100-word explanation of how this scholarship will further the practice of emergency nursing. Students who are more than 6 months beyond the completion of all formal course work and comprehensive examinations are not eligible. Selection is based on content and clarity of the goal statement (45%), professional association involvement (35%), presentation of the application (10%), and letters of reference (10%).

Financial Data The stipend is $5,000.

Duration 1 year; nonrenewable.

Number awarded Varies each year; recently, 3 of these scholarships were awarded.

Deadline May of each year.

[522]
ENA FOUNDATION SCHOLARSHIP IN HEALTHCARE OR RELATED FIELD

Emergency Nurses Association
Attn: ENA Foundation
915 Lee Street
Des Plaines, IL 60016-6569
(847) 460-4100   Toll Free: (800) 900-9659, ext. 4100
Fax: (847) 460-4004   E-mail: foundation@ena.org
Web: www.ena.org/foundation/scholarships

Summary To provide financial assistance to members of the Emergency Nurses Association (ENA) who are working on a master's degree in a field related to health care.

Eligibility This program is open to emergency nurses (R.N.) who are working on a master's degree in a field related to health care. Examples include (but are not limited to) business (M.B.A.), public health (M.P.H.), nurse education (N.Ed.), and informatics. Applicants must have been members of the association for at least 12 months and have a GPA of 3.0 or higher. They must submit a 1-page statement on their professional and educational goals and how this scholarship will help them attain those goals. Selection is based on content and clarity of the goal statement (45%), professional association involvement (35%), presentation of the application (10%), and letters of reference (10%).

Financial Data The stipend is $5,000.

Duration 1 year.

Number awarded 1 each year.

Deadline May of each year.

[523]
ENA FOUNDATION STATE CHALLENGE SCHOLARSHIPS

Emergency Nurses Association
Attn: ENA Foundation
915 Lee Street
Des Plaines, IL 60016-6569
(847) 460-4100   Toll Free: (800) 900-9659, ext. 4100
Fax: (847) 460-4004   E-mail: foundation@ena.org
Web: www.ena.org/foundation/scholarships

Summary To provide financial assistance to members of the Emergency Nurses Association (ENA) who are working on a master's degree.

Eligibility This program is open to emergency nurses (R.N.) who are working on a master's degree in nursing. Applicants must have been members of the association for at least 12 months and have a GPA of 3.0 or higher. They must submit a 1-page statement on their professional and educational goals and how this scholarship will help them attain those goals. Selection is based on content and clarity of the goal statement (45%), professional association involvement (35%), presentation of the application (10%), and letters of reference (10%).

Financial Data The stipend is $4,000 or $3,000.

Duration 1 year.

Number awarded 10 each year: 4 at $4,000 and 6 at $3,000.

Deadline May of each year.

[524]
END-OF-LIFE/PALLIATIVE CARE SMALL PROJECTS GRANTS

American Association of Critical-Care Nurses
Attn: Research Department
101 Columbia
Aliso Viejo, CA 92656-4109
(949) 362-2000, ext. 551
Toll Free: (800) 809-CARE, ext. 551
Fax: (949) 362-2020   E-mail: research@aacn.org
Web: www.aacn.org

Summary To provide funding to investigators, including students, who wish to conduct research on end of life and/or palliative care outcomes in critical care.

Eligibility This program is open to investigators who are proposing to conduct a research project focusing on end of life and/or palliative care outcomes in critical care. Eligible projects may focus on any age group (neonatal to elderly) in the critical care arena and may include patient education programs, staff development programs, CQI projects, outcomes evaluation projects, or small clinical research studies. Topics may include bereavement (e.g., family, patient, or caregiver); communication issues (e.g., verbal, non-verbal, written); caregiver needs (e.g., stress, education, emotional support); symptom management (e.g., nausea, vomiting, pain, anxiety, skin breakdown, dyspnea); advanced directives (e.g., staff/patient education, program development, ethical considerations); or life support withdrawal (e.g., ethical/legal concerns, clinical protocols). Funds may be awarded for new projects, projects in progress, or projects required for an academic degree. Collaborative projects are encouraged and may involve interdisciplinary teams, multiple nursing units, home health, subacute and transitional care, other institutions, or community agencies.

Financial Data The maximum grant is $500. Funds may be used to cover direct project expenses, such as printed materials, small equipment, supplies (including computer software), and assistive personnel. They may not be used for salaries or institutional overhead.

Number awarded   2 each year.
Deadline   September of each year.

[525]
ENVIRONMENT OF ELDER CARE NURSING RESEARCH GRANT

Sigma Theta Tau International
Attn: Research Services
550 West North Street
Indianapolis, IN 46202-3191
(317) 634-8171   Toll Free: (888) 634-7575
Fax: (317) 634-8188   E-mail: research@stti.iupui.edu
Web: www.nursingsociety.org

Summary   To provide funding to nurses interested in conducting research on elder care.
Eligibility   This program is open to registered nurses who have at least a master's or equivalent degree or are enrolled in a doctoral program. Applicants must be interested in conducting a research project focused on critical aspects of elder care, including clear lungs, no falls, safe skin, patient comfort, and ease-of-use. Applications from novice researchers who have received no other national research funds are encouraged. Preference is given to members of Sigma Theta Tau International, other qualifications being equal.
Financial Data   The maximum grant is $9,000.
Duration   1 year.
Additional data   Funding for this program is provided by Hill-Rom.
Number awarded   1 each year.
Deadline   June of each year.

[526]
EPILEPSY FOUNDATION BEHAVIORAL SCIENCES STUDENT FELLOWSHIPS

Epilepsy Foundation
Attn: Research Department
8301 Professional Place
Landover, MD 20785-2237
(301) 459-3700   Toll Free: (800) EFA-1000
Fax: (301) 577-2684   TDD: (800) 332-2070
E-mail: grants@efa.org
Web: www.epilepsyfoundation.org/research/grants.cfm

Summary   To provide funding to undergraduate and graduate students interested in working on a summer research training project in a behavioral science field relevant to epilepsy.
Eligibility   This program is open to undergraduate and graduate students in a behavioral science program relevant to epilepsy research or clinical care, including, but not limited to, sociology, social work, psychology, anthropology, nursing, economics, vocational rehabilitation, counseling, and political science. Applicants must be interested in working on an epilepsy research project under the supervision of a qualified mentor. Because the program is designed as a training opportunity, the quality of the training plans and environment are considered in the selection process. Other selection criteria include the quality of the proposed project, the relevance of the proposed work to epilepsy, the applicant's interest in the field of epilepsy, the applicant's qualifications, and the mentor's qualifications, including his or her commitment to the student and the project. U.S. citizenship is not required, but the project must be conducted in the United States. Applications from women, members of minority groups, and people with disabilities are especially encouraged. The program is not intended for students working on a dissertation research project.
Financial Data   The grant is $3,000.
Duration   3 months during the summer.
Additional data   This program is supported by the American Epilepsy Society, Abbott Laboratories, Ortho-McNeil Pharmaceutical Corporation, and Pfizer Inc.

Number awarded   Varies each year.
Deadline   February of each year.

[527]
ERNESTINE F. SHAW ENDOWED SCHOLARSHIP

Kansas State Nurses Association
Attn: Kansas Nurses Foundation
1109 S.W. Topeka Boulevard
Topeka, KS 66612-1602
(785) 233-8638   Fax: (785) 233-5222
E-mail: ksna@ksna.net
Web: www.nursingworld.org/SNAS/KS/Knf.htm

Summary   To provide financial assistance to residents of Kansas who are working on a degree in nursing at the undergraduate, master's, or doctoral level at a school in the state.
Eligibility   This program is open to students who are working on a nursing degree on the undergraduate or graduate level at a school in Kansas. Preference is given to residents of Sedgwick and Sumner counties. Applicants must have a GPA of 3.0 or higher. Along with their application, they must submit a personal narrative describing their anticipated role in nursing in the state of Kansas. Preference is given to full-time students. The following priority is used in awarding scholarships: 1) students enrolled in undergraduate R.N. nursing programs; 2) R.N.s working on B.S.N.s; and 3) graduate and postgraduate nursing students.
Financial Data   The stipend is $500.
Duration   1 year.
Additional data   This program was established in 2008.
Number awarded   1 each year.
Deadline   June of each year.

[528]
ESTELLE MASSEY OSBORNE SCHOLARSHIP

Nurses Educational Funds, Inc.
Attn: Scholarship Coordinator
304 Park Avenue South, 11th Floor
New York, NY 10010
(212) 590-2443   Fax: (212) 590-2446
E-mail: info@n-e-f.org
Web: www.n-e-f.org

Summary   To provide financial assistance to African Americans interested in earning a master's degree in nursing.
Eligibility   This program is open to African American registered nurses who are members of a national professional nursing organization and enrolled full or part time in an accredited master's degree program in nursing. Applicants must have completed at least 12 credits and have a cumulative GPA of 3.6 or higher. They must be U.S. citizens or have declared their official intention of becoming a citizen. Along with their application, they must submit an 800-word essay on their professional goals and potential for making a contribution to the nursing profession. Selection is based on academic excellence and the essay's content and clarity.
Financial Data   Stipends range from $2,500 to $10,000, depending on the availability of funds.
Duration   1 year; nonrenewable.
Additional data   There is a $20 application fee.
Number awarded   1 each year.
Deadline   February of each year.

[529]
EUNICE M. SMITH SCHOLARSHIPS

North Carolina Nurses Association
Attn: North Carolina Foundation for Nursing
103 Enterprise Street
P.O. Box 12025
Raleigh, NC 27605-2025
(919) 821-4250   Toll Free: (800) 626-2153
Fax: (919) 829-5807   E-mail: rns@ncnurses.org
Web: www.ncnurses.org/ncfn.asp

Summary To provide financial assistance to registered nurses in North Carolina who are interested in pursing additional education on a part-time basis.

Eligibility This program is open to registered nurses in North Carolina who are interested in pursuing additional education at the baccalaureate, master's, or doctoral level on a part-time basis. Applicants must be North Carolina residents (for at least 12 months prior to application), must be admitted to a program in North Carolina offering a nursing degree on the baccalaureate, master's, or Ph.D. level, must be enrolled part time but for at least 6 hours per semester, and must have a cumulative GPA of 3.0 or higher. Selection is based on GPA, professional involvement, community involvement, potential for contribution to the profession, and honors and certifications. Preference is given to members of the North Carolina Nurses Association.

Financial Data The stipend is $2,500 per year for graduate students or $1,000 per year for undergraduates.

Duration 1 year.

Additional data This program was established in 1995.

Number awarded 1 or more each year.

Deadline May of each year.

[530]
FADONA/LTC SCHOLARSHIP

Florida Association Directors of Nursing Administration/Long Term Care
200 Butler Street, Suite 305
West Palm Beach, FL 33407
(561) 659-2167   Fax: (561) 659-1291
E-mail: fadona@fadona.org
Web: www.fadona.org/scholarship.html

Summary To provide financial assistance to individuals employed in long-term care in Florida who are interested in continuing their education.

Eligibility This program is open to currently licensed R.N.s, L.P.N.s, or certified nursing assistants (C.N.A.s) employed in the long-term care industry in Florida. R.N.s must be currently accepted or enrolled in a baccalaureate or master's degree program in nursing, gerontology program, undergraduate or graduate program in health care management, or nurse practitioner program. L.P.N.s must be currently accepted or enrolled in an R.N. program or undergraduate health care management program. C.N.A.s must be currently accepted or enrolled in an R.N. or L.P.N. program. All applicants must have at least 2 years of employment in the long-term care field (a list of employers and dates of employment is required). They must be either a member of the Florida Association Directors of Nursing Administration/ Long Term Care or sponsored by a member. Financial need is not considered in the selection process.

Financial Data The stipend is at least $500. Funds are paid directly to the college, university, or accredited L.P.N. school.

Duration 1 year.

Number awarded 1 or more each year.

Deadline October of each year.

[531]
FILIPINO NURSES' ORGANIZATION OF HAWAII SCHOLARSHIP

Hawai'i Community Foundation
Attn: Scholarship Department
1164 Bishop Street, Suite 800
Honolulu, HI 96813
(808) 566-5570   Toll Free: (888) 731-3863
Fax: (808) 521-6286   E-mail: scholarships@hcf-hawaii.org
Web: www.hawaiicommunityfoundation.org

Summary To provide financial assistance to Hawaii residents of Filipino ancestry who are interested in preparing for a career as a nurse.

Eligibility This program is open to Hawaii residents of Filipino ancestry who are interested in studying in Hawaii or the mainland as full-time undergraduate or graduate students and majoring in nursing. They must be able to demonstrate academic achievement (GPA of 2.7 or higher), good moral character, and financial need. Along with their application, they must submit a short statement indicating their reasons for attending college, their planned course of study, and their career goals.

Financial Data The amounts of the awards depend on the availability of funds and the need of the recipient; recently, stipends averaged $1,000.

Duration 1 year.

Number awarded Varies each year; recently, 2 of these scholarships were awarded.

Deadline February of each year.

[532]
FLORENCE WHIPPLE SCHOLARSHIP

Idaho Nurses Association
Attn: Idaho Nurses Foundation
3525 Piedmont Road
Building 5, Suite 300
Atlanta, GA 30305
(404) 760-2803   Toll Free: (888) 721-8904
Fax: (404) 240-0998   E-mail: ed@idahonurses.org
Web: www.idahonurses.org

Summary To provide financial assistance to members of the Idaho Nurses Association (INA) and other residents of Idaho who are interested in obtaining training in nursing.

Eligibility This program is open to 1) INA members who are registered nurses and have been accepted to an accredited school of nursing to work on an advanced degree, and 2) residents of Idaho who are interesting in continuing their education at a school of nursing in or outside of Idaho. Applicants must be able to demonstrate financial need and a potential for making a definite contribution to nursing.

Financial Data The stipend varies; recently, it was $646.

Duration 1 year; may be renewed up to 2 additional years.

Additional data This program was established in 1956 as the Florence Whipple Scholarship and Loan Fund. The loan program was eventually closed.

Number awarded Varies each year; recently, 5 of these scholarships were awarded.

Deadline Deadline not specified.

[533]
FLORIDA ASSOCIATION OF NURSE ANESTHETISTS STUDENT SCHOLARSHIP AWARD

American Association of Nurse Anesthetists
Attn: AANA Foundation
222 South Prospect Avenue
Park Ridge, IL 60068-4001
(847) 655-1170   Fax: (847) 692-6968
E-mail: foundation@aana.com
Web: www.aanafoundation.com

Summary To provide financial assistance to members of the American Association of Nurse Anesthetists (AANA) from any state who are interested in obtaining further education at a program in Florida.

Eligibility This program is open to members of the association from any state who are currently enrolled in an accredited nurse anesthesia education program in Florida. Applicants must be second-year students who have completed 12 months of nurse anesthesia classes. Along with their application, they must submit a 200-word essay describing why they have chosen nurse anesthesia as a profession and their professional goals for the future. Financial need is also considered in the selection process.

Financial Data The stipend is $3,000.

Duration 1 year.

Additional data This scholarship, first awarded in 2009, is supported by the Florida Association of Nurse Anesthetists. The application processing fee is $25.

Number awarded 1 each year.

Deadline March of each year.

[534]
FLORIDA NURSES FOUNDATION SCHOLARSHIPS

Florida Nurses Association
Attn: Florida Nurses Foundation
1235 East Concord Street
P.O. Box 536985
Orlando, FL 32853-6985
(407) 896-3261   Fax: (407) 896-9042
E-mail: foundation@floridanurse.org
Web: www.floridanurse.org/foundationGrants/index.asp

Summary To provide financial assistance to Florida residents who are interested in working on an undergraduate or graduate degree in nursing.

Eligibility Applicants must have been Florida residents for at least 1 year and have completed at least 1 semester at an accredited nursing program in the state. They may be working on an associate, baccalaureate, master's, or doctoral degree. Undergraduates must have a GPA of 2.5 or higher and graduate students a GPA of 3.0 or higher. Along with their application, they must submit 1-page essays on 1) why it is necessary for them to receive this scholarship; and 2) their goals and their assessment of their potential for making a contribution to nursing and society.

Financial Data A stipend is awarded (amount not specified).

Duration 1 semester or year.

Additional data This program includes the following named programs open to all qualified applicants: the Edna Hicks Fund Scholarships, the Mary York Scholarships, the Undine Sams and Friends Scholarships, and the Ruth Finamore Scholarships.

Number awarded Varies each year.

Deadline May of each year.

[535]
FLORIDA ORGANIZATION OF NURSE EXECUTIVES RESEARCH GRANT

Florida Organization of Nurse Executives
Attn: Research Committee
307 Park Lake Circle
P.O. Box 533992
Orlando, FL 32853-3992
(407) 277-5515   Fax: (407) 277-5215
E-mail: fonexo@aol.com
Web: www.fonexo.com/committees/research.html

Summary To provide funding to members of the Florida Organization of Nurse Executives (FONE) who are interested in conducting a research project.

Eligibility This program is open to FONE members who qualify as a beginning researcher (i.e., have not been awarded more than $15,000 in external research funding and have not published

more than 3 research articles in peer-reviewed journals). Students in master's or doctoral programs are eligible, if a faculty mentor agrees to supervise the project. Applicants must be interested in conducting research on a nursing administration and leadership topic. The proposal should focus on a strategic priority of FONE: design of future patient care delivery systems, healthful practice environments, leadership, and/or positioning nurse leaders as valued health care executives and managers. The project must represent a new study or an enhancement to a study in process.

Financial Data The grant is $1,000. Funds may be used only for direct costs; investigator salary support and indirect costs are not supported.

Duration The project must be completed within 24 months.

Number awarded 1 each year.

Deadline March of each year.

[536]
FOUNDATION FOR NEONATAL RESEARCH AND EDUCATION RESEARCH GRANTS

Academy of Neonatal Nursing
Attn: Foundation for Neonatal Research and Education
200 East Holly Avenue
P.O. Box 56
Pitman, NJ 08071-0056
(856) 256-2343   Fax: (856) 589-7463
E-mail: FNRE@ajj.com
Web: www.inurse.com/fnre/grants.htm

Summary To provide funding to neonatal nurses and students interested in conducting a research project.

Eligibility Applicants must be professionally active neonatal nurses, engaged in a service, research, or educational role that contributes directly to the health care of neonates or to the neonatal nursing profession (includes all professional neonatal nursing roles and neonatal nursing students). They must be an active member of a professional association dedicated to enhancing neonatal nursing and the care of neonates. Participation in ongoing professional education in neonatal nursing must be demonstrated by at least 10 contact hours in neonatal content over the past 24 months.

Financial Data Grants up to $10,000 per project are available.

Duration 1 year or longer.

Additional data The Foundation for Neonatal Research and Education was established in 1992 by the National Association of Neonatal Nurses (NANN). Originally housed at the NANN office, it moved to its current location in 1998.

Number awarded Several each year.

Deadline April of each year.

[537]
FOUNDATION FOR NEONATAL RESEARCH AND EDUCATION SCHOLARSHIPS

Academy of Neonatal Nursing
Attn: Foundation for Neonatal Research and Education
200 East Holly Avenue
P.O. Box 56
Pitman, NJ 08071-0056
(856) 256-2343   Fax: (856) 589-7463
E-mail: FNRE@ajj.com
Web: www.inurse.com/fnre/scholarship.htm

Summary To provide financial assistance to neonatal nurses interested in working on a degree.

Eligibility Applicants must be professionally active neonatal nurses engaged in a service, research, or educational role that contributes directly to the health care of neonates or to the neonatal nursing profession. They must be an active member of a professional association dedicated to enhancing neonatal nursing and the care of neonates. Participation in ongoing professional education in neonatal nursing must be demonstrated by at least 10 contact hours in neonatal content over the past 24 months. Qualified nurses must have been admitted to a college or school of higher education to work on 1 of the following: bachelor of science in nursing, master of science in nursing for advanced practice in neonatal nursing, doctoral degree in nursing, or master's or post-master's degree in nursing administration or business management. They must have a GPA of 3.0 or higher. Along with their application, they must submit a 250-word statement on how they plan to make a significant difference in neonatal nursing practice. Financial need is not considered in the selection process.

Financial Data The stipends are $1,500 or $1,000.

Duration 1 year.

Additional data The Foundation for Neonatal Research and Education was established in 1992 by the National Association of Neonatal Nurses (NANN), 2270 Northpoint Parkway, Santa Rosa, CA 95407, (707) 568-2168. Originally housed at the NANN office, it moved to its current location in 1998.

Number awarded Varies each year.

Deadline April of each year.

[538]
FRANK T. MAZIARSKI, CRNA, MS SCHOLARSHIPS

American Association of Nurse Anesthetists
Attn: AANA Foundation
222 South Prospect Avenue
Park Ridge, IL 60068-4001
(847) 655-1170   Fax: (847) 692-6968
E-mail: foundation@aana.com
Web: www.aanafoundation.com

Summary To provide financial assistance to members of the American Association of Nurse Anesthetists (AANA) who are interested in obtaining further education, especially at schools in Washington.

Eligibility This program is open to members of the association who are currently enrolled in an accredited nurse anesthesia education program. Preference is given to students enrolled at schools in Washington. First-year students must have completed 6 months of nurse anesthesia classes; second-year students must have completed 12 months of nurse anesthesia classes. Along with their application, they must submit a 200-word essay describing why they have chosen nurse anesthesia as a profession and their professional goals for the future. Financial need is also considered in the selection process.

Financial Data The stipend is $3,000.

Duration 1 year.

Additional data This scholarship was first awarded in 2005. The application processing fee is $25.

Number awarded 1 each year.

Deadline March of each year.

[539]
FRIENDS OF NURSING SCHOLARSHIPS

Friends of Nursing
Attn: Scholarship Chair
P.O. Box 735
Englewood, CO 80151-0735
(303) 449-5318   E-mail: asmith2498@aol.com
Web: www.friendsofnursing.org/scholarships.htm

Summary To provide financial assistance to residents of any state who are working on an undergraduate or graduate degree in nursing at a school in Colorado.

Eligibility This program is open to registered nurses and nursing students who are residents of any state and working on a B.S.N. or higher degree at an NLN-accredited school of nursing in Colorado. Applicants must be enrolled at least as juniors and have a GPA of 3.0 or higher. Along with their application, they

must submit a 3-page essay in which they identify a health care issue in Colorado that they believe will have a major impact on nursing in the future, a discussion of their professional nursing beliefs, and a description of their career goals (including how they anticipate their education or research will contribute or help them achieve those goals). Financial need is considered in the selection process.

Financial Data A stipend is awarded (amount not specified).

Duration 1 year.

Number awarded 1 or more each year.

Deadline October of each year.

[540]
GALA SCHOLARSHIPS

American Association of Nurse Anesthetists
Attn: AANA Foundation
222 South Prospect Avenue
Park Ridge, IL 60068-4001
(847) 655-1170   Fax: (847) 692-6968
E-mail: foundation@aana.com
Web: www.aanafoundation.com

Summary To provide financial assistance to members of the American Association of Nurse Anesthetists (AANA) who are interested in obtaining further education in a program that respects and supports gay and lesbian people.

Eligibility This program is open to members of the association who are currently enrolled in an accredited nurse anesthesia education program that respects and supports gay and lesbian people. First-year students must have completed 6 months of nurse anesthesia classes; second-year students must have completed 12 months of nurse anesthesia classes. Along with their application, they must submit a 200-word essay describing why they have chosen nurse anesthesia as a profession and their professional goals for the future. Financial need is also considered in the selection process. The purpose of these scholarships is to honor gay and lesbian anesthetists.

Financial Data The stipend is $1,000.

Duration 1 year.

Additional data These scholarships were first awarded in 2001. The application processing fee is $25.

Number awarded 5 each year.

Deadline March of each year.

[541]
GANA SCHOLARSHIP

American Association of Nurse Anesthetists
Attn: AANA Foundation
222 South Prospect Avenue
Park Ridge, IL 60068-4001
(847) 655-1170   Fax: (847) 692-6968
E-mail: foundation@aana.com
Web: www.aanafoundation.com

Summary To provide financial assistance to members of the American Association of Nurse Anesthetists (AANA) from Georgia who are interested in obtaining further education.

Eligibility This program is open to members of the association who are registered nurses licensed to practice in Georgia and currently enrolled in an accredited nurse anesthesia education program in the state. Applicants must have completed 3 semesters as a full-time student. Along with their application, they must submit a 200-word essay describing why they have chosen nurse anesthesia as a profession and their professional goals for the future. Financial need is also considered in the selection process.

Financial Data The stipend is $1,000.

Duration 1 year.

Additional data Funding for this scholarship, first awarded in 2000, is provided by the Georgia Association of Nurse Anesthetists (GANA). The application processing fee is $25.

Number awarded 1 each year.
Deadline March of each year.

[542]
GARDNER FOUNDATION INS EDUCATION SCHOLARSHIP

Infusion Nurses Society
Attn: Gardner Foundation
315 Norwood Park South
Norwood, MA 02062
(781) 440-9408   Toll Free: (800) 694-0298
Fax: (781) 440-9409   E-mail: ins@ins1.org
Web: www.ins1.org/i4a/pages/index.cfm?pageid=3344

Summary To provide financial assistance to members of the Infusion Nurses Society (INS) who are interested in continuing their education.

Eligibility This program is open to INS members interested in a program of continuing education, including working on a college or graduate degree or attending a professional meeting or seminar. Applicants must demonstrate how the continuing education activity will enhance their infusion career, describe their professional goals, and explain how the scholarship will be used.

Financial Data The stipend is $1,000.
Duration This is a 1-time award.
Number awarded 2 each year.
Deadline January of each year.

[543]
GE HEALTHCARE DOCTORAL SCHOLARSHIP

Emergency Nurses Association
Attn: ENA Foundation
915 Lee Street
Des Plaines, IL 60016-6569
(847) 460-4100   Toll Free: (800) 900-9659, ext. 4100
Fax: (847) 460-4004   E-mail: foundation@ena.org
Web: www.ena.org

Summary To provide financial assistance for doctoral study to nurses who are members of the Emergency Nurses Association (ENA).

Eligibility This program is open to nurses (R.N.) who are working on a doctoral degree (Ph.D. or D.N.P.) to prepare for a career as a faculty member at a college of nursing. Applicants must have been members of the association for at least 12 months and have a GPA of 3.0 or higher. Along with their application, they must submit 1) a 100-word statement on their professional and educational goals and how this scholarship will help them attain those goals; and 2) a 100-word explanation of how this scholarship will further the practice of emergency nursing. Students who are more than 6 months beyond the completion of all formal course work and comprehensive examinations are not eligible. Selection is based on content and clarity of the goal statement (45%), professional association involvement (35%), presentation of the application (10%), and letters of reference (10%).

Financial Data The stipend is $5,000.
Duration 1 year; nonrenewable.
Additional data This program is sponsored by GE Healthcare.
Number awarded 1 each year.
Deadline May of each year.

[544]
GENEVIEVE SARAN RICHMOND AWARD

ExceptionalNurse.com
Attn: Scholarship Committee
13019 Coastal Circle
Palm Beach Gardens, FL 33410
(561) 627-9872   Fax: (561) 776-9254
TDD: (561) 776-9442   E-mail: ExceptionalNurse@aol.com
Web: www.ExceptionalNurse.com/scholarship.php

Summary To provide financial assistance to nursing students who have a disability.

Eligibility This program is open to students with a documented disability who have applied to, or have already been admitted to, a college or university nursing program on a full-time basis. Applicants must submit an essay on how they plan to contribute to the nursing profession and how their disability will influence their practice as a nurse. Selection is based on the essay, transcripts of high school and/or college courses completed, activities and honors received, 3 letters of recommendation, and financial need.

Financial Data The stipend is $500.
Duration 1 year; nonrenewable.
Number awarded 1 each year.
Deadline May of each year.

[545]
GEORGE B. BOLAND ADVANCED DEGREE PROGRAM OF NURSING EDUCATION

National Forty and Eight
Attn: Voiture Nationale
777 North Meridian Street
Indianapolis, IN 46204-1170
(317) 634-1804   Fax: (317) 632-9365
E-mail: voiturenationale@msn.com
Web: fortyandeight.org/40_8programs.htm

Summary To provide financial assistance to students working on an advanced degree in nursing.

Eligibility This program is open to students working full time on an advanced degree in nursing. Applications must be submitted to the local Voiture of the Forty and Eight in the county of the student's permanent residence; if the county organization has exhausted all of its nurses training funds, it will provide the student with an application for this scholarship. Students who are receiving assistance from the Eight and Forty Lung and Respiratory Disease Nursing Scholarship Program of the American Legion are not eligible. Financial need must be demonstrated.

Financial Data Grants may be used to cover tuition, required fees, room and board or similar living expenses, and other school-related expenses.

Additional data National Forty and Eight is the Honor Society of the American Legion. Students may not apply directly to the National Forty and Eight for these scholarships.

Number awarded Varies each year.
Deadline Deadline not specified.

[546]
GEORGE DEVANE CRNA ENDOWED SCHOLARSHIP

Kansas State Nurses Association
Attn: Kansas Nurses Foundation
1109 S.W. Topeka Boulevard
Topeka, KS 66612-1602
(785) 233-8638   Fax: (785) 233-5222
E-mail: ksna@ksna.net
Web: www.nursingworld.org/SNAS/KS/Knf.htm

Summary To provide financial assistance to residents of any state enrolled in a nurse anesthesia program in Kansas.

Eligibility This program is open to residents of any state currently enrolled in a Kansas nurse anesthesia program that is certified by the Council on Certification of the American Association of Nurse Anesthetists. CRNAs working toward a degree are not eligible. Preference is given to applicants in their second year of study, enrolled in school full time, and able to demonstrate greater financial need. Applicants must have a GPA of 3.0 or higher and must submit a personal narrative describing their anticipated role in nursing in the state.

Financial Data The stipend is $1,000.
Duration 1 year.

Number awarded   1 each year.
Deadline   June of each year.

[547]
GEORGE GUSTAFSON HSE MEMORIAL SCHOLARSHIP

American Society of Safety Engineers
Attn: ASSE Foundation
1800 East Oakton Street
Des Plaines, IL 60018
(847) 768-3435   Fax: (847) 768-3434
E-mail: agabanski@asse.org
Web: www.asse.org/foundation/scholarships/scholarships.php

Summary   To provide financial assistance to upper-division and graduate student members of the American Society of Safety Engineers (ASSE), especially those from Texas.

Eligibility   This program is open to ASSE student members who are working on an undergraduate or graduate degree in occupational safety, health, and environment or a closely-related field (e.g., industrial or environmental engineering, environmental science, industrial hygiene, occupational health nursing). Priority is given to residents of Texas or students attending a university in the state. Undergraduates must be full-time students who have completed at least 60 semester hours with a GPA of 3.0 or higher. Graduate students must also be enrolled full time, have completed at least 9 semester hours with a GPA of 3.5 or higher, and have earned a GPA of 3.0 or higher as an undergraduate. Along with their application, they must submit 2 essays of 300 words or less: 1) why they are seeking a degree in occupational safety and health or a closely-related field, a brief description of their current activities, and how those relate to their career goals and objectives; and 2) why they should be awarded this scholarship (including career goals and financial need). U.S. citizenship is not required.

Financial Data   The stipend is $2,500 per year.

Duration   1 year; recipients may reapply.

Additional data   This program, established in 2006, is supported by the Texas Safety Foundation.

Number awarded   1 each year.

Deadline   November of each year.

[548]
GEORGIA NURSES FOUNDATION SCHOLARSHIPS

Georgia Nurses Foundation, Inc.
Attn: Scholarship Committee
3032 Briarcliff Road, N.E.
Atlanta, GA 30329-2655
(404) 325-5536   Toll Free: (800) 324-0462
Fax: (404) 325-0407   E-mail: gnf@georgianurses.org
Web: www.georgianurses.org/scholarship_appl.htm

Summary   To provide financial assistance to Georgia residents who are working on a nursing degree, at any level, at an accredited school, college, or university.

Eligibility   This program is open to residents of Georgia who are currently enrolled (full or part time) in an NLN-accredited program in nursing. Applicants may be working on a degree at any level (including associate, baccalaureate, master's, or doctoral). They must have a GPA of 2.5 or higher and be able to document financial need. Priority is given to applicants who meet the following criteria: enrolled in a Georgia school, plan to practice professional nursing in Georgia following graduation, and belong to a professional organization (e.g., Georgia Association of Nursing Students, Georgia Nurses Association, Georgia Association for Nursing Education).

Financial Data   The stipend is at least $500. Funds may be sent directly to the recipient.

Duration   1 year.

Number awarded   Varies each year.
Deadline   June of each year.

[549]
GLENN AND GRETA SNELL ENDOWMENT FUND SCHOLARSHIP

Kansas State Nurses Association
Attn: Kansas Nurses Foundation
1109 S.W. Topeka Boulevard
Topeka, KS 66612-1602
(785) 233-8638   Fax: (785) 233-5222
E-mail: ksna@ksna.net
Web: www.nursingworld.org/SNAS/KS/Knf.htm

Summary   To provide financial assistance to residents of Kansas who are working on a degree in nursing at the undergraduate, master's, or doctoral level at a school in the state.

Eligibility   This program is open to students who are working on a nursing degree on the undergraduate or graduate level at a school in Kansas. Applicants must have a GPA of 3.0 or higher. Along with their application, they must submit a personal narrative describing their anticipated role in nursing in the state of Kansas. Preference is given to full-time students. The following priority is used in awarding scholarships: 1) students enrolled in undergraduate R.N. nursing programs and employed by Hutchinson Hospital; 2) R.N.s working on B.S.N.s and employed by Hutchinson Hospital; 3) R.N.s accepted by a nursing program to prepare for a faculty position in Kansas; and 4) R.N.s with a B.S.N. and accepted by a graduate program with a major in nursing supervision or administration for a position in Kansas.

Financial Data   The stipend is $1,000.

Duration   1 year.

Number awarded   1 each year.

Deadline   June of each year.

[550]
GLORIA SMITH AMERICAN NURSES FOUNDATION SCHOLAR AWARD

American Nurses Foundation
Attn: Nursing Research Grants Program
8515 Georgia Avenue, Suite 400
Silver Spring, MD 20910-3492
(301) 628-5227   Fax: (301) 628-5354
E-mail: anf@ana.org
Web: www.anfonline.org

Summary   To provide funding to nurses interested in conducting research on health care delivery to socioeconomic and ethnic minority populations.

Eligibility   This program is open to registered nurses who have earned a baccalaureate or higher degree. Applicants may be either beginning or experienced researchers. They must be interested in conducting research on accessibility or quality of health care delivery to socioeconomic and ethnic minority populations. Proposed research may be for a master's thesis or doctoral dissertation if the project has been approved by the principal investigator's thesis or dissertation committee.

Financial Data   The grant is $5,000. Funds may not be used as a salary for the principal investigator.

Duration   1 year.

Additional data   There is a $100 application fee.

Number awarded   Up to 4 each year.

Deadline   April of each year.

[551]
GOLD COUNTRY SECTION AND REGION II SCHOLARSHIP

American Society of Safety Engineers
Attn: ASSE Foundation
1800 East Oakton Street
Des Plaines, IL 60018
(847) 768-3435   Fax: (847) 768-3434
E-mail: agabanski@asse.org
Web: www.asse.org/foundation/scholarships/scholarships.php

Summary To provide financial assistance to upper-division and graduate student members of the American Society of Safety Engineers (ASSE) from designated western states.

Eligibility This program is open to ASSE student members who are working on an undergraduate or graduate degree in occupational safety, health, and environment or a closely-related field (e.g., industrial or environmental engineering, environmental science, industrial hygiene, occupational health nursing). Priority is given to residents of ASSE Region II (Arizona, Colorado, Idaho, Montana, Nevada, New Mexico, Utah, and Wyoming). Undergraduates must be full-time students who have completed at least 60 semester hours with a GPA of 3.0 or higher. Graduate students must also be enrolled full time, have completed at least 9 semester hours with a GPA of 3.5 or higher, and have had a GPA of 3.0 or higher as an undergraduate. Along with their application, they must submit 2 essays of 300 words or less: 1) why they are seeking a degree in occupational safety and health or a closely-related field, a brief description of their current activities, and how those relate to their career goals and objectives; and 2) why they should be awarded this scholarship (including career goals and financial need). U.S. citizenship is not required.

Financial Data The stipend is $1,000 per year.

Duration 1 year; recipients may reapply.

Number awarded 1 each year.

Deadline November of each year.

[552]
GONZALEZ PEDIATRIC NP STUDENT SCHOLARSHIP

American Academy of Nurse Practitioners
Attn: AANP Foundation
P.O. Box 12924
Austin, TX 78711-2924
(512) 276-5905   Fax: (512) 442-6469
E-mail: foundation@aanp.org
Web: aanp.org

Summary To provide financial assistance to members of the American Academy of Nurse Practitioners (AANP) who are working on a master's degree as a pediatric nurse practitioner (NP).

Eligibility This program is open to members of the academy who are enrolled in an M.S.N. degree program as a pediatric nurse practitioner. Applicants must have a GPA of 3.5 or higher. They must have completed at least 1 course for their master's program requirements but they cannot be finishing their degree during the current year. U.S. citizenship is required.

Financial Data The stipend is $1,000. Funds may be used only for educational expenses (tuition, books, equipment, etc.), not for expenses related to master's thesis and/or general research projects.

Duration 1 year.

Additional data This program was established in 2007. There is a $10 application fee.

Number awarded 1 each year.

Deadline October of each year.

[553]
GOOD SAMARITAN FOUNDATION SCHOLARSHIPS

Good Samaritan Foundation
5615 Kirby Drive, Suite 308
Houston, TX 77005
(713) 529-4646   Fax: (713) 521-1169
Web: www.gsftx.org/scholarships

Summary To provide financial assistance to student nurses enrolled in a program in nursing at an accredited university in Texas.

Eligibility This program is open to residents of Texas who have attained the clinical level of their nursing education. Applicants must be enrolled at an institution in Texas in an accredited nursing program at the L.V.N., Diploma, A.D.N., B.S.N., M.S.N., Ph.D., D.S.N., or D.N.P. level. They must be U.S. citizens or eligible to work in the United States and be planning to work as a nurse in Texas after graduation. Financial need is considered in the selection process. A personal interview is required.

Financial Data Scholarship awards may be used for clinical education expenses: tuition, fees, books, and some copying and seminars. Undergraduate awards are based on the amount of the tuition fees of that school and its nursing program. Graduate awards are paid on a reimbursement basis up to a pre-determined amount per semester.

Duration 1 year.

Additional data This program began in 1951.

Number awarded Varies each year. Since the program began, it has awarded more than 12,000 scholarships worth more than $14.6 million.

Deadline There are no formal deadlines, but applications should be received at least 8 weeks before the start of the semester.

[554]
GRADUATE SCHOLARSHIPS IN CANCER NURSING PRACTICE

American Cancer Society
Attn: Research Department
250 Williams Street, N.W.
Atlanta, GA 30303-1002
(404) 329-7558   Toll Free: (800) ACS-2345
Fax: (404) 321-4669   TDD: (866) 228-4327
E-mail: grants@cancer.org
Web: www.cancer.org

Summary To provide financial assistance to graduate students working on a master's degree or Doctor of Nursing Practice (D.N.P.) in cancer nursing.

Eligibility This program is open to registered nurses with a current license to practice who are enrolled in or applying to a master's degree or D.N.P. program in cancer nursing at an academic institution within the United States. Applicants must be U.S. citizens or permanent residents, be committed to preparing for a career full time, have had experience in professional nursing (as well as cancer nursing), be involved in professional and academic organizations, be involved in the American Cancer Society and other volunteer organizations, have published or contributed to publications and creative works, have received professional and personal awards and honors, have a focus for scholarly activity in a specific area of cancer nursing, have explicit and realistic professional goals, and be committed to a career in cancer nursing. They must be preparing to work in the following fields of cancer nursing: research, education, administration, or clinical practice.

Financial Data The stipend is $10,000 per year. Payments are made to the institution at the beginning of each semester.

Duration 1 to 2 years.

Number awarded Varies each year.

Deadline January of each year.

[555]
GREATER BOSTON CHAPTER LEADERSHIP AWARD

American Society of Safety Engineers
Attn: ASSE Foundation
1800 East Oakton Street
Des Plaines, IL 60018
(847) 768-3435   Fax: (847) 768-3434
E-mail: agabanski@asse.org
Web: www.asse.org/foundation/scholarships/scholarships.php

Summary   To provide financial assistance to upper-division and graduate students at colleges and universities in New England who are members or family of members of the American Society of Safety Engineers (ASSE).

Eligibility   This program is open to undergraduate and graduate students who are working on a degree in occupational safety, health, and environment or a closely-related field (e.g., industrial or environmental engineering, environmental science, industrial hygiene, occupational health nursing). Applicants must be 1) a member of an ASSE chapter in New England; 2) the spouse or child of an ASSE chapter member in New England; or 3) a member of an ASSE student section in New England. Undergraduates must be full-time students who have completed at least 60 semester hours with a GPA of 3.0 or higher. Graduate students must also be enrolled full time, have completed at least 9 semester hours with a GPA of 3.5 or higher, and have earned a GPA of 3.0 or higher as an undergraduate. Along with their application, they must submit 2 essays of 300 words or less: 1) why they are seeking a degree in occupational safety and health or a closely-related field, a brief description of their current activities, and how those relate to their career goals and objectives; and 2) why they should be awarded this scholarship (including career goals and financial need). U.S. citizenship is not required.

Financial Data   Stipends are $2,000 or $1,000 per year.

Duration   1 year; recipients may reapply.

Number awarded   2 each year: 1 at $2,000 and 1 at $1,000.

Deadline   November of each year.

[556]
GREATER CHICAGO CHAPTER SCHOLARSHIP

American Society of Safety Engineers
Attn: ASSE Foundation
1800 East Oakton Street
Des Plaines, IL 60018
(847) 768-3435   Fax: (847) 768-3434
E-mail: agabanski@asse.org
Web: www.asse.org/foundation/scholarships/scholarships.php

Summary   To provide financial assistance to upper-division and graduate student members of the American Society of Safety Engineers (ASSE) from designated midwestern states.

Eligibility   This program is open to ASSE student members who are working on an undergraduate or graduate degree in occupational safety, health, and environment or a closely-related field (e.g., industrial or environmental engineering, environmental science, industrial hygiene, occupational health nursing). Priority is given to students who reside or attend school in ASSE Region V (Illinois, Iowa, Kansas, Minnesota, Missouri, Nebraska, North Dakota, South Dakota, and Wisconsin). Undergraduates must be full-time students who have completed at least 60 semester hours with a GPA of 3.0 or higher. Graduate students must also be enrolled full time, have completed at least 9 semester hours with a GPA of 3.5 or higher, and have earned a GPA of 3.0 or higher as an undergraduate. Along with their application, they must submit 2 essays of 300 words or less: 1) why they are seeking a degree in occupational safety and health or a closely-related field, a brief description of their current activities, and how those relate to their career goals and objectives; and 2) why they should be awarded this scholarship (including career goals and financial need). U.S. citizenship is not required.

Financial Data   The stipend is $1,000 per year.

Duration   1 year; recipients may reapply.

Additional data   This program, established in 2008, is sponsored by the Greater Chicago Chapter of ASSE.

Number awarded   1 each year.

Deadline   November of each year.

[557]
HAROLD F. POLSTON SCHOLARSHIP

American Society of Safety Engineers
Attn: ASSE Foundation
1800 East Oakton Street
Des Plaines, IL 60018
(847) 768-3435   Fax: (847) 768-3434
E-mail: agabanski@asse.org
Web: www.asse.org/foundation/scholarships/scholarships.php

Summary   To provide financial assistance to upper-division and graduate student members of the American Society of Safety Engineers (ASSE), especially those in specified categories.

Eligibility   This program is open to ASSE student members who are working on an undergraduate or graduate degree in occupational safety, health, and environment or a closely-related field (e.g., industrial or environmental engineering, environmental science, industrial hygiene, occupational health nursing). Priority is given first to members of the Middle Tennessee Chapter of ASSE, second to students at Middle Tennessee State University in Murfreesboro, Tennessee or Murray State University in Murray, Kentucky, and third to residents of ASSE Region VII (Indiana, Kentucky, Michigan, Ohio, Tennessee, or West Virginia). Undergraduates must be full-time students who have completed at least 60 semester hours with a GPA of 3.0 or higher. Graduate students must also be enrolled full time, have completed at least 9 semester hours with a GPA of 3.5 or higher, and have earned a GPA of 3.0 or higher as an undergraduate. Along with their application, they must submit 2 essays of 300 words or less: 1) why they are seeking a degree in occupational safety and health or a closely-related field, a brief description of their current activities, and how those relate to their career goals and objectives; and 2) why they should be awarded this scholarship (including career goals and financial need). U.S. citizenship is not required.

Financial Data   The stipend is $2,000 per year.

Duration   1 year; recipients may reapply.

Additional data   This program, established in 2005, is supported by the Middle Tennessee Chapter of ASSE.

Number awarded   1 each year.

Deadline   November of each year.

[558]
HARRY TABACK 9/11 MEMORIAL SCHOLARSHIP

American Society of Safety Engineers
Attn: ASSE Foundation
1800 East Oakton Street
Des Plaines, IL 60018
(847) 768-3435   Fax: (847) 768-3434
E-mail: agabanski@asse.org
Web: www.asse.org/foundation/scholarships/scholarships.php

Summary   To provide financial assistance to upper-division and graduate student members of the American Society of Safety Engineers (ASSE).

Eligibility   This program is open to ASSE student members who are working on an undergraduate or graduate degree in occupational safety, health, and environment or a closely-related field (e.g., industrial or environmental engineering, environmental science, industrial hygiene, occupational health nursing). Undergraduates must be full-time students who have completed at least 60 semester hours with a GPA of 3.0 or higher. Graduate students must also be enrolled full time, have completed at least 9 semester hours with a GPA of 3.5 or higher, and have earned a GPA of

3.0 or higher as an undergraduate. Along with their application, they must submit 2 essays of 300 words or less: 1) why they are seeking a degree in occupational safety and health or a closely-related field, a brief description of their current activities, and how those relate to their career goals and objectives; and 2) why they should be awarded this scholarship (including career goals and financial need). U.S. citizenship is required.

Financial Data The stipend is $1,000 per year.

Duration 1 year; recipients may reapply.

Additional data This program was established to honor a victim of the attack on the World Trade Center on September 11, 2001.

Number awarded 1 each year.

Deadline November of each year.

[559]
HAZEL P. CURRIER MEMORIAL SCHOLARSHIP

American Association of Nurse Anesthetists
Attn: AANA Foundation
222 South Prospect Avenue
Park Ridge, IL 60068-4001
(847) 655-1170   Fax: (847) 692-6968
E-mail: foundation@aana.com
Web: www.aanafoundation.com

Summary To provide financial assistance to members of the American Association of Nurse Anesthetists (AANA) who are interested in obtaining further education.

Eligibility This program is open to members of the association who are currently enrolled in an accredited nurse anesthesia education program. First-year students must have completed 6 months of nurse anesthesia classes; second-year students must have completed 12 months of nurse anesthesia classes. Along with their application, they must submit a 200-word essay describing why they have chosen nurse anesthesia as a profession and their professional goals for the future. Financial need is also considered in the selection process.

Financial Data The stipend is $3,000.

Duration 1 year.

Additional data This program began in 2008. The application processing fee is $25.

Number awarded 1 each year.

Deadline March of each year.

[560]
HEALTH CARE FOR MONTANANS SCHOLARSHIP

New West Health Services
130 Neill Avenue
Helena, MT 59601
(406) 457-2200   Toll Free: (888) 500-3355
Fax: (406) 457-2299   E-mail: czipperian@nwhp.com
Web: www.newwesthealth.com/home/about/scholarships

Summary To provide financial assistance to Montana residents who are working on an undergraduate or graduate degree in a health-care related field at designated institutions in the state.

Eligibility This program is open to residents of Montana who are preparing for a career in health care at a designated institution within the state. Applicants must be enrolled in 1) their second year at a 2-year college, 2) their junior or senior year at a 4-year college or university, or 3) a graduate program in public health and/or nursing. They must have a GPA of 3.0 or higher and be able to demonstrate financial need (expected family financial contribution of $7,500 or less). Along with their application, they must submit a 250-word essay on their concept of an ideal health care job in 5 years and how that would fit their vision of what Montana's health care delivery should look like.

Financial Data The stipend for students working on a bachelor's or master's degree is $2,000. The stipend for students working on an associate degree is $1,000.

Duration 1 year; nonrenewable.

Additional data This program was established in 2008. The designated institutions are Montana State University at Bozeman, Montana State University at Billings, Montana State University-Northern, University of Montana at Missoula, Montana Tech of the University of Montana at Butte, Carroll College, University of Great Falls, Rocky Mountain College, Helena College of Technology, and Flathead Valley Community College.

Number awarded Up to 9 each year.

Deadline April of each year.

[561]
HELEN LAIDLAW FOUNDATION NURSING AND HEALTH CARE SCHOLARSHIPS

Helen Laidlaw Foundation
c/o Nancy E. Huck, President
314 Newman Street
East Tawas, MI 48730-1214
(989) 362-9117   Fax: (989) 362-7675

Summary To provide financial assistance to Michigan residents interested in preparing for a health care-related career at a school in any state.

Eligibility This program is open to high school seniors and students who are currently enrolled full time in an undergraduate or graduate degree or nondegree program at a school in any state. Applicants must be preparing for a career in a health care field. Nursing candidates receive preference. In the selection process, consideration is given first to residents of northeastern Michigan and second to those from the entire state.

Financial Data Stipends range from $500 to $1,500 per year. Funds are paid directly to the recipient's school.

Duration 1 year; may be renewed.

Deadline February of each year.

[562]
HERTA GAST AWARD FOR CHILD/ADOLESCENT PSYCHIATRIC NURSING RESEARCH

International Society of Psychiatric-Mental Health Nurses
Attn: ISPN Foundation
2810 Crossroads Drive, Suite 3800
Madison, WI 53718
(608) 443-2463   Toll Free: (866) 330-7227
Fax: (608) 443-2474   E-mail: info@ispn-psych.org
Web: www.ispn-psych.org/html/foundation.html

Summary To provide funding to members of the International Society of Psychiatric-Mental Health Nurses (ISPN) who are interested in conducting research in psychiatric mental health nursing.

Eligibility This program is open to psychiatric nurses who 1) are active members of the association's Association of Child and Adolescent Psychiatric Nurses Division, and 2) already have a master's or doctoral degree in nursing or are working on a master's or doctoral degree in nursing. Applicants must be interested in conducting research (qualitative or quantitative) related to psychiatric mental health nursing. Proposals (no more than 5 single-spaced pages) must include: title and purpose, background and significance, hypotheses and research questions, methods, budget, timeline, and references.

Financial Data The grant is $1,500.

Duration 1 year.

Number awarded 1 each year.

Deadline December of each year.

[563]
HILDEGARD E. PEPLAU AMERICAN NURSES FOUNDATION SCHOLAR AWARD

American Nurses Foundation
Attn: Nursing Research Grants Program
8515 Georgia Avenue, Suite 400
Silver Spring, MD 20910-3492
(301) 628-5227 Fax: (301) 628-5354
E-mail: anf@ana.org
Web: www.anfonline.org

Summary To provide funding to nurses interested in conducting research on psychiatric-mental health nursing.

Eligibility This program is open to registered nurses who have earned a baccalaureate or higher degree. Applicants may be either beginning or experienced researchers. They must be interested in conducting research on psychiatric-mental health nursing with an interpersonal relations focus. The research outcomes should advance the clinical practice of nursing and contribute to knowledge about psycho-social phenomena in nursing. Proposed research may be for a master's thesis or doctoral dissertation, if the project has been approved by the principal investigator's thesis or dissertation committee.

Financial Data The grant is $3,500. Funds may not be used as a salary for the principal investigator.

Duration 1 year.

Additional data This program was established in 1995. There is a $100 application fee.

Number awarded 1 each year.

Deadline April of each year.

[564]
H.M. MUFFLY MEMORIAL SCHOLARSHIP

Colorado Nurses Foundation
7400 East Arapahoe Road, Suite 211
Centennial, CO 80112
(303) 694-4728 Fax: (303) 694-4869
E-mail: mail@cnfound.org
Web: www.cnfound.org/scholarships.html

Summary To provide financial assistance to residents of Colorado who are working on a bachelor's or higher degree in nursing at a college or university in the state.

Eligibility This program is open to Colorado residents who have been accepted as a student in an approved nursing program in the state. Applicants must be working on a bachelor's or higher degree. Undergraduates must have a GPA of 3.25 or higher and graduate students must have a GPA of 3.5 or higher. Selection is based on professional philosophy and goals, dedication to the improvement of patient care in Colorado, demonstrated commitment to nursing, critical thinking skills, potential for leadership, involvement in community and professional organizations, recommendations, GPA, and financial need.

Financial Data The stipend is $3,000.

Duration 1 year.

Number awarded 2 each year.

Deadline October of each year.

[565]
HOSPICE AND PALLIATIVE NURSES FOUNDATION EDUCATIONAL SCHOLARSHIP

Hospice and Palliative Nurses Foundation
Attn: Director of Development
One Penn Center West, Suite 229
Pittsburgh, PA 15276-0100
(412) 787-9301 Fax: (412) 787-9305
Web: www.hpnf.org/DisplayPage.aspx?Title=Scholarships

Summary To provide financial assistance to members of the Hospice and Palliative Nurses Association (HPNA) who are interested in working on an academic degree.

Eligibility This program is open to HPNA members providing end-of-life care. Applicants must be enrolled in a school of nursing or doctoral program and have successfully completed at least 1 semester of course work. Along with their application, they must submit a 1-page essay on how they would use the funds if they are selected, their career plans following completion of this degree program, and how they plan to use their education to advance end-of-life care.

Financial Data The stipend is $500. Funds may be used for tuition, books, computer software, or supplies related to nursing education.

Duration 1 year; nonrenewable.

Additional data This program began in 2004.

Number awarded 4 each year: 1 in each degree program (associate, bachelor's, master's, doctoral).

Deadline May of each year.

[566]
HPNF CERTIFICATION RESEARCH GRANT

Hospice and Palliative Nurses Foundation
Attn: Director of Development
One Penn Center West, Suite 229
Pittsburgh, PA 15276-0100
(412) 787-9301 Fax: (412) 787-9305
Web: www.hpnf.org

Summary To provide funding to doctoral candidates and other scholarships who are interested in conducting research related to certification in the field of hospice and palliative nursing.

Eligibility This program is open to students enrolled in a doctoral program and to scholars who have a master's or doctoral degree. Applicants must be interested in conducting a research project that involves the impact of certification within the field of hospice and palliative nursing. They must currently be actively involved in some aspect of hospice and palliative care practice, education, or research.

Financial Data The grant is $15,000.

Duration Research must be completed within 1 year.

Number awarded 1 each year.

Deadline May of each year.

[567]
ILLINOIS ASSOCIATION OF NURSE ANESTHETISTS SCHOLARSHIPS

American Association of Nurse Anesthetists
Attn: AANA Foundation
222 South Prospect Avenue
Park Ridge, IL 60068-4001
(847) 655-1170 Fax: (847) 692-6968
E-mail: foundation@aana.com
Web: www.aanafoundation.com

Summary To provide financial assistance to members of the American Association of Nurse Anesthetists (AANA) from any state who are interested in obtaining further education at a program in Illinois.

Eligibility This program is open to members of the association from any state who are currently enrolled in an accredited nurse anesthesia education program in Illinois. First-year students must have completed 6 months of nurse anesthesia classes; second-year students must have completed 12 months of nurse anesthesia classes. Along with their application, they must submit a 200-word essay describing why they have chosen nurse anesthesia as a profession and their professional goals for the future. Financial need is also considered in the selection process.

Financial Data The stipend is $3,000.

Duration 1 year.

Additional data Funding for this scholarship, first awarded in 2010, is provided by the Illinois Association of Nurse Anesthetists. The application processing fee is $25.

Number awarded 1 each year.
Deadline March of each year.

[568]
ILLINOIS NURSE EDUCATOR SCHOLARSHIP PROGRAM

Illinois Student Assistance Commission
Attn: Scholarship and Grant Services
1755 Lake Cook Road
Deerfield, IL 60015-5209
(847) 948-8550   Toll Free: (800) 899-ISAC
Fax: (847) 831-8549   TDD: (800) 526-0844
E-mail: collegezone@isac.org
Web: www.collegezone.com/studentzone/596_8833.htm

Summary To provide scholarship/loans to residents of Illinois working on a graduate degree in nursing at a school in the state and interested in becoming a nurse educator after graduation.

Eligibility This program is open to Illinois residents who are enrolled or accepted for enrollment at least half time in a graduate program in professional nursing education at an approved institution of higher education in the state. Applicants must be planning to teach in Illinois in the field of nursing education. U.S. citizenship or eligible non-citizenship status is required.

Financial Data Students who attend a public college or university receive a scholarship that covers tuition and fees. Students who attend a private college or university receive a scholarship equal to the amount paid for the most expensive comparable program at an Illinois public institution. In addition, all students receive a stipend of up to $10,000 to cover the cost of attendance, including living expenses. This is a scholarship/loan program; recipients must sign an agreement to teach nursing in Illinois. If the teaching commitment is not fulfilled, the recipient must repay the entire amount received plus interest and reasonable collection costs.

Duration Up to 4 calendar years.
Number awarded Varies each year.
Deadline February of each year.

[569]
ILLINOIS NURSES ASSOCIATION CENTENNIAL SCHOLARSHIP

Illinois Nurses Association
Attn: Illinois Nurses Foundation
105 West Adams Street, Suite 2101
Chicago, IL 60603
(312) 419-2900   Fax: (312) 419-2920
E-mail: info@illinoisnurses.com
Web: www.illinoisnurses.com

Summary To provide financial assistance to nursing undergraduate and graduate students who are members of underrepresented groups.

Eligibility This program is open to students working on an associate, bachelor's, or master's degree at an accredited NLNAC or CCNE school of nursing. Applicants must be members of a group underrepresented in nursing (African Americans, Hispanics, American Indians, Asians, and males). Undergraduates must have earned a passing grade in all nursing courses taken to date and have a GPA of 2.85 or higher. Graduate students must have completed at least 12 semester hours of graduate work and have a GPA of 3.0 or higher. All applicants must be willing to 1) act as a spokesperson to other student groups on the value of the scholarship to continuing their nursing education, and 2) be profiled in any media or marketing materials developed by the Illinois Nurses Foundation. Along with their application, they must submit a narrative of 250 to 500 words on how they, as a nurse, plan to affect policy at either the state or national level that impacts on nursing or health care generally, or how they believe they will impact the nursing profession in general.

Financial Data A stipend is awarded (amount not specified).
Duration 1 year.
Number awarded 1 or more each year.
Deadline March of each year.

[570]
ILLINOIS STATE COUNCIL "THE LAND OF LINCOLN" SCHOLARSHIP

Emergency Nurses Association
Attn: ENA Foundation
915 Lee Street
Des Plaines, IL 60016-6569
(847) 460-4100   Toll Free: (800) 900-9659, ext. 4100
Fax: (847) 460-4004   E-mail: foundation@ena.org
Web: www.ena.org

Summary To provide financial assistance to members of the Emergency Nurses Association (ENA) who are working on a master's degree.

Eligibility This program is open to emergency nurses (R.N.) who are working on a master's degree. Applicants must have been members of the association for at least 12 months and have a GPA of 3.0 or higher. They must submit a 1-page statement on their professional and educational goals and how this scholarship will help them attain those goals. Selection is based on content and clarity of the goal statement (45%), professional association involvement (35%), presentation of the application (10%), and letters of reference (10%).

Financial Data The stipend is $5,000.
Duration 1 year.
Additional data This program is funded by the Illinois ENA State Council.
Number awarded 1 each year.
Deadline May of each year.

[571]
IMOGENE KING RESEARCH GRANT

Florida Nurses Association
Attn: Florida Nurses Foundation
1235 East Concord Street
P.O. Box 536985
Orlando, FL 32853-6985
(407) 896-3261   Fax: (407) 896-9042
E-mail: foundation@floridanurse.org
Web: www.floridanurse.org/foundationGrants/index.asp

Summary To provide funding to graduate nursing students in Florida who are interested in conducting a research project.

Eligibility This program is open to registered nurses licensed to practice in Florida and interested in conducting a research project. Applicants must be graduate students working on a master's thesis or doctoral dissertation. They may not have received more than a cumulative total of $5,000 in research funding during the past 3 years. Selection is based on significance to nursing, scientific merit, innovation, appropriateness of the methodology to the research question, qualifications of the investigator, adequacy of human subjects and animal protection, and appropriateness of budget, environment, support, and time frame.

Financial Data Grants range from $500 to $750. Funds may be used only for direct research expenses. The following are not covered: salary, educational assistance expenses (such as tuition or textbooks), costs related to travel, expenses associated with presenting a paper or attending a conference, or purchase of personal computers and other equipment.

Duration 1 year.
Additional data There is a $25 application fee.
Number awarded 1 each year.
Deadline May of each year.

[572]
IMOGENE WARD NURSING SCHOLARSHIP

Florida Association Directors of Nursing Administration/Long
  Term Care
200 Butler Street, Suite 305
West Palm Beach, FL 33407
(561) 659-2167   Fax: (561) 659-1291
E-mail: fadona@fadona.org
Web: www.fadona.org/scholarship-ward.html

Summary To provide financial assistance to employees of long-term care facilities in Florida who are interested in becoming a registered nurse.

Eligibility This program is open to employees of long-term care facilities in Florida who are nominated by their employer. If their employer is not a member of Florida Association Directors of Nursing Administration/Long Term Care, the nomination must be endorsed by a member. Nominees must be enrolled at an accredited Florida nursing program and working on certification as an R.N. They must be willing to pledge at least 2 years working full-time in long-term care in Florida. Along with their application, they must submit a 300-word essay on what it takes to be an exceptional nurse. Nominees may be interviewed.

Financial Data A stipend is awarded (amount not specified).

Duration 1 year.

Number awarded 1 or more each year.

Deadline October of each year.

[573]
INDIANA ASSOCIATION OF NURSE ANESTHETISTS SCHOLARSHIP

American Association of Nurse Anesthetists
Attn: AANA Foundation
222 South Prospect Avenue
Park Ridge, IL 60068-4001
(847) 655-1170   Fax: (847) 692-6968
E-mail: foundation@aana.com
Web: www.aanafoundation.com

Summary To provide financial assistance to members of the American Association of Nurse Anesthetists (AANA) from Indiana who are interested in obtaining further education and working in that state.

Eligibility This program is open to members of the association from Indiana who are currently enrolled in an accredited nurse anesthesia education program in any state. First-year students must have completed 6 months of nurse anesthesia classes; second-year students must have completed 12 months of nurse anesthesia classes. Preference is given to applicants who are interested in returning to Indiana after graduation and being involved in the Indiana Association of Nurse Anesthetists. Along with their application, they must submit a 200-word essay describing why they have chosen nurse anesthesia as a profession and their professional goals for the future. Financial need is also considered in the selection process.

Financial Data The stipend is $1,000.

Duration 1 year.

Additional data Funds for this scholarship, first awarded in 2005, are provided by the Indiana Association of Nurse Anesthetists. The application processing fee is $25.

Number awarded 2 each year.

Deadline March of each year.

[574]
INSTITUTE FOR NURSING GENERAL SCHOLARSHIPS

New Jersey State Nurses Association
Attn: Institute for Nursing
1479 Pennington Road
Trenton, NJ 08618-2661
(609) 883-5335   Toll Free: (888) UR-NJSNA
Fax: (609) 883-5343   E-mail: institute@njsna.org
Web: www.njsna.org/displaycommon.cfm?an=5

Summary To provide financial assistance to New Jersey residents who are preparing for a career as a nurse at a school in the state.

Eligibility Applicants must be New Jersey residents currently enrolled in a diploma, associate, baccalaureate, or master's nursing program located in the state. Applicants who are R.N.s must be members of the New Jersey State Nurses Association. Selection is based on financial need, GPA, and leadership potential.

Financial Data The stipend is $1,000.

Duration 1 year.

Number awarded Varies each year; recently, 2 of these scholarships were awarded.

Deadline January of each year.

[575]
INTERNATIONAL ORGANIZATION OF MULTIPLE SCLEROSIS NURSES RESEARCH GRANT

International Organization of Multiple Sclerosis Nurses
Attn: Research Committee
359 Main Street, Suite A
Hackensack, NJ 07601
(201) 487-1050   Fax: (201) 678-2291
E-mail: info@iomsn.org
Web: www.iomsn.org/Research_Grant.htm

Summary To provide financial assistance to student and professional members of the International Organization of Multiple Sclerosis Nurses (IOMSN) who are interested in conducting a research project.

Eligibility This program is open to IOMSN members who are registered nurses active in or demonstrating interest in multiple sclerosis nursing; graduate student researchers are also eligible. Applicants must be interested in conducting a quantitative or qualitative research project that addresses clinical practice dimensions of multiple sclerosis nursing.

Financial Data The grant is $5,000.

Duration Projects must be completed within 2 years.

Additional data This program is supported by Teva Neuroscience. Recipients must submit a publishable manuscript presenting the research to an appropriate refereed journal and present a paper or poster pertaining to the research at a multiple sclerosis, neuroscience, or rehabilitation conference within 2 to 3 years of initial funding.

Number awarded 1 each year.

Deadline Applications may be submitted at any time.

[576]
IOWA HEALTH CARE ASSOCIATION FOUNDATION SCHOLARSHIP

Iowa Health Care Association
Attn: Iowa Health Care Association Foundation
1775 90th Street
West Des Moines, IA 50266-1563
(515) 978-2204   Toll Free: (800) 422-3106
Fax: (515) 978-2209   E-mail: ihca@iowahealthcare.org
Web: www.iowahealthcare.org

Summary To provide financial assistance to employees of facilities that belong to the Iowa Health Care Association (IHCA) or Iowa Center for Assisted Living (ICAL) who are interested in attending college in any state to prepare for a career in the long-term care field.

Eligibility This program is open to employees of IHCA or ICAL member nursing homes, assisted living residencies, or residential care facilities. Applicants must be interested in attending college in any state to work on a bachelor's or master's degree in nursing (R.N. or L.P.N.), health care administration, physical therapy, or occupational therapy with the goal of employment in the long-term care field. Along with their application, they must submit an essay on their work history in long-term care, their personal qualities that enable them to fulfill the responsibility of providing quality care to facility residents or tenants, the rewards they gain from working in long-term care, and their career plans once their educational goal is achieved. Financial need is not considered in the selection process.

Financial Data The stipend is $1,000. Funds are paid to the recipient's educational institution.

Duration 1 year.

Additional data IHCA and ICAL represent 576 long-term care facilities in Iowa.

Number awarded Up to 25 each year.

Deadline May of each year.

[577]
IOWA NURSES FOUNDATION SCHOLARSHIPS

Iowa Nurses Association
Attn: Iowa Nurses Foundation
1501 42nd Street, Suite 471
West Des Moines, IA 50266
(515) 225-0495   Fax: (515) 225-2201
E-mail: info@iowanurses.org
Web: www.iowanurses.org/Default.aspx?tabid=2050

Summary To provide financial assistance to members of the Iowa Nurses Association who are working on an undergraduate or graduate nursing degree at a school in any state.

Eligibility This program is open to practicing R.N.s who are members of the association. Pre-licensure students are not eligible. Applicants must have completed at least 50% of the requirements for a bachelor's degree or at least 12 semester hours of graduate work leading to a master's degree in nursing or doctoral studies in nursing or a related field. They may be attending school in any state but must have a career plan to work in Iowa. Along with their application, they must submit brief essays on their career goals, the areas of nursing practice where they believe they have something special to offer, their interest in that area, how their interest and goals will enhance the delivery of quality health care in Iowa, and how this assistance would impact their ability to meet their educational goals. Financial need is not considered in the selection process.

Financial Data The stipend is $500.

Duration 1 year.

Number awarded 4 each year: 2 to students working on an R.N. to B.S.N. degree and 2 to graduate students.

Deadline February of each year.

[578]
IRENE AND DAISY MACGREGOR MEMORIAL SCHOLARSHIP

National Society Daughters of the American Revolution
Attn: Committee Services Office, Scholarships
1776 D Street, N.W.
Washington, DC 20006-5303
(202) 628-1776
Web: www.dar.org/natsociety/edout_scholar.cfm

Summary To provide financial assistance to graduate students working on a degree in medicine or psychiatric nursing.

Eligibility This program is open to students who have been accepted into or are enrolled in an approved program of graduate

psychiatric nursing or medicine. Applicants must be U.S. citizens and attend an accredited medical school, college, or university in the United States. They must obtain a letter of sponsorship from a local Daughters of the American Revolution (DAR) chapter. Preference is given to women applicants if they are "equally qualified." Selection is based on academic excellence, commitment to the field of study, and financial need.

Financial Data The stipend is $5,000 per year.

Duration 1 year; may be renewed for up to 3 additional years.

Number awarded 1 or more each year.

Deadline April of each year.

[579]
ISPN FOUNDATION PSYCHIATRIC NURSING RESEARCH AWARD

International Society of Psychiatric-Mental Health Nurses
Attn: ISPN Foundation
2810 Crossroads Drive, Suite 3800
Madison, WI 53718
(608) 443-2463   Toll Free: (866) 330-7227
Fax: (608) 443-2474   E-mail: info@ispn-psych.org
Web: www.ispn-psych.org/html/foundation.html

Summary To provide funding to members of the International Society of Psychiatric-Mental Health Nurses (ISPN) who are interested in conducting research in psychiatric mental health nursing.

Eligibility This program is open to psychiatric nurses who 1) are active members of the association and 2) already have a master's or doctoral degree in nursing or are working on a master's or doctoral degree in nursing. Applicants must be interested in conducting research (qualitative or quantitative) related to psychiatric mental health nursing. Proposals (no more than 5 single-spaced pages) must include: title and purpose, background and significance, hypotheses and research questions, methods, budget, timeline, and references.

Financial Data The grant is $1,000.

Duration 1 year.

Number awarded 1 each year.

Deadline December of each year.

[580]
JAMES P. KOHN MEMORIAL SCHOLARSHIP

American Society of Safety Engineers
Attn: ASSE Foundation
1800 East Oakton Street
Des Plaines, IL 60018
(847) 768-3435   Fax: (847) 768-3434
E-mail: agabanski@asse.org
Web: www.asse.org/foundation/scholarships/scholarships.php

Summary To provide financial assistance to graduate student members of the American Society of Safety Engineers (ASSE).

Eligibility This program is open to student members who are working on a graduate degree in occupational safety and health or a closely-related field (e.g., industrial or environmental engineering, environmental science, industrial hygiene, occupational health nursing). Applicants must be full-time students who have completed at least 9 semester hours with a GPA of 3.5 or higher. Their undergraduate GPA must have been 3.0 or higher. Along with their application, they must submit 2 essays of 300 words or less: 1) why they are seeking a degree in occupational safety and health or a closely-related field, a brief description of their current activities, and how those relate to their career goals and objectives; and 2) why they should be awarded this scholarship (including career goals and financial need). U.S. citizenship is not required.

Financial Data The stipend is $1,000 per year.

Duration 1 year; recipients may reapply.

Number awarded 1 each year.

Deadline November of each year.

[581]
JANEL PARKER CAREER MOBILITY SCHOLARSHIP

American Nephrology Nurses' Association
Attn: ANNA National Office
200 East Holly Avenue
P.O. Box 56
Pitman, NJ 08071-0056
(856) 256-2320   Toll Free: (888) 600-2662
Fax: (856) 589-7463   E-mail: annascholarships@ajj.com
Web: www.annanurse.org

Summary To provide financial assistance to members of the American Nephrology Nurses' Association (ANNA) who are interested in working on a baccalaureate or advanced degree in nursing.

Eligibility Applicants must be current association members, have been members for at least 2 years, be actively involved in nephrology nursing related health care services, and be accepted or enrolled in a baccalaureate or higher degree program in nursing. Along with their application, they must submit a 250-word essay on their career and educational goals that includes the expected time frame for completing their degree, the application of the award to meet expected expenses, and the impact of the completion of the degree program on their nephrology nursing practice.

Financial Data The stipend is $2,500.

Duration 1 year.

Additional data These scholarships, first awarded in 1993, are sponsored by Anthony J. Jannetti, Inc.

Number awarded 1 each year.

Deadline October of each year.

[582]
JANKY FOUNDATION SCHOLARSHIP

Minnesota Nurses Association
Attn: Minnesota Nurses Association Foundation
1625 Energy Park Drive, Suite 200
St. Paul, MN 55108
(651) 414-2822   Toll Free: (800) 536-4662, ext. 122
Fax: (651) 695-7000   E-mail: linda.owens@mnnurses.org
Web: www.mnnurses.org

Summary To provide financial assistance to members of the Minnesota Nurses Association (MNA) who are interested in working on a graduate degree in nursing.

Eligibility This program is open to MNA members who have a current R.N. licensure and have been accepted into an approved program of study leading to a graduate academic degree in nursing. Applicants must submit a brief description of their career goals following their graduate education. Selection is based on that statement, professional activities, demonstrated leadership ability, scholarship in nursing, MNA activities, and community involvement.

Financial Data The stipend is $2,000 per year.

Duration 1 year; may be renewed.

Number awarded 1 each year.

Deadline May of each year.

[583]
JAPANESE WOMEN'S SOCIETY FOUNDATION ACADEMIC SCHOLARSHIP

Japanese Women's Society Foundation
Attn: Scholarship Committee
P.O. Box 3233
Honolulu, HI 96801
(808) 547-9192
Web: www.jwsonline.org/scholarships

Summary To provide financial assistance to graduate students from Hawaii working on a degree in a field related to gerontology or geriatrics.

Eligibility This program is open to graduate students who are residents of Hawaii or attending a college or university in the state. Applicants may be studying medicine, nursing, public health, social work, or the arts and sciences, but they must be able to demonstrate an interest and commitment in the field of gerontology or geriatrics based on course work, research, and/or volunteerism. Along with their application, they must submit a brief description of their plans for further academic training and how this will help them to achieve their career goals of working on behalf of Hawaii's elderly. Preference is given to citizens of the United States, although citizens of other countries may apply. Financial need is considered in the selection process.

Financial Data The stipend is $2,500.

Duration 1 year.

Number awarded 2 each year.

Deadline March of each year.

[584]
JEAN E. JOHNSON AMERICAN NURSES FOUNDATION SCHOLAR AWARD

American Nurses Foundation
Attn: Nursing Research Grants Program
8515 Georgia Avenue, Suite 400
Silver Spring, MD 20910-3492
(301) 628-5227   Fax: (301) 628-5354
E-mail: anf@ana.org
Web: www.anfonline.org

Summary To provide funding to nurses interested in conducting research on reducing the impact of physical illness.

Eligibility This program is open to registered nurses who have earned a baccalaureate or higher degree. Applicants may be either beginning or experienced researchers. They must be interested in conducting research on reducing the negative impact of physical illness, especially cancer. Proposed research may be for a master's thesis or doctoral dissertation, if the project has been approved by the principal investigator's thesis or dissertation committee.

Financial Data The grant is $3,500. Funds may not be used as a salary for the principal investigator.

Duration 1 year.

Additional data This program was established in 1999. There is a $100 application fee.

Number awarded 1 each year.

Deadline April of each year.

[585]
JEANETTE ASH MEMORIAL SCHOLARSHIP

Emergency Nurses Association
Attn: ENA Foundation
915 Lee Street
Des Plaines, IL 60016-6569
(847) 460-4100   Toll Free: (800) 900-9659, ext. 4100
Fax: (847) 460-4004   E-mail: foundation@ena.org
Web: www.ena.org

Summary To provide financial assistance to members of the Emergency Nurses Association (ENA) who are working on a master's degree.

Eligibility This program is open to emergency nurses (R.N.) who are working on a master's degree. Applicants must have been members of the association for at least 12 months and have a GPA of 3.0 or higher. They must submit a 1-page statement on their professional and educational goals and how this scholarship will help them attain those goals. Selection is based on content and clarity of the goal statement (45%), professional association involvement (35%), presentation of the application (10%), and letters of reference (10%).

Financial Data The stipend is $5,000.

Duration 1 year.

Additional data This program is funded by the New Jersey West Central Chapter of ENA.

Number awarded 1 each year.

Deadline May of each year.

[586]
JILL LAURA CREEDON SCHOLARSHIP AWARD

ExceptionalNurse.com
Attn: Scholarship Committee
13019 Coastal Circle
Palm Beach Gardens, FL 33410
(561) 627-9872   Fax: (561) 776-9254
TDD: (561) 776-9442   E-mail: ExceptionalNurse@aol.com
Web: www.ExceptionalNurse.com/scholarship.php

Summary To provide financial assistance to nursing students who have a disability.

Eligibility This program is open to students with a documented disability or medical challenge who have applied to, or have already been admitted to, a college or university nursing program on a full-time basis. Applicants must submit an essay on how they plan to contribute to the nursing profession and how their disability will influence their practice as a nurse. Selection is based on the essay, transcripts of high school and/or college courses completed, activities and honors received, 3 letters of recommendation, and financial need.

Financial Data The stipend is $500.

Duration 1 year; nonrenewable.

Additional data This program is funded by the Johnson & Johnson Campaign for Nursing's Future.

Number awarded 1 each year.

Deadline May of each year.

[587]
JOAN K. STOUT, RN, RESEARCH GRANT

Sigma Theta Tau International
Attn: Research Services
550 West North Street
Indianapolis, IN 46202-3191
(317) 634-8171   Toll Free: (888) 634-7575
Fax: (317) 634-8188   E-mail: research@stti.iupui.edu
Web: www.nursingsociety.org

Summary To provide funding to nurses interested in conducting research on the impact of the practice of simulation education.

Eligibility This program is open to registered nurses with a current license who have a master's degree and/or are enrolled in a doctoral program. Applicants must be interested in conducting a research project on the impact of the practice of simulation education in schools of nursing and clinical care settings.

Financial Data The grant is $5,000.

Duration 1 year.

Additional data This program is supported by a donation from the Hugoton Foundation.

Number awarded 1 each year.

Deadline June of each year.

[588]
JOHN E. O'CONNOR MEMORIAL SCHOLARSHIP

American Association of Nurse Anesthetists
Attn: AANA Foundation
222 South Prospect Avenue
Park Ridge, IL 60068-4001
(847) 655-1170   Fax: (847) 692-6968
E-mail: foundation@aana.com
Web: www.aanafoundation.com

Summary To provide financial assistance to members of the American Association of Nurse Anesthetists (AANA) who are interested in obtaining further education.

Eligibility This program is open to members of the association who are currently enrolled in an accredited nurse anesthesia education program. Applicants must be second-year students who have completed 12 months of nurse anesthesia classes. Along with their application, they must submit a 200-word essay describing why they have chosen nurse anesthesia as a profession and their professional goals for the future. Financial need is also considered in the selection process.

Financial Data The stipend is $3,000.

Duration 1 year.

Additional data Funds for this scholarship, first awarded in 1994, are provided by the David L. Jelinek Agency, LLC. The application processing fee is $25.

Number awarded 1 each year.

Deadline March of each year.

[589]
JOHN F. GARDE SCHOLARSHIP

American Association of Nurse Anesthetists
Attn: AANA Foundation
222 South Prospect Avenue
Park Ridge, IL 60068-4001
(847) 655-1170   Fax: (847) 692-6968
E-mail: foundation@aana.com
Web: www.aanafoundation.com

Summary To provide financial assistance to members of the American Association of Nurse Anesthetists (AANA) who are interested in obtaining further education.

Eligibility This program is open to members of the association who are currently enrolled in an accredited nurse anesthesia education program. First-year students must have completed 6 months of nurse anesthesia classes; second-year students must have completed 12 months of nurse anesthesia classes. Along with their application, they must submit a 200-word essay describing why they have chosen nurse anesthesia as a profession and their professional goals for the future. Financial need is also considered in the selection process.

Financial Data The stipend is $1,000.

Duration 1 year.

Additional data This scholarship, first awarded in 2001, is sponsored by the Council on Accreditation of Nurse Anesthesia Educational Programs. The application processing fee is $25.

Number awarded 1 each year.

Deadline March of each year.

[590]
JOHNSON & JOHNSON CAMPAIGN FOR NURSING'S FUTURE-AMERICAN ASSOCIATION OF COLLEGES OF NURSING MINORITY NURSE FACULTY SCHOLARS PROGRAM

American Association of Colleges of Nursing
One Dupont Circle, N.W., Suite 530
Washington, DC 20036
(202) 463-6930   Fax: (202) 785-8320
E-mail: scholarship@aacn.nche.edu
Web: www.aacn.nche.edu/Education/financialaid.htm

Summary To provide scholarship/loans to minority students who are working on a graduate degree in nursing to prepare for a career as a faculty member.
Eligibility This program is open to members of racial and ethnic minority groups (Alaska Native, American Indian, Black or African American, Native Hawaiian or other, Pacific Islander, Hispanic or Latino, or Asian American) who are enrolled full time at a school of nursing. Applicants must be working on 1) a doctoral nursing degree (e.g., Ph.D., D.N.P.), or 2) a clinically-focused master's degree in nursing (e.g., M.S.N., M.S.). They must commit to 1) serve in a teaching capacity at a nursing school for a minimum of 1 year for each year of support they receive; 2) provide 6-month progress reports to the American Association of Colleges of Nursing (AACN) throughout the entire funding process and during the payback period; 3) agree to work with an assigned mentor throughout the period of the scholarship grant; and 4) attend an annual leadership training conference to connect with their mentor, fellow scholars, and colleagues. Selection is based on ability to contribute to nursing education; leadership potential; development of goals reflecting education, research, and professional involvement; ability to work with a mentor/adviser throughout the award period; proposed research and/or practice projects that are significant and show commitment to improving nursing education and clinical nursing practice in the United States; and evidence of commitment to a career in nursing education and to recruiting, mentoring, and retaining future underrepresented minority nurses. Preference is given to students enrolled in doctoral nursing programs. Applicants must be U.S. citizens, permanent residents, refugees, or qualified immigrants.
Financial Data The stipend is $18,000 per year. The award includes $1,500 that is held in escrow to cover the costs for the recipient to attend the leadership training conference. Recipients are required to sign a letter of commitment that they will provide 1 year of service in a teaching capacity at a nursing school in the United States for at least 1 year for each year of support received; if they fail to complete that service requirement, they must repay all funds received.
Duration 1 year; may be renewed 1 additional year.
Additional data This program, established in 2007, is sponsored by the Johnson & Johnson Campaign for Nursing's Future.
Number awarded 5 each year.
Deadline May of each year.

[591]
JOHNSON & JOHNSON SCHOLARSHIP FUND

American Assembly for Men in Nursing
AAMN Foundation
6700 Oporto-Madrid Boulevard
P.O. Box 130220
Birmingham, AL 35213
(205) 956-0146   Fax: (205) 956-0149
E-mail: aamn@aamn.org
Web: www.aamn.org

Summary To provide financial assistance to men working on a pre-R.N. licensure or graduate degree in nursing.
Eligibility This program is open to male students currently enrolled in an accredited pre-R.N. licensure or graduate degree program in nursing. Applicants must have a GPA of 2.75 or higher. Along with their application, they must submit an essay of 250 to 300 words that covers why they want to be a nurse, how they might contribute to the nursing profession, and their current career plans. Financial need is not considered in the selection process.
Financial Data The stipend is $1,000.
Duration 1 year.
Additional data This program was established in 2004 with funding from Johnson & Johnson's Campaign for Nursing's Future.

Number awarded 20 each year: 16 for pre-R.N. licensure students and 4 for graduate students. Of the 20 scholarships, 4 are reserved for minority students.
Deadline March of each year.

[592]
JOSH GOTTHEIL MEMORIAL BONE MARROW TRANSPLANT CAREER DEVELOPMENT AWARDS

Oncology Nursing Society
Attn: ONS Foundation
125 Enterprise Drive
Pittsburgh, PA 15275-1214
(412) 859-6100   Toll Free: (866) 257-4ONS
Fax: (412) 859-6163   E-mail: foundation@ons.org
Web: www.ons.org

Summary To provide funding for further education to professional registered nurses who can demonstrate meritorious practice in bone marrow transplant (BMT) nursing.
Eligibility This program is open to professional registered nurses who are interested in pursuing education at the bachelor's or master's degree level. Applicants must be currently employed as a registered nurse working in BMT (at least 75% of time must be devoted to patient care) or in the position of nurse manager, nurse practitioner, clinical nurse specialist, BMT coordinator, or equivalent position. They must have at least 2 years in BMT nursing practice. Candidates are evaluated on the following criteria: 1) clarity of professional goal statement; 2) demonstrated commitment to professional development in BMT nursing; 3) demonstrated commitment to continuing professional practice in BMT nursing; 4) recommendations; and 5) contributions and/or professional nursing practice. Applicants must not have previously received this career development award from the foundation.
Financial Data The stipend is $2,000. Funds may be used to support a continuing education program or to supplement tuition in a bachelor's or master's program.
Duration 1 year.
Additional data These awards were first presented in 1995.
Number awarded 4 each year.
Deadline November of each year.

[593]
JOSIE KING FOUNDATION RESEARCH GRANT

American Nurses Foundation
Attn: Nursing Research Grants Program
8515 Georgia Avenue, Suite 400
Silver Spring, MD 20910-3492
(301) 628-5227   Fax: (301) 628-5354
E-mail: anf@ana.org
Web: www.anfonline.org

Summary To provide funding to nurses interested in conducting research related to patient safety.
Eligibility This program is open to registered nurses who have earned a baccalaureate or higher degree. Applicants may be either beginning or experienced researchers. They must be planning to conduct research that is related to patient safety. Proposed research may be for a master's thesis or doctoral dissertation, if the project has been approved by the principal investigator's thesis or dissertation committee.
Financial Data The grant is $5,000. Funds may not be used as a salary for the principal investigator.
Duration 1 year.
Additional data This program, established in 2010, is sponsored by the Josie King Foundation. There is a $100 application fee.
Number awarded 1 each year.
Deadline April of each year.

[594]
JOYCE OLSON ENDOWED SCHOLARSHIP

Kansas State Nurses Association
Attn: Kansas Nurses Foundation
1109 S.W. Topeka Boulevard
Topeka, KS 66612-1602
(785) 233-8638   Fax: (785) 233-5222
E-mail: ksna@ksna.net
Web: www.nursingworld.org/SNAS/KS/Knf.htm

Summary To provide financial assistance to students in Kansas who are working on a nursing degree at the undergraduate, master's, or doctoral level at a school in the state.

Eligibility This program is open to residents of Kansas who are working on a nursing degree on the undergraduate or graduate level at a school in the state. Applicants must have a GPA of 3.0 or higher. Along with their application, they must submit a personal narrative describing their anticipated role in nursing in the state of Kansas. Preference is given to full-time students. The following priority is used in awarding scholarships: 1) R.N.s working on B.S.N.s; 2) graduate and postgraduate nursing students; 3) students enrolled in certificate nursing programs (e.g., advanced registered nurse practitioner); and 4) students enrolled in undergraduate nursing programs.

Financial Data The stipend is $500.

Duration 1 year.

Number awarded 1 each year.

Deadline June of each year.

[595]
JOYCE W. KELLY SCHOLARSHIP

American Association of Nurse Anesthetists
Attn: AANA Foundation
222 South Prospect Avenue
Park Ridge, IL 60068-4001
(847) 655-1170   Fax: (847) 692-6968
E-mail: foundation@aana.com
Web: www.aanafoundation.com

Summary To provide financial assistance to members of the American Association of Nurse Anesthetists (AANA) who are interested in obtaining further education.

Eligibility This program is open to members of the association who are currently enrolled in an accredited nurse anesthesia education program. First-year students must have completed 6 months of nurse anesthesia classes; second-year students must have completed 12 months of nurse anesthesia classes. Along with their application, they must submit a 200-word essay describing why they have chosen nurse anesthesia as a profession and their professional goals for the future. Financial need is also considered in the selection process. Students attending Kaiser Permanente School of Anesthesia are not eligible.

Financial Data The stipend is $4,000.

Duration 1 year.

Additional data Funding for this scholarship, first awarded in 1998, is provided by Kaiser Permanente School of Anesthesia. The application processing fee is $25.

Number awarded 1 each year.

Deadline March of each year.

[596]
JSM ANESTHESIA LOUISIANA SCHOLARSHIP

American Association of Nurse Anesthetists
Attn: AANA Foundation
222 South Prospect Avenue
Park Ridge, IL 60068-4001
(847) 655-1170   Fax: (847) 692-6968
E-mail: foundation@aana.com
Web: www.aanafoundation.com

Summary To provide financial assistance to members of the American Association of Nurse Anesthetists (AANA) from Louisiana who are interested in obtaining further education at a school in the state.

Eligibility This program is open to members of the association who are residents of Louisiana attending a nurse anesthesia program in the state. First-year students must have completed 6 months of nurse anesthesia classes; second-year students must have completed 12 months of nurse anesthesia classes. Along with their application, they must submit a 200-word essay describing why they have chosen nurse anesthesia as a profession and their professional goals for the future. Financial need is also considered in the selection process.

Financial Data The stipend is $2,000.

Duration 1 year.

Additional data Funding for this scholarship, first awarded in 2004, is provided by J. Stephens Mayhugh & Associates, Inc. The application processing fee is $25.

Number awarded 1 each year.

Deadline March of each year.

[597]
JUDY KNOX SCHOLARSHIP

North Carolina Nurses Association
Attn: North Carolina Foundation for Nursing
103 Enterprise Street
P.O. Box 12025
Raleigh, NC 27605-2025
(919) 821-4250   Toll Free: (800) 626-2153
Fax: (919) 829-5807   E-mail: rns@ncnurses.org
Web: www.ncnurses.org/ncfn.asp

Summary To provide financial assistance to registered nurses in North Carolina who are interested in working on a bachelor's or master's degree.

Eligibility This program is open to registered nurses in North Carolina who are working part time on a bachelor's or master's degree at a school in the state. Applicants must have been North Carolina residents for at least 12 months prior to application and have a cumulative GPA of 3.0 or higher. Along with their application, they must submit a 500-word essay on their reasons for pursuing additional education and for doing so on a part-time basis. Selection is based on that essay (25 points), GPA (15 points), professional involvement (20 points), community involvement (5 points), honors (15 points), certifications (15 points), and letters of reference (5 points).

Financial Data The stipend is $1,000.

Duration 1 year.

Additional data This program was established in 2009.

Number awarded 1 or more each year.

Deadline May of each year.

[598]
JULIA HARDY AMERICAN NURSES FOUNDATION SCHOLAR AWARD

American Nurses Foundation
Attn: Nursing Research Grants Program
8515 Georgia Avenue, Suite 400
Silver Spring, MD 20910-3492
(301) 628-5227   Fax: (301) 628-5354
E-mail: anf@ana.org
Web: www.anfonline.org

Summary To provide funding to nurses interested in conducting research on health care systems.

Eligibility This program is open to registered nurses who have earned a baccalaureate or higher degree. Applicants must be beginning researchers who have had no more than 3 research-based publications in refereed journals and have received, as a principal investigator, no more than $15,000 in extramural funding in any 1 research area. They must be interested in conducting research related to health care systems. Proposed research may be for a master's thesis or doctoral dissertation, if the project has been approved by the principal investigator's thesis or dissertation committee.

Financial Data The grant is $5,000. Funds may not be used as a salary for the principal investigator.

Duration 1 year.

Additional data There is a $100 application fee.

Number awarded 2 each year.

Deadline April of each year.

[599]
KANSAS HOSPITAL EDUCATION AND RESEARCH FOUNDATION SCHOLARSHIPS

Kansas Hospital Association
Attn: Kansas Hospital Education and Research Foundation
215 S.E. Eighth Avenue
Topeka, KS 66603-3906
(785) 233-7436   Fax: (795) 233-6955
Web: www.kha-net.org

Summary To provide financial assistance to employees of Kansas hospitals and other students in Kansas who are enrolled in a course of study leading to a certificate or degree in a health care program.

Eligibility This program is open to students enrolled or planning to enroll full or part time at an area technical school, 2-year college, or 4-year college or university in Kansas. Applicants must be 1) employees of Kansas hospitals working on a certificate, degree, or credential in an allied health or nursing program that is accredited by its respective governing body; 2) employees of Kansas hospitals working on a master's or doctoral degree in a field of health care; 3) future nursing or allied health education faculty members working on a master's degree or certification; 4) undergraduate or graduate students working on a health care human resources degree; or 5) juniors, seniors, or graduate students working on a degree in health care administration. Priority is given to professions and geographic areas experiencing shortages in Kansas, applicants furthering their knowledge base in health care by working toward a degree or certificate not currently held, students working on a degree to enable them to teach in health care, applicants demonstrating leadership on a project or institutional level, and applicants committed to pursuing their health care career in Kansas.

Financial Data Stipends are $500 for undergraduate hospital employees, $1,000 for graduate hospital employees, $1,000 for students preparing to become a faculty member, $500 for health care human resources students, and $500 for health care administration students.

Duration 1 year.

Additional data Funding for the scholarship in health care human resources is provided by the Kansas Hospital Human Resources' Association. Funding for the scholarships in health care administration is provided by the Kansas Association of Health Care Executives.

Number awarded 16 each year: 6 for undergraduate and graduate students in fields of health care, 3 for students working on a master's degree or a final certification to enable them to teach in a health care field, 1 for a student working on a degree in human resources in health care, and 6 for students working on a degree in health care administration.

Deadline February of each year.

[600]
KANSAS NURSES FOUNDATION GENERAL SCHOLARSHIPS

Kansas State Nurses Association
Attn: Kansas Nurses Foundation
1109 S.W. Topeka Boulevard
Topeka, KS 66612-1602
(785) 233-8638   Fax: (785) 233-5222
E-mail: ksna@ksna.net
Web: www.nursingworld.org/SNAS/KS/Knf.htm

Summary To provide financial assistance to students in Kansas who are working on a nursing degree on the undergraduate, master's, or doctoral level at a school in the state.

Eligibility This program is open to residents of Kansas who are working on a nursing degree on the undergraduate or graduate level at a school in the state. Applicants must have a GPA of 3.0 or higher. Along with their application, they must submit a personal narrative describing their anticipated role in nursing in the state of Kansas. Preference is given to full-time students. The following priority is used in awarding scholarships: 1) R.N.s working on B.S.N.s; 2) graduate and postgraduate nursing students; 3) students enrolled in certificate nursing programs (e.g., advanced registered nurse practitioner); and 4) students enrolled in undergraduate nursing programs.

Financial Data The stipend is $500.

Duration 1 year.

Number awarded 3 each year.

Deadline June of each year.

[601]
KAREN O'NEILL MEMORIAL SCHOLARSHIP

Emergency Nurses Association
Attn: ENA Foundation
915 Lee Street
Des Plaines, IL 60016-6569
(847) 460-4100   Toll Free: (800) 900-9659, ext. 4100
Fax: (847) 460-4004   E-mail: foundation@ena.org
Web: www.ena.org

Summary To provide financial assistance to members of the Emergency Nurses Association (ENA) who are working on a master's degree.

Eligibility This program is open to emergency nurses (R.N.) who are working on a master's degree. Applicants must have been members of the association for at least 12 months and have a GPA of 3.0 or higher. They must submit a 1-page statement on their professional and educational goals and how this scholarship will help them attain those goals. Selection is based on content and clarity of the goal statement (45%), professional association involvement (35%), presentation of the application (10%), and letters of reference (10%).

Financial Data The stipend is $3,000.

Duration 1 year.

Number awarded 1 each year.

Deadline May of each year.

[602]
KATHARINE DENSFORD DREVES RESEARCH GRANTS

Minnesota Nurses Association
Attn: Minnesota Nurses Association Foundation
1625 Energy Park Drive, Suite 200
St. Paul, MN 55108
(651) 414-2822   Toll Free: (800) 536-4662, ext. 122
Fax: (651) 695-7000   E-mail: linda.owens@mnnurses.org
Web: www.mnnurses.org

Summary To provide funding to members of the Minnesota Nurses Association (MNA) who are interested in conducting a research project.

Eligibility This program is open to MNA members who have at least a master's degree or are enrolled in a master's program. Applicants must be interested in conducting a research project related to nursing practice. They are encouraged to address issues pertaining to the inclusion of women and girls, ethnic minorities, and children under 21 years of age. Preference is given to first-time applicants.

Financial Data The maximum grant is $10,000.

Duration Research must be completed within 2 years.

Number awarded 1 or more each year.

Deadline March, May, September, or December of each year.

[603]
KATHERINE POPE SCHOLARSHIP

Georgia Nurses Foundation, Inc.
Attn: Scholarship Committee
3032 Briarcliff Road, N.E.
Atlanta, GA 30329-2655
(404) 325-5536   Toll Free: (800) 324-0462
Fax: (404) 325-0407   E-mail: gnf@georgianurses.org
Web: www.georgianurses.org/scholarship_appl.htm

Summary To provide financial assistance to Georgia residents who are working on a nursing degree, at any level, at an accredited school, college, or university.

Eligibility This program is open to residents of Georgia who are currently enrolled (full or part time) in an NLN-accredited program in nursing. Applicants may be working on a degree at any level (including associate, baccalaureate, master's, or doctoral). They must have a GPA of 2.5 or higher and be able to document financial need. Priority is given to applicants who meet the following criteria: enrolled in a Georgia school, plan to practice professional nursing in Georgia following graduation, and a member of a professional organization (e.g., Georgia Association of Nursing Students, Georgia Nurses Association, Georgia Association for Nursing Education).

Financial Data The stipend is at least $500. Funds may be sent directly to the recipient.

Duration 1 year.

Number awarded 1 each year.

Deadline June of each year.

[604]
KAY WAGNER, CRNA SCHOLARSHIP

American Association of Nurse Anesthetists
Attn: AANA Foundation
222 South Prospect Avenue
Park Ridge, IL 60068-4001
(847) 655-1170   Fax: (847) 692-6968
E-mail: foundation@aana.com
Web: www.aanafoundation.com

Summary To provide financial assistance to members of the American Association of Nurse Anesthetists (AANA) from any state who are interested in obtaining further education at a program in Pennsylvania.

Eligibility This program is open to members of the association from any state who are currently enrolled in an accredited nurse anesthesia education program in Pennsylvania. Applicants must have a GPA of 4.0. First-year students must have completed 6 months of nurse anesthesia classes; second-year students must have completed 12 months of nurse anesthesia classes. Along with their application, they must submit a 200-word essay describing why they have chosen nurse anesthesia as a profession and their professional goals for the future. Financial need is also considered in the selection process.

Financial Data The stipend is $3,000.

Duration 1 year.

Additional data This scholarship, first awarded in 2010, is supported by the Pennsylvania Association of Nurse Anesthetists. The application processing fee is $25.

Number awarded 1 each year.

Deadline March of each year.

[605]
KEITH BAIN SCHOLARSHIP

American Society of Safety Engineers
Attn: ASSE Foundation
1800 East Oakton Street
Des Plaines, IL 60018
(847) 768-3435   Fax: (847) 768-3434
E-mail: agabanski@asse.org
Web: www.asse.org/foundation/scholarships/scholarships.php

Summary To provide financial assistance to upper-division and graduate student members of the American Society of Safety Engineers (ASSE), especially those in specified categories.

Eligibility This program is open to ASSE student members who are working on an undergraduate or graduate degree in occupational safety, health, and environment or a closely-related field (e.g., industrial or environmental engineering, environmental science, industrial hygiene, occupational health nursing). Priority is given first to members of the Middle Tennessee Chapter of ASSE, second to students at Middle Tennessee State University in Murfreesboro, Tennessee or Murray State University in Murray, Kentucky, and third to residents of ASSE Region VII (Indiana, Kentucky, Michigan, Ohio, Tennessee, or West Virginia). Undergraduates must be full-time students who have completed at least 60 semester hours with a GPA of 3.0 or higher. Graduate students must also be enrolled full time, have completed at least 9 semester hours with a GPA of 3.5 or higher, and have earned a GPA of 3.0 or higher as an undergraduate. Along with their application, they must submit 2 essays of 300 words or less: 1) why they are seeking a degree in occupational safety and health or a closely-related field, a brief description of their current activities, and how those relate to their career goals and objectives; and 2) why they should be awarded this scholarship (including career goals and financial need). U.S. citizenship is not required.

Financial Data The stipend is $2,000 per year.

Duration 1 year; recipients may reapply.

Additional data This program, established in 2008, is supported by the Middle Tennessee Chapter of ASSE.

Number awarded 1 each year.

Deadline November of each year.

[606]
KENTUCKY NURSING INCENTIVE SCHOLARSHIP FUND

Kentucky Board of Nursing
Attn: Nursing Incentive Scholarship Fund
312 Whittington Parkway, Suite 300
Louisville, KY 40222-5172
(502) 429-7180   Toll Free: (800) 305-2042, ext. 7180
Fax: (502) 429-7011
Web: kbn.ky.gov/education/nisf

Summary To provide scholarship/loans to residents of Kentucky interested in preparing for a career as a nurse and working in the state.

Eligibility This program is open to Kentucky residents who will be attending approved prelicensure nursing programs (registered nurse or practical nurse) or graduate nursing programs in any state. Applicants must be interested in working as a nurse in Kentucky following graduation. Preference is given to applicants with financial need, licensed practical nurses pursuing registered nursing education, and registered nurses pursuing graduate nursing education.

Financial Data The stipend is $3,000 per year. This is a scholarship/loan program. Recipients must work as a nurse in Kentucky for 1 year for each academic year funded. If a recipient does not complete the nursing program within the specified time period, or does not complete the required employment, then the recipient is required to repay any monies awarded plus accrued interest at 8%.

Duration 1 year; may be renewed if the recipient maintains normal academic progress (15 credit hours per year for prelicensure and B.S.N. students; 9 credit hours per year for graduate nursing students).

Number awarded Varies each year.

Deadline May of each year.

[607]
KENTUCKY STATE COUNCIL FOUNDERS SCHOLARSHIP

Emergency Nurses Association
Attn: ENA Foundation
915 Lee Street
Des Plaines, IL 60016-6569
(847) 460-4100   Toll Free: (800) 900-9659, ext. 4100
Fax: (847) 460-4004   E-mail: foundation@ena.org
Web: www.ena.org

Summary To provide financial assistance to members of the Emergency Nurses Association (ENA) who are working on a master's degree.

Eligibility This program is open to emergency nurses (R.N.) who are working on a master's degree. Applicants must have been members of the association for at least 12 months and have a GPA of 3.0 or higher. They must submit a 1-page statement on their professional and educational goals and how this scholarship will help them attain those goals. Selection is based on content and clarity of the goal statement (45%), professional association involvement (35%), presentation of the application (10%), and letters of reference (10%).

Financial Data The stipend is $5,000.

Duration 1 year.

Additional data This program is funded by the Kentucky ENA State Council.

Number awarded 1 each year.

Deadline May of each year.

[608]
LAKEVIEW SCHOLARSHIP

American Association of Nurse Anesthetists
Attn: AANA Foundation
222 South Prospect Avenue
Park Ridge, IL 60068-4001
(847) 655-1170   Fax: (847) 692-6968
E-mail: foundation@aana.com
Web: www.aanafoundation.com

Summary To provide financial assistance to members of the American Association of Nurse Anesthetists (AANA) who are interested in obtaining further education.

Eligibility This program is open to members of the association who are currently enrolled in an accredited nurse anesthesia education program. Applicants must be second-year students who have completed 12 months of nurse anesthesia classes. Along with their application, they must submit a 200-word essay describing why they have chosen nurse anesthesia as a profession and their professional goals for the future. Financial need is also considered in the selection process.

Financial Data The stipend is $3,000.

Duration 1 year.

Additional data This scholarship was first awarded in 1995. The application processing fee is $25.

Number awarded 1 each year.

Deadline March of each year.

[609]
LAURA JEAN ARMSTRONG SCHOLARSHIP

Hawai'i Community Foundation
Attn: Scholarship Department
1164 Bishop Street, Suite 800
Honolulu, HI 96813
(808) 566-5570   Toll Free: (888) 731-3863
Fax: (808) 521-6286   E-mail: scholarships@hcf-hawaii.org
Web: www.hawaiicommunityfoundation.org

Summary To provide financial assistance to Hawaii residents who are interested in working on a graduate degree in nursing.

Eligibility This program is open to Hawaii residents who are studying nursing as full-time graduate students. Applicants must be able to demonstrate academic achievement (GPA of 2.7 or higher), good moral character, and financial need. Along with their application, they must submit a short statement indicating their reasons for attending college, their planned course of study, and their career goals.

Financial Data The amounts of the awards depend on the availability of funds and the need of the recipient; recently, the stipend was $4,000.

Duration 1 year.

Additional data Recipients may attend college in Hawaii or on the mainland.

Number awarded Varies each year; recently, 1 of these scholarships was awarded.

Deadline February of each year.

[610]
LESLIE GROY SCHOLARSHIP

Public Health Nurses Association of Colorado
Attn: Scholarship Chair
c/o The Alliance
800 Grant Street, Suite 335
Denver, CO 80203
E-mail: gjmiller@jeffco.us
Web: www.phnac.org/index.php?s=18&item=35

Summary To provide financial assistance to members of the Public Health Nurses Association of Colorado (PHNAC) who are interested in working on an undergraduate or advanced degree.

Eligibility This program is open to PHNAC members who are interested in taking courses that will help them attain an undergraduate or advanced degree in public health or public health nursing.

Financial Data The stipend is $1,000. Funds are paid as reimbursement for courses taken, upon receipt of documentation of completion of the course with a passing grade and a short summary paper of the course. Applicants must submit a letter that includes their educational goals and 5-year career goals related to public health nursing in Colorado, a current resume, verification of acceptance to the program, a letter of reference, and an estimate of expenses for the courses to be funded.

Duration 1 academic year.

Number awarded 1 or more each year.

Deadline January or July of each year.

[611]
LILLIAN SHOLTIS BRUNNER FELLOWSHIP FOR HISTORICAL RESEARCH IN NURSING

University of Pennsylvania
School of Nursing
Attn: Barbara Bates Center for the Study of the History of
    Nursing
307 Nursing Education Building
Philadelphia, PA 19104-6096
(215) 898-4502   Fax: (215) 573-2168
E-mail: dantonio@nursing.upenn.edu
Web: www.nursing.upenn.edu/history/research.htm

Summary   To provide funding to pre- and postdoctoral scholars interested in conducting research at the Barbara Bates Center for the Study of the History of Nursing in Philadelphia, Pennsylvania.

Eligibility   This program is open to scholars interested in conducting research on the history of nursing at the center. Although postdoctoral candidates are preferred, the fellowship is also available to those at the predoctoral level. Proposals should cover aims, background significance, previous work, methods, facilities needed, other research support needed, budget, and professional accomplishments. Selection is based on evidence of preparation and/or productivity in historical research related to nursing.

Financial Data   The grant is $2,500.

Duration   2 weeks.

Additional data   Scholars must be in residence at the Barbara Bates Center for the Study of the History of Nursing for the duration of the program. They are expected to participate in Center activities and present their research at a Center seminar.

Number awarded   1 each year.

Deadline   December of each year.

[612]
LINCOLN COMMUNITY FOUNDATION MEDICAL RESEARCH SCHOLARSHIP

Lincoln Community Foundation
215 Centennial Mall South, Suite 100
Lincoln, NE 68508
(402) 474-2345   Toll Free: (888) 448-4668
Fax: (402) 476-8532   E-mail: lcf@lcf.org
Web: www.lcf.org/page29412.cfm

Summary   To provide financial assistance to residents of Nebraska who are interested in working on an advanced degree in nursing or another medical field at a school in any state.

Eligibility   This program is open to residents of Nebraska who are working on an advanced degree in a medical field (nursing students may apply as undergraduates or graduate students). Applicants must submit an essay explaining their progress toward completing their education, why they have chosen to prepare for a career in a medical field, and their future career goals once they complete their degree. Preference is given to 1) female applicants; 2) students preparing for careers as physicians and nurses; and 3) applicants who demonstrate financial need.

Financial Data   Stipends provided by the foundation generally range from $500 to $2,000.

Duration   1 year; may be renewed up to 3 additional years.

Number awarded   1 or more each year.

Deadline   May of each year.

[613]
LISA GLENNON MEMORIAL SCHOLARSHIP

Emergency Nurses Association
Attn: ENA Foundation
915 Lee Street
Des Plaines, IL 60016-6569
(847) 460-4100   Toll Free: (800) 900-9659, ext. 4100
Fax: (847) 460-4004   E-mail: foundation@ena.org
Web: www.ena.org

Summary   To provide financial assistance to members of the Emergency Nurses Association (ENA) who are working on a master's degree.

Eligibility   This program is open to emergency nurses (R.N.) who are working on a master's degree. Applicants must have been members of the association for at least 12 months and have a GPA of 3.0 or higher. They must submit a 1-page statement on their professional and educational goals and how this scholarship will help them attain those goals. Selection is based on content and clarity of the goal statement (45%), professional association involvement (35%), presentation of the application (10%), and letters of reference (10%).

Financial Data   The stipend is $5,000.

Duration   1 year.

Additional data   This program is funded by the New Jersey ENA State Council.

Number awarded   1 each year.

Deadline   May of each year.

[614]
LORETTA FORD SCHOLARSHIP

North Carolina Nurses Association
Attn: North Carolina Foundation for Nursing
103 Enterprise Street
P.O. Box 12025
Raleigh, NC 27605-2025
(919) 821-4250   Toll Free: (800) 626-2153
Fax: (919) 829-5807   E-mail: rns@ncnurses.org
Web: www.ncnurses.org/ncfn.asp

Summary   To provide financial assistance to registered nurses in North Carolina and other states who are interested in becoming nurse practitioners.

Eligibility   This program is open to registered nurses who are interested in working on a graduate degree so they can become nurse practitioners. Applicants must be registered nurses with previous work experience in a medically underserved population in a nonmetropolitan area. They must have been accepted into an approved master's degree nurse practitioner program in North Carolina. Financial need must be demonstrated. Priority is given to North Carolina residents and to those registered nurses who are active in their local and statewide professional nursing association. Special consideration is give to applicants who plan to practice in a medically underserved area.

Financial Data   The stipend ranges from $500 to $1,000.

Duration   1 year.

Additional data   This program was established by the North Carolina Nurses Association Council of Nurse Practitioners and is administered by the North Carolina Foundation for Nursing. Funding for the scholarship is provided by Pratt Pharmaceutical.

Deadline   Deadline not specified.

[615]
LOUISIANA HEALTH CARE EDUCATOR LOAN FORGIVENESS PROGRAM

Louisiana Office of Student Financial Assistance
1885 Wooddale Boulevard
P.O. Box 91202
Baton Rouge, LA 70821-9202
(225) 922-1012   Toll Free: (800) 259-LOAN, ext. 1012
Fax: (225) 922-0790   E-mail: custserv@osfa.state.la.us
Web: www.osfa.state.la.us

Summary   To provide forgivable loans to students working on a graduate degree in nursing or allied health at a school in Louisiana and planning to become a teacher of those subjects.

Eligibility   This program is open to students working on a master's or doctoral degree in nursing or allied health at a college or university in Louisiana. Applicants must be willing to agree that they will teach in the field of registered nursing or in a top demand allied health education program at a participating postsecondary institution in Louisiana. They must be nominated by their institution of higher education.

Financial Data   The program provides loans of $20,000 per year. For each year that the recipient teaches nursing or allied health at a postsecondary institution in Louisiana, $10,000 of the loan is forgiven. Students who fail to comply with the agreement to teach must remain the loan.

Duration   1 year; may be renewed for 1 additional year for master's degree students or 2 additional years for doctoral students.

Number awarded   Varies each year.

Deadline   Deadline not specified.

[616]
LUCILE V. LUKENS AMERICAN NURSES FOUNDATION SCHOLAR AWARD

American Nurses Foundation
Attn: Nursing Research Grants Program
8515 Georgia Avenue, Suite 400
Silver Spring, MD 20910-3492
(301) 628-5227   Fax: (301) 628-5354
E-mail: anf@ana.org
Web: www.anfonline.org

Summary   To provide funding to nurses interested in conducting research.

Eligibility   This program is open to registered nurses who have earned a baccalaureate or higher degree. Applicants may be either beginning or experienced researchers. Proposed research may be for a master's thesis or doctoral dissertation if the project has been approved by the principal investigator's thesis or dissertation committee. There are no restrictions on the research topic.

Financial Data   The grant is $10,000. Funds may not be used as a salary for the principal investigator.

Duration   1 year.

Additional data   This program was established in 2006. There is a $100 application fee.

Number awarded   1 each year.

Deadline   April of each year.

[617]
LUCILLE JOEL SCHOLARSHIP

New Jersey State Nurses Association
Attn: Institute for Nursing
1479 Pennington Road
Trenton, NJ 08618-2661
(609) 883-5335   Toll Free: (888) UR-NJSNA
Fax: (609) 883-5343   E-mail: institute@njsna.org
Web: www.njsna.org/displaycommon.cfm?an=5

Summary   To provide financial assistance to New Jersey residents who are working on a master's degree in nursing at a school in the state.

Eligibility   This program is open to New Jersey residents currently enrolled in a master's degree program in the state. Applicants must be R.N.s and members of the New Jersey State Nurses Association. They must be able to document an interest in health policy or psychiatric/mental health nursing. Selection is based on financial need, GPA, and leadership potential.

Financial Data   The stipend is $1,000.

Duration   1 year.

Number awarded   1 each year.

Deadline   January of each year.

[618]
LUCY C. AYERS SCHOLARSHIPS

Lucy C. Ayers Foundation, Inc.
The Summit South
300 Centerville Road, Suite 300S
Warwick, RI 02886-0203

Summary   To provide financial assistance to nursing students in Rhode Island.

Eligibility   This program is open to students enrolled in an accredited Rhode Island nursing program leading to licensure as a registered nurse (R.N.). Applicants may be working on a diploma or an associate, bachelor's, master's, or doctoral degree. They must submit a brief statement describing their reasons for requesting financial aid.

Financial Data   The stipend is $1,000.

Duration   1 year.

Additional data   This program was established in 1998 with funds from the sale of the Lucy C. Ayers Residence For Nurses, originally chartered in 1926 as the Lucy C. Ayers Home for Nurses. It had served as a residence for retired or temporarily inactive graduate nurses of Rhode Island Hospital and its school of nursing. The program also provides assistance to graduates of the Rhode Island Hospital School of Nursing who need financial aid for continuing education or other purposes.

Number awarded   1 or more per year.

Deadline   Deadline not specified.

[619]
M. ELIZABETH CARNEGIE SCHOLARSHIP

Nurses Educational Funds, Inc.
Attn: Scholarship Coordinator
304 Park Avenue South, 11th Floor
New York, NY 10010
(212) 590-2443   Fax: (212) 590-2446
E-mail: info@n-e-f.org
Web: www.n-e-f.org

Summary   To provide financial assistance to African Americans who wish to work on a doctoral degree in nursing.

Eligibility   This program is open to African American registered nurses who are members of a national professional nursing organization and enrolled in a nursing or nursing-related program at the doctoral level. Applicants must have a GPA of 3.6 or higher. They must be U.S. citizens or have declared their official intention of becoming a citizen. Along with their application, they must submit an 800-word essay on their professional goals and potential for making a contribution to the nursing profession. Selection is based on academic excellence and the essay's content and clarity.

Financial Data   Stipends range from $2,500 to $10,000, depending on the availability of funds.

Duration   1 year; nonrenewable.

Additional data   There is a $20 application fee.

Number awarded   1 each year.

Deadline   February of each year.

[620]
M. LOUISE CARPENTER GLOECKNER, M.D. SUMMER RESEARCH FELLOWSHIP

Drexel University College of Medicine
Attn: Director, Archives and Special Collections on Women in
  Medicine
Hagerty Library
33rd and Market Streets
Philadelphia, PA 19104
(215) 895-6661   Fax: (215) 895-6660
E-mail: archives@drexelmed.edu
Web: archives.drexelmed.edu/fellowship.php

Summary To provide funding to scholars and students interested in conducting research during the summer on the history of women in medicine at the Archives and Special Collections on Women in Medicine at Drexel University in Philadelphia.

Eligibility This program is open to students at all levels, scholars, and general researchers. Applicants must be interested in conducting research utilizing the archives, which emphasize the history of women in medicine, nursing, medical missionaries, the American Medical Women's Association, American Women's Hospital Service, and other women in medicine organizations. Selection is based on research background of the applicant, relevance of the proposed research project to the goals of the applicant, overall quality and clarity of the proposal, appropriateness of the proposal to the holdings of the collection, and commitment of the applicant to the project.

Financial Data The grant is $4,000.

Duration 4 to 6 weeks during the summer.

Number awarded 1 each year.

Deadline January of each year.

[621]
MAINE ASSOCIATION OF NURSE ANESTHETISTS SCHOLARSHIP

American Association of Nurse Anesthetists
Attn: AANA Foundation
222 South Prospect Avenue
Park Ridge, IL 60068-4001
(847) 655-1170   Fax: (847) 692-6968
E-mail: foundation@aana.com
Web: www.aanafoundation.com

Summary To provide financial assistance to members of the American Association of Nurse Anesthetists (AANA) who are residents of Maine pursuing further education at a program in the state.

Eligibility This program is open to members of the association who are residents of Maine attending a nurse anesthesia program in the state. First-year students must have completed 6 months of nurse anesthesia classes; second-year students must have completed 12 months of nurse anesthesia classes. Along with their application, they must submit a 200-word essay describing why they have chosen nurse anesthesia as a profession and their professional goals for the future. Financial need is also considered in the selection process.

Financial Data The stipend is $1,000.

Duration 1 year.

Additional data Funding for this scholarship, first awarded in 1997, is provided by the Maine Association of Nurse Anesthetists (MEANA). The application processing fee is $25.

Number awarded 1 each year.

Deadline March of each year.

[622]
MARCH OF DIMES GRADUATE NURSING SCHOLARSHIPS

March of Dimes Foundation
Attn: Vice President for Research
1275 Mamaroneck Avenue
White Plains, NY 10605
(914) 997-4488   Fax: (914) 997-4560
E-mail: mlavan@marchofdimes.com
Web: www.marchofdimes.com/professionals/685.asp

Summary To provide financial assistance to registered nurses enrolled in graduate programs in maternal and child nursing.

Eligibility This program is open to registered nurses who are enrolled in graduate programs in maternal and child nursing and have at least 1 academic term to complete. Applicants must be a member of the American College of Nurse-Midwives (ACNM), the National Association of Neonatal Nurses (NANN), or the Association of Women's Health, Obstetric and Neonatal Nurses (AWHONN). They must submit a 500-word essay on their educational plan; their career goals and how they correlate with the mission of the March of Dimes to improve the health of babies by preventing birth defects and infant mortality; their past, current, and planned involvement in nursing for mothers and infants; and why they should be awarded the scholarship. Financial need is not considered in the selection process.

Financial Data The stipend is $5,000.

Duration 1 year; nonrenewable.

Additional data This program was established in 1997.

Number awarded Varies each year; recently, 8 of these scholarships were awarded.

Deadline January of each year.

[623]
MARCIA GRANUCCI SCHOLARSHIP

Visiting Nurse Association of Central Jersey
Attn: Director of Development
176 Riverside Avenue
Red Bank, NJ 07701
(732) 224-6760   Toll Free: (800) VNA-3330
Web: www.vnacj.org

Summary To provide financial assistance to residents of New Jersey working on a graduate degree in mental health or community health nursing at a school in any state.

Eligibility This program is open to New Jersey residents who are currently licensed as a nurse. Applicants must have been accepted into an NLN-accredited graduate program in any state in mental health or community health nursing. They must have a GPA of 3.0 or higher. Along with their application, they must submit a 300-word statement on why they have chosen psychiatric/mental health or community health as their educational concentration.

Financial Data The stipend is $2,000. Funds are paid directly to the recipient's college or university.

Duration 1 year.

Additional data This scholarship has been awarded since 1996.

Number awarded 1 each year.

Deadline May of each year.

[624]
MARGARET JONES MEMORIAL NURSING FUND

Hawai'i Community Foundation
Attn: Scholarship Department
1164 Bishop Street, Suite 800
Honolulu, HI 96813
(808) 566-5570   Toll Free: (888) 731-3863
Fax: (808) 521-6286   E-mail: scholarships@hcf-hawaii.org
Web: www.hawaiicommunityfoundation.org

Summary To provide financial assistance to Hawaii residents who are interested in preparing for a career in nursing.
Eligibility This program is open to students enrolled as juniors, seniors, or graduate students in 1) a B.S.N. or M.S.N. program in Hawaii, or 2) a Ph.D. program in nursing in Hawaii or on the U.S. mainland. Preference may be given to members of the Hawai'i Nurses Association. Applicants must be residents of the state of Hawaii; be able to demonstrate financial need; be interested in attending an accredited 2- or 4-year college or university as full-time students; and be able to demonstrate academic achievement (3.0 GPA or above).
Financial Data The amounts of the awards depend on the availability of funds and the need of the recipient; recently, stipends averaged $888.
Duration 1 year.
Additional data This fund was established in 1917 to honor Margaret Jones, a nurse killed when the S.S. *Lusitania* was sunk by a German submarine during World War I.
Number awarded Varies each year; recently, 13 of these scholarships were awarded.
Deadline February of each year.

[625]
MARGRETTA MADDEN STYLES CREDENTIALING SCHOLARS GRANTS

American Nurses Credentialing Center
Attn: Institute for Credentialing Innovation
8515 Georgia Avenue, Suite 400
Silver Spring, MD 20910-3492
(301) 628-5250   Toll Free: (800) 284-2378
Web: www.nursecredentialing.org

Summary To provide funding to registered nurses interested in conducting research related to credentialing for nurses.
Eligibility This program is open to registered nurses who have earned a baccalaureate or higher degree. Applicants may be either beginning or experienced researchers. They must be interested in conducting research on the impact of credentialing practices in nursing for consumers, health care employers and employees, policymakers, nurses, and the nursing profession. Proposed research may be for a master's thesis or doctoral dissertation, if the project has been approved by the principal investigator's thesis or dissertation committee.
Financial Data Grants range up to $25,000.
Duration 1 year.
Additional data Applications must be submitted to the American Nurses Foundation, Attn: Nursing Research Grants Program, 8515 Georgia Avenue, Suite 400, Silver Spring, MD 20910-3492. Applications must be accompanied by a $35 fee.
Number awarded 1 each year.
Deadline April of each year.

[626]
MARIA ROACH, CRNA SCHOLARSHIP

American Association of Nurse Anesthetists
Attn: AANA Foundation
222 South Prospect Avenue
Park Ridge, IL 60068-4001
(847) 655-1170   Fax: (847) 692-6968
E-mail: foundation@aana.com
Web: www.aanafoundation.com

Summary To provide financial assistance to members of the American Association of Nurse Anesthetists (AANA) who are residents of any state pursuing further education at a program in Louisiana.
Eligibility This program is open to members of the association who are residents of any state attending a nurse anesthesia program in Louisiana. First-year students must have completed 6 months of nurse anesthesia classes; second-year students must

have completed 12 months of nurse anesthesia classes. Along with their application, they must submit a 200-word essay describing why they have chosen nurse anesthesia as a profession and their professional goals for the future. Financial need is also considered in the selection process.
Financial Data The stipend is $1,500.
Duration 1 year.
Additional data This program began in 2008. The application processing fee is $25.
Number awarded 1 each year.
Deadline March of each year.

[627]
MARTHA E. BRILL AMERICAN NURSES FOUNDATION SCHOLAR AWARD

American Nurses Foundation
Attn: Nursing Research Grants Program
8515 Georgia Avenue, Suite 400
Silver Spring, MD 20910-3492
(301) 628-5227   Fax: (301) 628-5354
E-mail: anf@ana.org
Web: www.anfonline.org

Summary To provide funding to nurses interested in conducting research.
Eligibility This program is open to registered nurses who have earned a baccalaureate or higher degree. Applicants must be beginning researchers who have had no more than 3 research-based publications in refereed journals and have received, as a principal investigator, no more than $15,000 in extramural funding in any 1 research area. Proposed research may be for a master's thesis or doctoral dissertation, if the project has been approved by the principal investigator's thesis or dissertation committee. There are no restrictions on the research topic.
Financial Data The grant is $10,000. Funds may not be used as a salary for the principal investigator.
Duration 1 year.
Additional data This program was established in 2006. There is a $100 application fee.
Number awarded 1 each year.
Deadline April of each year.

[628]
MARY BARKER APN NURSING SCHOLARSHIP

Wisconsin Nurses Association
Attn: Nurses Foundation of Wisconsin, Inc.
6117 Monona Drive, Suite 1
Madison, WI 53716
(608) 221-0383   Fax: (608) 221-2788
E-mail: info@wisconsinnurses.org
Web: www.wisconsinnurses.org

Summary To provide financial assistance to registered nurses in Wisconsin who are interested in working on a graduate degree with preparation as an Advanced Practice Nurse (APN) at a school in any state.
Eligibility This program is open to registered nurses in Wisconsin who are interested in working on a graduate degree in nursing with preparation as an APN. Applicants must be members of the Wisconsin Nurses Association. They must provide verification of enrollment in a master's degree nursing program, a post-master's nurse practitioner certificate program, or a Ph.D. program or D.N.P. program at an NLN or CCNE accredited school of nursing in any state. Selection is based on financial need and potential to make a contribution to nursing in Wisconsin.
Financial Data The stipend is $2,000.
Duration 1 year.
Number awarded 2 each year.
Deadline April of each year.

[629]
MARY BETH HAYWARD SCHOLARSHIP FOR RNS PREPARING TO TEACH NURSING

Ohio Nurses Association
Attn: Ohio Nurses Foundation
4000 East Main Street
Columbus, OH 43213-2983
(614) 237-5414   Fax: (614) 237-6074
E-mail: gharsheymeade@ohnurses.org
Web: www.ohnurses.org

Summary   To provide financial assistance to registered nurses in Ohio who are working on a nursing degree as preparation for a career in teaching nursing.

Eligibility   This program is open to Ohio residents who have a valid Ohio nursing license. Applicants must have a GPA of 2.5 or higher as an undergraduate or 3.5 or higher if working on a graduate degree. They must be planning to enroll full time at a school in any state to prepare for a career as a teacher in an accredited Ohio nursing program. Along with their application, they must submit a personal statement on why they wish to teach nursing in Ohio. Selection is based on that statement, college academic records, school activities, and community services. Priority is given to members of the Ohio Nurses Association.

Financial Data   A stipend is awarded (amount not specified).

Duration   1 year; recipients may reapply for 1 additional year if they maintain a cumulative GPA of 2.5 or higher.

Number awarded   1 or more each year.

Deadline   January of each year.

[630]
MARY ELIZABETH CARNEGIE AMERICAN NURSES FOUNDATION SCHOLAR AWARD

American Nurses Foundation
Attn: Nursing Research Grants Program
8515 Georgia Avenue, Suite 400
Silver Spring, MD 20910-3492
(301) 628-5227   Fax: (301) 628-5354
E-mail: anf@ana.org
Web: www.anfonline.org

Summary   To provide funding to nurses, especially members of the National Black Nurses' Association (NBNA), interested in conducting research.

Eligibility   This program is open to registered nurses who have earned a baccalaureate or higher degree. Preference is given to NBNA members. Applicants may be either beginning or experienced researchers. They must be interested in conducting research on a topic related to nursing. Proposed research may be for a master's thesis or doctoral dissertation, if the project has been approved by the principal investigator's thesis or dissertation committee.

Financial Data   The grant is $8,500. Funds may not be used as a salary for the principal investigator.

Duration   1 year.

Additional data   This award was first presented in 2007. There is a $100 application fee.

Number awarded   1 each year.

Deadline   April of each year.

[631]
MARY ELLEN HATFIELD SCHOOL NURSING SCHOLARSHIPS

South Carolina Nurses Foundation, Inc.
Attn: Awards Committee Chair
1821 Gadsden Street
Columbia, SC 29201
(803) 252-4781   Fax: (803) 779-3870
E-mail: brownk1@aol.com
Web: www.scnursesfoundation.org/index_files/Page316.htm

Summary   To provide financial assistance to school nurses in South Carolina who are interested in working on an associate, bachelor's, or graduate degree in nursing at a school in any state.

Eligibility   This program is open to nurses who are currently practicing in a school setting (K-12) in South Carolina and have a valid nursing license. Applicants may be 1) L.P.N.s who are enrolled in an A.D.N. or B.S.N. program and have successfully completed 10 hours of undergraduate work; or 2) R.N.s who are enrolled in a B.S.N. program or a graduate program in nursing or public health and have successfully completed 10 hours of undergraduate work or 12 hours of graduate course work. They must be a current member of a professional organization and have career goals that include making a contribution to school nursing. Along with their application, they must submit a 2-page statement describing what they like about school nursing and how furthering their education will assist them in improving service to school-aged children and youth. Financial need is not considered in the selection process.

Financial Data   The stipend is $500.

Duration   1 year.

Additional data   These scholarships, first presented in 2006, are offered in conjunction with the South Carolina Department of Health and Environmental Control, Division of Women and Children's Services, Attn: Cathy Young-Jones, Mills/Jarrett Complex, Box 101106, Columbia, SC 29211, (803) 898-0767.

Number awarded   2 each year: 1 to an L.P.N. student and 1 to an R.N. student.

Deadline   August of each year.

[632]
MARY GRAY SCHOLARSHIP

Arkansas Nurses Association
Attn: Arkansas Nurses Foundation
1123 South University, Suite 1015
Little Rock, AR 72204
(501) 244-2363   Fax: (501) 244-9903
E-mail: arna@arna.org
Web: www.arna.org/snas/ar/fdtn/info.htm

Summary   To provide financial assistance to residents of Arkansas interested in working on a degree in advanced practice nursing in any state.

Eligibility   This program is open to residents of Arkansas who have a current nursing license and have graduated from a regionally-accredited program (i.e., L.P.N., R.N., B.S.N., M.S.N., or A.P.N.). Applicants must be interested in working on an advanced degree as an advanced nurse practitioner, clinical nurse specialist, certified nurse midwife, or certified nurse anesthetist at a school in any state. Along with their application, they must submit a cover letter describing their desire for the scholarship and intended use of funds, a statement regarding institutional financial assistance, a current resume, 2 letters of recommendation, official transcripts, a letter of acceptance into an advanced degree program accredited by NLNAC or CCNE (except doctoral programs), and a list of extracurricular activities.

Financial Data   A stipend is awarded (amount not specified).

Duration   1 year.

Number awarded   1 each year.

Deadline   May of each year.

[633]
MARY LEWIS WYCHE FELLOWSHIP

North Carolina Nurses Association
Attn: North Carolina Foundation for Nursing
103 Enterprise Street
P.O. Box 12025
Raleigh, NC 27605-2025
(919) 821-4250   Toll Free: (800) 626-2153
Fax: (919) 829-5807   E-mail: rns@ncnurses.org
Web: www.ncnurses.org/ncfn.asp

Summary To provide financial assistance to registered nurses in North Carolina who are interested in working on a graduate degree.

Eligibility This program is open to registered nurses in North Carolina who are working full time on a master's or doctoral degree in nursing education, practice, or administration at a school in the state. Applicants must have been North Carolina residents for at least 12 months prior to application and have a cumulative GPA of 3.0 or higher. Along with their application, they must submit a 300-word essay on their reasons for pursuing additional education and for doing so on a full-time basis. Selection is based on that essay (25 points), GPA (15 points), professional involvement (20 points), community involvement (5 points), honors (15 points), certifications (15 points), and letters of reference (5 points). Preference is given to members of the North Carolina Nurses Association.

Financial Data The stipend is $5,000.

Duration 1 year.

Additional data This program was established in 2003.

Number awarded 1 or more each year.

Deadline May of each year.

[634]
MARY OPAL WOLANIN GRADUATE SCHOLARSHIP

National Gerontological Nurses Association
7794 Grow Drive
Pensacola, FL 32514-7072
(850) 473-1174   Toll Free: (800) 723-0560
Fax: (850) 484-8762   E-mail: ngna@dancyamc.com
Web: www.ngna.org/awards-amp-scholarships.html

Summary To provide financial assistance to graduate student members of the National Gerontological Nurses Association (NGNA).

Eligibility This program is open to members of the association who are majoring in gerontology/geriatric nursing and carrying at least 6 units at a school accredited by the NLN. Applicants must submit 2 letters of recommendation, a transcript (at least a 3.0 GPA is required), and a 300-word statement of professional and educational goals with emphasis on contributions they expect to make to improve nursing care for older adults.

Financial Data The stipend is $500.

Duration 1 year.

Number awarded 1 or more each year.

Deadline April of each year.

[635]
MARYLAND GRADUATE AND PROFESSIONAL SCHOOL SCHOLARSHIPS

Maryland Higher Education Commission
Attn: Office of Student Financial Assistance
839 Bestgate Road, Suite 400
Annapolis, MD 21401-3013
(410) 260-4565   Toll Free: (800) 974-1024, ext. 4565
Fax: (410) 260-3200   TDD: (800) 735-2258
E-mail: osfamail@mhec.state.md.us
Web: www.mhec.state.md.us

Summary To provide financial assistance to professional and graduate students in Maryland who are interested in preparing for a career in the legal or medical professions.

Eligibility This program is open to students enrolled at designated universities in graduate and professional programs in dentistry, law, medicine, nursing, pharmacy, social work, or veterinary medicine. Applicants must be Maryland residents and able to demonstrate financial need.

Financial Data Stipends range from $1,000 to $5,000 per year.

Duration 1 year; may be renewed for up to 3 additional years if the recipient remains enrolled in an eligible program, maintains satisfactory academic progress, and continues to demonstrate financial need.

Additional data The selected institutions are the University of Maryland at Baltimore Schools of Medicine, Dentistry, Law, Pharmacy, or Social Work; the University of Baltimore School of Law, the Johns Hopkins University School of Medicine; the Virginia-Maryland Regional College of Veterinary Medicine; or certain Maryland institutions offering a master's degree in nursing or social work or a first professional degree in pharmacy.

Number awarded Varies each year.

Deadline February of each year.

[636]
MARYLAND GRADUATE NURSING SCHOLARSHIP AND LIVING EXPENSES GRANTS

Maryland Higher Education Commission
Attn: Office of Student Financial Assistance
839 Bestgate Road, Suite 400
Annapolis, MD 21401-3013
(410) 260-4594   Toll Free: (800) 974-1024, ext. 4594
Fax: (410) 260-3200   TDD: (800) 735-2258
E-mail: dsmith@mhec.state.md.us
Web: www.mhec.state.md.us

Summary To provide scholarship/loans to graduate students in Maryland who are interested in preparing for a career as a nursing faculty member.

Eligibility This program is open to Maryland residents enrolled as a graduate student at a college or university in the state. Applicants must be working on a master's of science in nursing (M.S.N.) degree or another graduate-level nursing program to prepare for a career as a nursing faculty member. They must be sponsored by a nursing school in Maryland that affirms that a nursing faculty position will be available for them upon completion of their graduate program, either at the sponsoring school or at another school of nursing in Maryland. Financial need is not considered in selection of Graduate Nursing Scholarships. Recipients who can also demonstrate financial need are eligible to apply for an additional Living Expenses Grant. Priority is given to students who are 1) participating in Competitive Institutional Grant projects funded by the state, or 2) enrolled in programs that prepare faculty for positions that historically have been difficult to fill.

Financial Data The stipend for Graduate Nursing Scholarships is for the amount of tuition and mandatory fees, to a maximum of $13,000 per year. The amount of the Living Expenses Grant varies up to $25,000 per year. Recipients must agree to work as a full-time nurse faculty member at a school of nursing in Maryland for 2 years for each year the award was received as a full-time student or for 1 and a half years for each year the award was received as a part-time student. They must begin the service obligation within 6 months of graduation.

Duration 1 year; may be renewed for 3 additional years, but the total available for Graduate Nursing Scholarships is $26,000 and the total available for Living Expenses Grants is $50,000. Renewal is available if the recipient maintains a GPA of 3.0 or higher, remains enrolled in an eligible program, maintains satisfactory academic progress as defined by their institution, and, if receiving a Living Expenses Grant, continues to demonstrate financial need.

Number awarded Varies each year.
Deadline July of each year for fall semester; November of each year for spring semester; April of each year for summer semester.

[637]
MARYLAND HOSPITAL ASSOCIATION SCHOLARS PROGRAM

Maryland Hospital Association
Attn: Catherine Crowley, Vice President
6820 Deerpath Road
Elkridge, MD 21075
(410) 379-6200
Web: www.mdhospitals.org

Summary To provide financial assistance to employees and volunteers at hospitals in Maryland who are interested in attending college in the state to work on an undergraduate or graduate degree in a health-related field.
Eligibility This program is open to residents of Maryland who are employees or active volunteers at hospitals in the state. Applicants must be accepted to or enrolled at a college or university in the state in a program leading to an undergraduate or graduate degree or certificate in life sciences, nursing, or allied health. They must be within 1 to 2 years of completing educational requirements and have a GPA of 3.0 or higher.
Financial Data The stipend is $2,500.
Duration 1 year.
Additional data This program, established in 2002, is jointly sponsored by Care First, PRIME, The Chesapeake Registry, and the Maryland Hospital Association.
Number awarded Varies each year. Recently, 17 of these scholarships were awarded: 10 to undergraduate nursing students, 3 to master's degree nursing students, 1 to a doctoral degree nursing student, 2 to students working on an associated degree in allied health, and 1 to a student working on a bachelor's degree in allied health.
Deadline May of each year.

[638]
MARYLAND ORGANIZATION OF NURSE EXECUTIVES SCHOLARSHIP AWARD

Maryland Organization of Nurse Executives
c/o Terri Gaffney, Scholarship Committee Chair
Nursing Spectrum
803 West Broad Street, Suite 500
Falls Church, VA 22046
(703) 237-6515   E-mail: tgaffney@nursingspectrum.com
Web: www.mdone.org

Summary To provide financial assistance to nurses working on a graduate degree in nursing administration or management in Maryland.
Eligibility This program is open to registered nurses practicing in Maryland who have a bachelor's degree in nursing and have completed at least 12 hours of graduate credits. Applicants must be working on an initial graduate degree in nursing administration or management. Along with their application, they must submit a short essay describing their planned career path, professional goals, and proposed use of the award monies.
Financial Data The stipend is $1,500.
Duration 1 year.
Number awarded 1 or more each year.
Deadline July of each year.

[639]
MARYLAND WORKFORCE SHORTAGE STUDENT ASSISTANCE GRANT PROGRAM

Maryland Higher Education Commission
Attn: Office of Student Financial Assistance
839 Bestgate Road, Suite 400
Annapolis, MD 21401-3013
(410) 260-4565   Toll Free: (800) 974-1024, ext. 4565
Fax: (410) 260-3200   TDD: (800) 735-2258
E-mail: osfamail@mhec.state.md.us
Web: www.mhec.state.md.us

Summary To provide scholarship/loans to Maryland residents interested in a career in nursing and other specified workforce shortage areas.
Eligibility This program is open to residents of Maryland who are high school seniors, undergraduates, or graduate students. Applicants must be enrolled or planning to enroll at a 2-year or 4-year Maryland college or university. They may major in the following service areas: 1) child development or early childhood education, for students who plan to become full-time employees as a director or senior staff member in a licensed Maryland child care center or as a licensed family day care provider in the state; 2) human services degree programs, for students who plan to become employees of Maryland community-based programs and are interested in working on a degree in aging services, counseling, disability services, mental health, nursing, occupational therapy, physical therapy, psychology, rehabilitation, social work, special education, supported employment, vocational rehabilitation, or other program providing support services to individuals with special needs; 3) education, for students who become teachers in the following areas of certification: technology education (secondary), chemistry (secondary), computer science (secondary), earth and space science (secondary), English for speakers of other languages (elementary and secondary), foreign languages (German, Italian, Japanese, Latin, or Spanish), mathematics, (secondary), physical science (secondary), physics (secondary), or special education (infant/primary, elementary/middle, secondary/adult, severely and profoundly disabled, hearing impaired, or visually impaired); 4) nursing, for students who become employed as a nurse in a licensed hospital, adult day care center, nursing home, public health agency, home health agency, eligible institution of postsecondary education that awards nursing degrees or diplomas, or other approved organization; 5) physical therapy or occupational therapy, for students who plan to become employed as a therapist or therapy assistant to handicapped children in a public school in Maryland, in an approved non-public education program, or in a state therapeutic hospital; 6) law, for students interested in preparing for a career in providing legal services to low-income residents in the state; 7) social work; or 8) public sector, for employment in services in the public or non-profit sectors in which there is a shortage of qualified practitioners to low-income or underserved residents or areas of the state. Applicants are ranked by GPA and then by need within each occupational field. Students with the greatest need within each GPA range are awarded first.
Financial Data Awards are $4,000 per year for full-time undergraduate and graduate students at 4-year institutions, $2,000 per year for part-time undergraduate and graduate students at 4-year institutions, $2,000 per year for full-time students at community colleges, or $1,000 per year for part-time students at community colleges. Within 1 year of graduation, recipients must provide 1 year of service in Maryland in their field of study for each year of financial aid received under this program; failure to comply with that service obligation will require them to repay the scholarship money with interest.
Duration 1 year; may be renewed up to 4 additional years, provided the recipient continues to meet eligibility requirements.
Additional data This program was established in 2007 as a replacement for several programs previously offered by the Mary-

land Higher Education Commission. Awards in the human services degree programs area are designated the Ida G. and L. Leonard Rubin Scholarship. Awards in the service area of education are designated the Sharon Christa McAuliffe Scholarship. Awards in the service areas of nursing, social work, and public service are designated the Parren J. Mitchell Public Service Scholarship. Awards in the service area of law are designated the William Donald Schaefer Scholarship.

Number awarded Varies each year.

Deadline June of each year.

[640]
MASSACHUSETTS ASSOCIATION OF NURSE ANESTHETISTS

American Association of Nurse Anesthetists
Attn: AANA Foundation
222 South Prospect Avenue
Park Ridge, IL 60068-4001
(847) 655-1170   Fax: (847) 692-6968
E-mail: foundation@aana.com
Web: www.aanafoundation.com

Summary To provide financial assistance to members of the American Association of Nurse Anesthetists (AANA) from Massachusetts who are interested in obtaining further education.

Eligibility This program is open to members of the association who are residents of Massachusetts enrolled in a nurse anesthesia program at a school in any state. Applicants must show leadership qualities and support of their state nurse anesthesia organization. First-year students must have completed 6 months of nurse anesthesia classes; second-year students must have completed 12 months of nurse anesthesia classes. Along with their application, they must submit a 200-word essay describing why they have chosen nurse anesthesia as a profession and their professional goals for the future. Financial need is also considered in the selection process.

Financial Data The stipend is $1,000.

Duration 1 year.

Additional data This scholarship was first awarded in 2007. The application processing fee is $25.

Number awarded 1 each year.

Deadline March of each year.

[641]
MASSACHUSETTS LABOR RELATIONS SCHOLARSHIPS

Massachusetts Nurses Association
Attn: Massachusetts Nurses Foundation
340 Turnpike Street
Canton, MA 02021
(781) 830-5745   Toll Free: (800) 882-2056, ext. 745
Fax: (781) 821-4445   E-mail: cmessia@mnarn.org
Web: www.massnurses.org/about-man/mns/scholarships

Summary To provide financial assistance to members of the Massachusetts Nurses Association (MNA) who are working on an undergraduate or graduate degree in nursing, labor relations, or a related field.

Eligibility This program is open to MNA members who are registered nurses or health care professionals with at least 1 year of professional experience. Applicants must have been accepted into an NLN-accredited baccalaureate or master's degree program in nursing or a baccalaureate or master's degree program in labor relations or a related field. Along with their application, they must submit a 500-word essay on their career goals, how education will enhance those goals, and their contribution to the profession of nursing or health care through practice, education, research, and/or labor relations. Selection is based on the essay, professional development activities, community work, and 2 professional references. Minorities are specifically encouraged to apply.

Financial Data The stipend is $1,000.

Duration 1 year.

Number awarded 2 each year.

Deadline May of each year.

[642]
MASSACHUSETTS NURSES ASSOCIATION UNIT 7 SCHOLARSHIPS

Massachusetts Nurses Association
Attn: Massachusetts Nurses Foundation
340 Turnpike Street
Canton, MA 02021
(781) 830-5745   Toll Free: (800) 882-2056, ext. 745
Fax: (781) 821-4445   E-mail: cmessia@mnarn.org
Web: www.massnurses.org/about-man/mns/scholarships

Summary To provide financial assistance to registered nurses and health care professionals who are members of the Massachusetts Nurses Association (MNA) and planning to work on an undergraduate or graduate degree.

Eligibility This program is open to MNA members in Unit 7 who are either registered nurses or other health care professionals with at least 2 years of professional experience. Applicants must have been accepted into an NLN-accredited undergraduate or graduate degree program in their respective field. Along with their application, they must submit a 500-word essay on their career goals, how education will enhance those goals, and their contribution to their profession. Selection is based on the essay, 2 professional references, community work, and professional development activities. Minorities are specifically encouraged to apply.

Financial Data The stipend is $1,000.

Duration 1 year.

Additional data Unit 7 is a bargaining unit that represents registered nurses, public health nurses, nurse practitioners, nursing instructors, community psychiatric mental health nurses, community mental health nursing advisers, health care facility inspectors, psychologists, physical therapists, occupational therapists, and audiologists.

Number awarded 2 each year: 1 to a nurse and 1 to a health care professional.

Deadline May of each year.

[643]
MASSACHUSETTS SENIOR CARE FOUNDATION SCHOLARSHIP PROGRAM

Massachusetts Senior Care Association
Attn: Massachusetts Senior Care Foundation
2310 Washington Street, Suite 300
Newton Lower Falls, MA 02462
(617) 558-0202   Toll Free: (800) CARE-FOR
Fax: (617) 558-3546   E-mail: info@maseniorcare.org
Web: www.maseniorcarefoundation.org

Summary To provide financial assistance to employees of nursing facilities or assisted living residences in Massachusetts interested in further study in a field related to long-term care at a school in any state.

Eligibility This program is open to current employees of nursing facilities and assisted living residences in Massachusetts who have been working in long-term care for at least 1 year and have received above-average performance evaluations from their supervisors. Applicants must be working toward certification, licensure, or an advanced degree in a field related to long-term care or taking prerequisite courses in order to enroll in an advanced degree program (e.g., biology or other courses needed in order to enter a nursing program). Along with their application, they must submit an essay describing their personal background, why they chose a career in long-term care, and how they view their career goals in long-term care.

Financial Data Stipends up to $2,000 are available.

Duration 1 year.

Number awarded Varies each year; recently, 53 of these scholarships were awarded.

Deadline April of each year.

[644]
MEDICAL PROFESSIONS SCHOLARSHIPS OF STRAIGHTFORWARD MEDIA

StraightForward Media
508 Seventh Street, Suite 202
Rapid City, SD 57701
(605) 348-3042   Fax: (605) 348-3043
E-mail: info@straightforwardmedia.com
Web: www.straightforwardmedia.com

Summary To provide financial assistance to students working on a degree in a medical-related profession.

Eligibility This program is open to students who are working on or planning to work on a degree in a medical-related profession (including physicians, technicians, physician's assistants, nurses, therapists, and other health professionals). Applicants must submit online essays (no minimum or maximum word limit) on 1) why they chose a medical profession over other educational opportunities and what contribution they will make to the medical world, and 2) how this scholarship will help them meet their educational and professional goals. Financial need is not considered in the selection process.

Financial Data The stipend is $500. Funds are paid directly to the student.

Duration 1 year.

Number awarded 4 each year: 1 for each award cycle.

Deadline February, May, August, or November of each year.

[645]
MEDICAL-SURGICAL NURSES CAREER MOBILITY SCHOLARSHIP

Academy of Medical-Surgical Nurses
Attn: Foundation
200 East Holly Avenue
P.O. Box 56
Pitman, NJ 08071-0056
Toll Free: (866) 877-AMSN   E-mail: AMSN@ajj.com
Web: www.medsurgnurse.org

Summary To provide financial assistance to members of the Academy of Medical-Surgical Nurses (AMSN) who are interested in furthering their education.

Eligibility This program is open to AMSN members who are enrolled or planning to enroll in a program of additional training, including L.P.N. to R.N., R.N. to B.S.N., R.N. to M.S.N., or M.S.N. to doctorate. Applicants must submit a brief statement describing how additional education will enhance their care of adult medical-surgical patients.

Financial Data The stipend is $1,000.

Duration 1 year; nonrenewable.

Number awarded 1 each year.

Deadline May of each year.

[646]
MEDINA SCHOLARSHIP FOR HISPANICS IN SAFETY

American Society of Safety Engineers
Attn: ASSE Foundation
1800 East Oakton Street
Des Plaines, IL 60018
(847) 768-3435   Fax: (847) 768-3434
E-mail: agabanski@asse.org
Web: www.asse.org/foundation/scholarships/scholarships.php

Summary To provide financial assistance to Hispanic upper-division and graduate student members of the American Society of Safety Engineers (ASSE).

Eligibility This program is open to ASSE student members who are working on an undergraduate or graduate degree in occupational safety, health, and environment or a closely-related field (e.g., industrial or environmental engineering, environmental science, industrial hygiene, occupational health nursing). Applicants must be bilingual (Spanish-English); Hispanic ethnicity is preferred. Students attending an ABET-accredited school also receive preference. Undergraduates must be full-time students who have completed at least 60 semester hours with a GPA of 3.0 or higher. Graduate students must also be enrolled full time, have completed at least 9 semester hours with a GPA of 3.5 or higher, and have earned a GPA of 3.0 or higher as an undergraduate. Along with their application, they must submit 2 essays of 300 words or less: 1) why they are seeking a degree in occupational safety and health or a closely-related field, a brief description of their current activities, and how those relate to their career goals and objectives; and 2) why they should be awarded this scholarship (including career goals and financial need). U.S. citizenship is not required.

Financial Data The stipend is $3,000 per year.

Duration 1 year; recipients may reapply.

Additional data This program was established in 2005.

Number awarded 1 each year.

Deadline November of each year.

[647]
MERIDIAN HEALTH CARE SYSTEMS JEAN MARSHALL SCHOLARSHIP

New Jersey State Nurses Association
Attn: Institute for Nursing
1479 Pennington Road
Trenton, NJ 08618-2661
(609) 883-5335   Toll Free: (888) UR-NJSNA
Fax: (609) 883-5343   E-mail: institute@njsna.org
Web: www.njsna.org/displaycommon.cfm?an=5

Summary To provide financial assistance to New Jersey residents who are working on a master's or higher degree in nursing at a school in the state.

Eligibility Applicants must be New Jersey residents who are registered nurses currently enrolled in a master's or higher degree program in nursing located in the state. They must be members of the New Jersey State Nurses Association. Selection is based on financial need, GPA, and leadership potential.

Financial Data The stipend is $1,000.

Duration 1 year.

Number awarded 1 each year.

Deadline January of each year.

[648]
MERLE MAPES SCHOLARSHIP FUND

Nebraska Association of Nurse Anesthetists
625 South 14th Street, Suite A
Lincoln, NE 68508
(402) 436-2165   Fax: (402) 436-2169
Web: www.neana.org

Summary To provide financial assistance to graduate nurse anesthesia students who are interested in practicing in Nebraska.
Eligibility This program is open to senior graduate students enrolled in a nurse anesthesia program. Applicants must be interested in practicing in rural or medical shortage areas of Nebraska. Along with their application, they must submit a personal letter describing their qualifications and specific area or hospital where they will be working.
Financial Data The stipend is $1,000.
Duration 1 year.
Number awarded 1 each year.
Deadline January of each year.

[649]
MICHAEL KELLY SMITH MEMORIAL SCHOLARSHIP

American Association of Nurse Anesthetists
Attn: AANA Foundation
222 South Prospect Avenue
Park Ridge, IL 60068-4001
(847) 655-1170   Fax: (847) 692-6968
E-mail: foundation@aana.com
Web: www.aanafoundation.com

Summary To provide financial assistance to male members of the American Association of Nurse Anesthetists (AANA) who are residents of Kansas and interested in obtaining further education.
Eligibility This program is open to male members of the association who are currently enrolled in the second or third year of an accredited nurse anesthesia education program and planning to work on a D.N.P. Applicants must be residents of Kansas and have a GPA of 3.5 or higher. They must have expressed an interest in leadership in national professional organizations, including (but not limited to) AANA and Sigma Theta Tau. Along with their application, they must submit a 200-word essay describing why they have chosen nurse anesthesia as a profession and their professional goals for the future. Financial need is also considered in the selection process.
Financial Data The stipend is $1,500.
Duration 1 year.
Additional data This scholarship was first awarded in 2004. The application processing fee is $25.
Number awarded 1 each year.
Deadline March of each year.

[650]
MICHIGAN ASSOCIATION OF NURSE ANESTHETISTS SCHOLARSHIPS

American Association of Nurse Anesthetists
Attn: AANA Foundation
222 South Prospect Avenue
Park Ridge, IL 60068-4001
(847) 655-1170   Fax: (847) 692-6968
E-mail: foundation@aana.com
Web: www.aanafoundation.com

Summary To provide financial assistance to members of the American Association of Nurse Anesthetists (AANA) from any state who are interested in obtaining further education at a program in Michigan.
Eligibility This program is open to members of the association from any state who are currently enrolled in an accredited nurse anesthesia education program in Michigan. First-year students must have completed 6 months of nurse anesthesia classes; second-year students must have completed 12 months of nurse anesthesia classes. Along with their application, they must submit a 200-word essay describing why they have chosen nurse anesthesia as a profession and their professional goals for the future. Financial need is also considered in the selection process.
Financial Data The stipend is $1,000.

Duration 1 year.
Additional data Funding for this scholarship, first awarded in 1997, is provided by the Michigan Association of Nurse Anesthetists. The application processing fee is $25.
Number awarded 5 each year: 1 at each of the 5 schools in Michigan with an accredited nurse anesthesia program.
Deadline March of each year.

[651]
MICHIGAN NURSE ANESTHESIA RESEARCH GRANT

American Association of Nurse Anesthetists
Attn: AANA Foundation
222 South Prospect Avenue
Park Ridge, IL 60068-4001
(847) 655-1170   Fax: (847) 692-6968
E-mail: foundation@aana.com
Web: www.aanafoundation.com

Summary To provide funding to student members of the American Association of Nurse Anesthetists who are interested in conducting research.
Eligibility This program is open to nurse anesthesia students in good academic standing who are members of the association. Applicants must be proposing a research project related to their field. Along with their application, they must submit a letter of support from their research adviser and a 100-word statement on how their research impacts nurse anesthesia practice and/or education. Preference is given to CRNAs.
Financial Data Grants are currently limited to $1,000.
Duration 1 year.
Number awarded 1 each year.
Deadline April of each year.

[652]
MICHIGAN NURSES ASSOCIATION CONDUCT AND UTILIZATION OF RESEARCH IN NURSING AWARD

Michigan Nurses Association
Attn: Michigan Nurses Foundation
2310 Jolly Oak Road
Okemos, MI 48864-4599
(517) 349-5640, ext. 213   Toll Free: (888) MI-NURSE
Fax: (517) 349-5818   E-mail: Pam.Wojtowicz@minurses.org
Web: www.michigannursesfoundation.org/awards.shtml

Summary To provide funding for research to members of the Michigan Nurses Association.
Eligibility The principal investigator must be a registered nurse who is licensed to practice in Michigan, is a Michigan resident, is a member of the association, and has earned or is working on a master's or doctoral degree. Proposals for clinical nursing studies that have direct impact on patient care receive priority. Multidisciplinary studies with a nursing focus will be considered, but basic or laboratory research is not eligible. Applications requesting budgets totaling more than $5,000 will not be reviewed.
Financial Data The grant is $5,000.
Duration 1 year.
Additional data Recipients are asked to present their research at the association's conference or to write an article for the association's journal, the *Michigan Nurse.*. An interim report is due in October and a final report is due upon completion of the project.
Number awarded 1 or more each year.
Deadline July of each year.

[653]
MICHIGAN NURSES FOUNDATION SCHOLARSHIP PROGRAM

Michigan Nurses Association
Attn: Michigan Nurses Foundation
2310 Jolly Oak Road
Okemos, MI 48864-4599
(517) 349-5640, ext. 213   Toll Free: (888) MI-NURSE
Fax: (517) 349-5818   E-mail: Pam.Wojtowicz@minurses.org
Web: www.michigannursesfoundation.org/awards.shtml

Summary To provide financial assistance to undergraduate or graduate nursing students at schools in Michigan.

Eligibility This program is open to students enrolled at a Michigan school of nursing that grants a certificate for practical nursing or an associate, baccalaureate, or higher degree in nursing. Applicants must submit brief statements on their vision of their future nursing practice and how they intend to use the scholarship monies if awarded. Selection is based on community involvement, financial need, and participation in the Michigan Nursing Student Association or Michigan Nurses Association.

Financial Data The stipend is $500.

Duration 1 year.

Number awarded At least 4 each year.

Deadline July of each year.

[654]
MIDWEST NURSING RESEARCH SOCIETY/ AMERICAN NURSES FOUNDATION SCHOLAR AWARD

American Nurses Foundation
Attn: Nursing Research Grants Program
8515 Georgia Avenue, Suite 400
Silver Spring, MD 20910-3492
(301) 628-5227   Fax: (301) 628-5354
E-mail: anf@ana.org
Web: www.anfonline.org

Summary To provide funding to members of the Midwest Nursing Research Society (MNRS) who are interested in conducting research.

Eligibility This program is open to registered nurses who have earned a baccalaureate or higher degree. Applicants may be either beginning or experienced researchers. Proposed research may be for a master's thesis or doctoral dissertation if the project has been approved by the principal investigator's thesis or dissertation committee. There are no restrictions on the research topic, but applicants must be current MNRS members.

Financial Data The grant is $7,500. Funds may not be used as a salary for the principal investigator.

Duration 1 year.

Additional data Funding for this program is provided by the MNRS. There is a $100 application fee.

Number awarded 1 each year.

Deadline April of each year.

[655]
MINNESOTA ANA-ASSEMBLY OF PAST PRESIDENTS SCHOLARSHIP

American Association of Nurse Anesthetists
Attn: AANA Foundation
222 South Prospect Avenue
Park Ridge, IL 60068-4001
(847) 655-1171   Fax: (847) 692-7137
E-mail: foundation@aana.com
Web: www.aanafoundation.com

Summary To provide financial assistance to members of the American Association of Nurse Anesthetists (AANA) from Minnesota who are interested in obtaining further education at a program in the state.

Eligibility This program is open to members of the association who are currently enrolled in an accredited nurse anesthesia education program in Minnesota. Applicants must agree to remain in Minnesota for at least 2 years after graduation. First-year students must have completed 6 months of nurse anesthesia classes; second-year students must have completed 12 months of nurse anesthesia classes. Along with their application, they must submit a 200-word essay describing why they have chosen nurse anesthesia as a profession and their professional goals for the future. Financial need is also considered in the selection process.

Financial Data The stipend is $1,000.

Duration 1 year.

Additional data This scholarship, first awarded in 2003, is sponsored by the Assembly of Past Presidents of the Minnesota Association of Nurse Anesthetists. The application processing fee is $25.

Number awarded 1 each year.

Deadline March of each year.

[656]
MINNESOTA ASSOCIATION OF NURSE ANESTHETISTS SCHOLARSHIP

American Association of Nurse Anesthetists
Attn: AANA Foundation
222 South Prospect Avenue
Park Ridge, IL 60068-4001
(847) 655-1170   Fax: (847) 692-6968
E-mail: foundation@aana.com
Web: www.aanafoundation.com

Summary To provide financial assistance to members of the American Association of Nurse Anesthetists (AANA) from any state who are interested in obtaining further education at a program in Minnesota.

Eligibility This program is open to members of the association from any state who are currently enrolled in an accredited nurse anesthesia education program in Minnesota. First-year students must have completed 6 months of nurse anesthesia classes; second-year students must have completed 12 months of nurse anesthesia classes. Along with their application, they must submit a 200-word essay describing why they have chosen nurse anesthesia as a profession and their professional goals for the future. Financial need is also considered in the selection process.

Financial Data The stipend is $3,000.

Duration 1 year.

Additional data This scholarship, first awarded in 2009, is sponsored by the Minnesota Association of Nurse Anesthetists. The application processing fee is $25.

Number awarded 2 each year.

Deadline March of each year.

[657]
MINNESOTA NURSES ASSOCIATION FOUNDATION RESEARCH GRANTS

Minnesota Nurses Association
Attn: Minnesota Nurses Association Foundation
1625 Energy Park Drive, Suite 200
St. Paul, MN 55108
(651) 414-2822   Toll Free: (800) 536-4662, ext. 122
Fax: (651) 695-7000   E-mail: linda.owens@mnnurses.org
Web: www.mnnurses.org

Summary To provide funding to members of the Minnesota Nurses Association (MNA) who are interested in conducting a research project.

Eligibility This program is open to MNA members who have at least a master's degree or are enrolled in a master's program. Applicants must be interested in conducting a research project related to nursing practice. They are encouraged to address issues pertaining to the inclusion of women and girls, ethnic minorities, and children under 21 years of age. Preference is given to first-time applicants.

Financial Data The maximum grant is $5,000.

Duration Research must be completed within 2 years.

Number awarded 1 or more each year.

Deadline March, May, September, or December of each year.

[658]
MINNESOTA STATE COUNCIL "PATHWAYS II" SCHOLARSHIP

Emergency Nurses Association
Attn: ENA Foundation
915 Lee Street
Des Plaines, IL 60016-6569
(847) 460-4100   Toll Free: (800) 900-9659, ext. 4100
Fax: (847) 460-4004   E-mail: foundation@ena.org
Web: www.ena.org

Summary To provide financial assistance to members of the Emergency Nurses Association (ENA) who are working on a master's degree.

Eligibility This program is open to emergency nurses (R.N.) who are working on a master's degree. Applicants must have been members of the association for at least 12 months and have a GPA of 3.0 or higher. They must submit a 1-page statement on their professional and educational goals and how this scholarship will help them attain those goals. Selection is based on content and clarity of the goal statement (45%), professional association involvement (35%), presentation of the application (10%), and letters of reference (10%).

Financial Data The stipend is $5,000.

Duration 1 year.

Additional data This program is funded by the Minnesota ENA State Council.

Number awarded 1 each year.

Deadline May of each year.

[659]
MINUTECLINIC FAMILY NP STUDENT SCHOLARSHIP

American Academy of Nurse Practitioners
Attn: AANP Foundation
P.O. Box 12924
Austin, TX 78711-2924
(512) 276-5905   Fax: (512) 442-6469
E-mail: foundation@aanp.org
Web: aanp.org

Summary To provide financial assistance to members of the American Academy of Nurse Practitioners (AANP) who are working on a master's degree as a family nurse practitioner (NP).

Eligibility This program is open to members of the academy who are enrolled in an M.S.N. degree program as a family nurse practitioner. Applicants must have a GPA of 3.5 or higher. They must have completed at least 1 course for their master's program requirements. but they cannot be finishing their degree during the current year. U.S. citizenship is required.

Financial Data The stipend is $1,000. Funds may be used only for educational expenses (tuition, books, equipment, etc.), not for expenses related to master's thesis and/or general research projects.

Duration 1 year.

Additional data This program is sponsored by MinuteClinic, L.L.C. There is a $10 application fee.

Number awarded 1 each year.

Deadline October of each year.

[660]
MISSISSIPPI GRADUATE CAR TAG STIPEND PROGRAM

Mississippi Nurses Association
Attn: Mississippi Nurses Foundation
31 Woodgreen Place
Madison, MS 39110
(601) 898-0850   Fax: (601) 898-0190
E-mail: foundation@msnurses.org
Web: msnursesfoundation.com/scholarships

Summary To provide scholarship/loans to residents of Mississippi who are working on a graduate degree in nursing at a school in the state and have a license plate for nursing on their car.

Eligibility This program is open to residents of Mississippi who have a current registered nurse (R.N.) license and are currently enrolled full or part time in a master's or doctoral nursing program in the state. Applicants must have a special nursing license plate on their personal vehicle at the time of application and during receipt of funding. They must have a GPA of 3.0 or higher. Along with their application, they must submit an essay of 1,500 to 2,500 words on the value of nursing leadership to 1 of the following: health care reform, health care ethics in a technological society, or health policy. Selection is based on that essay, transcripts, school of nursing activities, community activities, awards and honors, and 3 letters of reference.

Financial Data The stipend is $6,000. Funds are paid directly to students at the rate of $500 per month for 12 months for full-time students or $250 per month for 24 months for part-time students. Students must sign a contract to work in Mississippi within the first 2 years following completion of the program. If they fail to comply with that contract, they must repay all funds received, plus interest.

Duration 1 year for full-time students; 2 years for part-time students.

Number awarded Varies each year. Recently, 4 of these stipends were awarded: 3 to master's degree students and 1 to a doctoral student.

Deadline June of each year.

[661]
MISSISSIPPI NURSES FOUNDATION RESEARCH SEED GRANTS

Mississippi Nurses Association
Attn: Mississippi Nurses Foundation
31 Woodgreen Place
Madison, MS 39110
(601) 898-0850   Fax: (601) 898-0190
E-mail: foundation@msnurses.org
Web: msnursesfoundation.com/scholarships

Summary To provide funding to members of the Mississippi Nurses Association (MNA) who are interested in conducting a research project.

Eligibility This program is open to registered nurses currently licensed in Mississippi who are MNA members. Applicants may be a graduate nursing student in a master's or doctoral program in Mississippi or a nurse clinician, educator, or administrator working in a health care facility in the state. They must be interested in conducting a research project whose goal is relevant to the purpose of the MNA research grant program to 1) deliver health and nursing care to a specified community or population about prevalent health care issues in Mississippi, or 2) provide evidence-based or outcomes-based focus for health care delivery and/or nursing practice within the state. Applications for graduate student projects are accepted only if the study has been approved by the applicant's graduate adviser. Residents of Mississippi who are attending graduate programs out of state may be considered on a case-by-case basis. Applications for work-related projects are accepted only if the study has been approved by a colleague, supervisor, or administrator of the facility. U.S. citizenship is required.

Financial Data   The grant is $500.

Duration   1 year.

Additional data   These grants were first awarded in 2010.

Number awarded   2 each year.

Deadline   May of each year.

[662]
MISSISSIPPI NURSES FOUNDATION SCHOLARLY WRITING AWARD

Mississippi Nurses Association
Attn: Mississippi Nurses Foundation
31 Woodgreen Place
Madison, MS 39110
(601) 898-0850   Fax: (601) 898-0190
E-mail: foundation@msnurses.org
Web: msnursesfoundation.com/scholarships

Summary   To recognize and reward members of the Mississippi Nurses Association (MNA) who are working on a doctoral degree and submit outstanding manuscripts on a relevant topic.

Eligibility   This award is available to registered nurses currently licensed in Mississippi who are MNA members. Applicants must be enrolled in a doctoral program in nursing or a related area. They must submit a manuscript, up to 3,600 words in length, that has not been previously published but is publishable as submitted. The manuscript should be written on 1 of the following topics: 1) report of a nursing project or research; 2) description of an innovative practice in nursing; or 3) scholarly essay related to nursing.

Financial Data   The award is $1,000.

Duration   The award is presented annually.

Additional data   This award is sponsored by the Arthur L. Davis Publishing Agency.

Number awarded   1 each year.

Deadline   November of each year.

[663]
MISSISSIPPI NURSING EDUCATION LOAN/ SCHOLARSHIP PROGRAM-MSN

Mississippi Office of Student Financial Aid
3825 Ridgewood Road
Jackson, MS 39211-6453
(601) 432-6997   Toll Free: (800) 327-2980 (within MS)
Fax: (601) 432-6527   E-mail: sfa@ihl.state.ms.us
Web: www.mississippi.edu/riseupms/financialaid-state.php

Summary   To provide scholarship/loans to Mississippi residents who are interested in working on a master's degree in nursing.

Eligibility   This program is open to current Mississippi residents who are licensed registered nurses and have completed a B.S.N. degree. Applicants must be interested in working on an M.S.N. degree and have a GPA of 3.0 or higher. They must have been fully admitted at an accredited school of nursing in Mississippi.

Financial Data   Scholarship/loans are $4,000 per academic year for up to 2 years or a total of $8,000 (prorated over 3 years for part-time participants). For each year of service in Mississippi as a professional nurse (patient care), 1 year's loan will be forgiven. For nurses who received prorated funding over 3 years, the time of service required is 2 years. In the event the recipient fails to fulfill the service obligation, repayment of principal and interest is required.

Duration   1 year; may be renewed up to 1 additional year of full-time study or 2 years of part-time study provided the recipient maintains a GPA of 3.0 or higher each semester.

Additional data   The service requirement may not be deferred to work on a Ph.D. degree.

Number awarded   Varies each year, depending on the availability of funds; awards are granted on a first-come, first-served basis.

Deadline   March of each year.

[664]
MISSISSIPPI NURSING EDUCATION LOAN/ SCHOLARSHIP PROGRAM-PHD

Mississippi Office of Student Financial Aid
3825 Ridgewood Road
Jackson, MS 39211-6453
(601) 432-6997   Toll Free: (800) 327-2980 (within MS)
Fax: (601) 432-6527   E-mail: sfa@ihl.state.ms.us
Web: www.mississippi.edu/riseupms/financialaid-state.php

Summary   To provide scholarship/loans to Mississippi residents who are interested in working on a doctoral degree in nursing.

Eligibility   This program is open to current Mississippi residents who are licensed registered nurses and have completed an M.S.N. degree. Applicants must be interested in working on a doctoral degree and have a GPA of 3.0 or higher. They must have been fully admitted at an accredited school of nursing in Mississippi.

Financial Data   Scholarship/loans are $5,000 per academic year for up to 2 years or a total of $10,000 (prorated over 4 years for part-time participants). For each year of service in Mississippi as a professional nurse (patient care) or a full-time teacher in an accredited school of nursing, 1 year's loan will be forgiven. For nurses who received prorated funding over 4 years, the time of service required is 2 years. In the event the recipient fails to fulfill the service obligation, repayment of principal and interest is required.

Duration   1 year; may be renewed up to 1 additional year of full-time study or 3 years of part-time study provided the recipient maintains a GPA of 3.0 or higher each semester.

Number awarded   Varies each year, depending on the availability of funds; awards are granted on a first-come, first-served basis.

Deadline   March of each year.

[665]
MISSISSIPPI NURSING TEACHER STIPEND PROGRAM

Mississippi Office of Student Financial Aid
3825 Ridgewood Road
Jackson, MS 39211-6453
(601) 432-6997   Toll Free: (800) 327-2980 (within MS)
Fax: (601) 432-6527   E-mail: sfa@ihl.state.ms.us
Web: www.mississippi.edu/riseupms/financialaid-state.php

Summary   To provide scholarship/loans to Mississippi licensed registered nurses who are interested in preparing for a career in teaching nursing.

Eligibility   This program is open to Mississippi residents who have a current nursing license and have been admitted into 1) an M.S.N. program at a graduate school of nursing in Mississippi or 2) the Ph.D. nursing program at the University of Southern Mississippi or the University of Mississippi Medical Center. Applicants must be full-time students with a GPA of 3.0 or higher. They must also be participating in the Mississippi Nursing Education Loan/Scholarship Program.

Financial Data   Under this program, students working on an M.S.N. or Ph.D. are eligible to receive up to $1,000 per month. This is a scholarship/loan program. Obligation can be discharged by full-time teaching in Mississippi in professional nursing for 2 years for every year of scholarship assistance received. In the event the recipient fails to fulfill the service obligation, repayment of principal and interest is required.

Duration   Up to 1 calendar year for M.S.N. students; up to 2 calendar years for Ph.D. students.

Number awarded Varies each year, depending on the availability of funds; awards are granted on a first-come, first-served basis.

Deadline March of each year.

[666]
MISSOURI ASSOCIATION OF NURSE ANESTHETISTS SCHOLARSHIP

American Association of Nurse Anesthetists
Attn: AANA Foundation
222 South Prospect Avenue
Park Ridge, IL 60068-4001
(847) 655-1170   Fax: (847) 692-6968
E-mail: foundation@aana.com
Web: www.aanafoundation.com

Summary To provide financial assistance to members of the American Association of Nurse Anesthetists (AANA) who are residents of Missouri pursuing further education at a program in the state.

Eligibility This program is open to members of the association who are residents of Missouri attending a nurse anesthesia program in the state. First-year students must have completed 6 months of nurse anesthesia classes; second-year students must have completed 12 months of nurse anesthesia classes. Along with their application, they must submit a 200-word essay describing why they have chosen nurse anesthesia as a profession and their professional goals for the future. Financial need is also considered in the selection process.

Financial Data The stipend is $3,000.

Duration 1 year.

Additional data This program is sponsored by the Missouri Association of Nurse Anesthetists. The application processing fee is $25.

Number awarded 1 each year.

Deadline March of each year.

[667]
MNA SCHOOL NURSE SCHOLARSHIP

Massachusetts Nurses Association
Attn: Massachusetts Nurses Foundation
340 Turnpike Street
Canton, MA 02021
(781) 830-5745   Toll Free: (800) 882-2056, ext. 745
Fax: (781) 821-4445   E-mail: cmessia@mnarn.org
Web: www.massnurses.org/about-man/mns/scholarships

Summary To provide financial assistance to members of the Massachusetts Nurses Association (MNA) who are working on an advanced degree in school health services.

Eligibility This program is open to MNA members who are currently employed as school nurses. Applicants must be working on an advanced degree in school health issues or a related field. They must be able to demonstrate a serious intent to advance school nursing practice. Along with their application, they must submit a 500-word essay on their career goals, how education will enhance those goals, and their contribution to their profession. Selection is based on the essay, professional development activities, community work, and 2 professional references. Minorities are specifically encouraged to apply.

Financial Data A stipend is awarded (amount not specified).

Duration 1 year.

Number awarded 1 each year.

Deadline May of each year.

[668]
MNAF GRADUATE DEGREE SCHOLARSHIP

Minnesota Nurses Association
Attn: Minnesota Nurses Association Foundation
1625 Energy Park Drive, Suite 200
St. Paul, MN 55108
(651) 414-2822   Toll Free: (800) 536-4662, ext. 122
Fax: (651) 695-7000   E-mail: linda.owens@mnnurses.org
Web: www.mnnurses.org

Summary To provide financial assistance to members of the Minnesota Nurses Association (MNA) who are interested in working on a graduate degree in nursing.

Eligibility This program is open to MNA members who have a current R.N. licensure and have been accepted into an approved program of study leading to a graduate academic degree in nursing. Applicants must submit a brief description of their career goals following their graduate education. Selection is based on that statement, professional activities, demonstrated leadership ability, scholarship in nursing, MNA activities, and community involvement.

Financial Data The stipend is $2,000 per year.

Duration 1 year; may be renewed.

Number awarded 1 each year.

Deadline May of each year.

[669]
MNRS/CANS DISSERTATION RESEARCH GRANT

Midwest Nursing Research Society
Attn: Executive Director
10200 West 44th Avenue, Suite 304
Wheat Ridge, CO 80033-2840
(720) 898-4831   Toll Free: (866) 908-8716
Fax: (303) 422-8894   E-mail: mnrs@resourcenter.com
Web: www.mnrs.org/i4a/pages/index.cfm?pageid=3529

Summary To provide funding for dissertation research to candidates for a doctorate in nursing who are members of the Midwest Nursing Research Society (MNRS) and the Council for the Advancement of Nursing Science (CANS).

Eligibility This program is open to nursing doctoral candidates at universities in the Midwest who are members of both MNRS and CANS. Applicants must be proposing to conduct quantitative or qualitative dissertation research on a topic relevant to nursing science. Preference is given to projects that present research purposes and aims that are sufficiently distinct for review and evaluation based on their own scientific merits.

Financial Data The grant is $2,500.

Duration 1 year.

Number awarded 4 each year.

Deadline December of each year.

[670]
MOLN MEMBER SCHOLARSHIPS

Minnesota Organization of Leaders in Nursing
1821 University Avenue West, Suite S256
St. Paul, MN 55104
(651) 999-5344   Fax: (651) 917-1835
E-mail: office@moln.org
Web: www.moln.org/sections/scholarships.php

Summary To provide financial assistance to members of the Minnesota Organization of Leaders in Nursing (MOLN) who are interested in returning to school to earn an additional degree in nursing.

Eligibility This program is open to MOLN members (must have been voting members for at least 12 months) who are currently enrolled or have been admitted to a relevant bachelor's, master's, or doctoral degree program. Applicants must have a GPA of 3.0 or higher in their current academic work. Along with their application, they must submit a 2-page essay on their goals in returning to school to complete a degree, how attainment of this degree will facilitate their professional development as a leader in nursing, and how their educational and career goals relate to the goals of MOLN. Selection is based on the essay, a letter of recommendation, and transcripts. Financial need is not considered.

Financial Data The stipend is $500.

Duration 1 year.

Number awarded Up to 6 each year.

Deadline June of each year.

[671]
MORGAN-SANDERS ENDOWED SCHOLARSHIP

Kansas State Nurses Association
Attn: Kansas Nurses Foundation
1109 S.W. Topeka Boulevard
Topeka, KS 66612-1602
(785) 233-8638   Fax: (785) 233-5222
E-mail: ksna@ksna.net
Web: www.nursingworld.org/SNAS/KS/Knf.htm

Summary To provide financial assistance to students in Kansas who are working on an undergraduate or graduate degree in nursing at a school in the state.

Eligibility This program is open to residents of Kansas who have a GPA of 3.0 or higher. The award is given according to the following priorities, in descending order: 1) R.N.s working on a B.S.N. degree; 2) graduate students in nursing education, nursing administration, or adult education programs (with priority given to master's and then doctoral level); 3) nonacademic nursing or nursing-related programs leading to a certificate; 4) students enrolled in undergraduate B.S.N. programs; and 5) students enrolled in undergraduate A.D.N. programs. Students enrolled in graduate or certificate program preparation for clinical nurse specialists, nurse practitioners, nurse midwives, and nurse anesthetists are not eligible. Preference is given to students engaged in full-time study. Along with their application, they must submit a personal narrative describing their anticipated role in nursing in the state.

Financial Data The stipend is $500.

Duration 1 year.

Number awarded 1 each year.

Deadline June of each year.

[672]
MYASTHENIA GRAVIS FOUNDATION NURSING FELLOWSHIPS

Myasthenia Gravis Foundation of America, Inc.
355 Lexington Avenue, 15th Floor
New York, NY 10017
(212) 297-2156   Toll Free: (800) 541-5454
Fax: (212) 370-9047   E-mail: mgfa@myasthenia.org
Web: www.myasthenia.org/hp_fellowships.cfm

Summary To provide funding to nurses and nursing students interested in conducting research on problems encountered by patients with Myasthenia Gravis.

Eligibility This program is open to nurses and nursing students who are interested in conducting research on the problems encountered by patients with Myasthenia Gravis or related neuromuscular conditions. Applicants must submit a budget, 10-page research plan, and biographical sketch.

Financial Data The grant is $5,000.

Duration Up to 1 year.

Number awarded Varies each year.

Deadline October of each year.

[673]
NADONA OF NORTH DAKOTA NURSING SCHOLARSHIP

NADONA of North Dakota
c/o Julie Hanson, President
750 Main Street East
Mayville, ND 58277
(701) 786-3401   Fax: (701) 789-9022
E-mail: jhanson-lhm@polarcomm.com
Web: www.ndnadona.org

Summary To provide financial assistance to employees of long-term care facilities in North Dakota who are interested in working on a degree in nursing at a school in any state.

Eligibility This program is open to employees of long-term care facilities in North Dakota that also have a member of NADONA of North Dakota on the staff. Applicants must be a licensed R.N., L.P.N., or certified nursing assistant. They must be planning to attend a school in any state to work on to work on an R.N. or L.P.N. in nursing management or gerontology or a master's degree in nursing, health care administration, or nurse practitioner. Along with their application, they must submit brief statements on 1) their future professional plans and interests unique to long-term care; and 2) any personal or professional experiences in long-term care that have led to their decision to prepare for a career in long-term care administration and the challenges they believe the long-term care profession holds.

Financial Data A stipend is awarded (amount not specified).

Duration 1 year.

Additional data The sponsor is the North Dakota affiliate of National Association Directors of Nursing Administration in Long Term Care (NADONA).

Number awarded 1 or more each year.

Deadline August of each year.

[674]
NAPNAP FOUNDATION GRADUATE STUDENT RESEARCH GRANT

National Association of Pediatric Nurse Practitioners
Attn: NAPNAP Foundation
20 Brace Road, Suite 200
Cherry Hill, NJ 08034-2634
(856) 857-9700   Toll Free: (877) 662-7627
Fax: (856) 857-1600   E-mail: info@napnap.org
Web: www.napnap.org

Summary To provide funding to graduate student members of the National Association of Pediatric Nurse Practitioners (NAPNAP) who are interested in conducting research.

Eligibility This program is open to graduate student members of the association who are interested in conducting research related to pediatric nursing. The proposed research should deal with a significant problem regarding children and families.

Financial Data The maximum grant is $1,000.

Duration 1 year.

Number awarded 1 each year.

Deadline March of each year.

[675]
NASN EDUCATIONAL ADVANCEMENT AWARDS

National Association of School Nurses
Attn: Scholarship Chair
8484 Georgia Avenue, Suite 420
Silver Spring, MD 20910
(240) 821-1130   Toll Free: (866) 627-6767
Fax: (301) 585-1791   E-mail: nasn@nasn.org
Web: www.nasn.org/Default.aspx?tabid=86

Summary To provide funding to members of the National Association of School Nurses (NASN) who are interested in advancing their education.

Eligibility This program is open to licensed registered nurses who are employed as a school nurse. Applicants must have been active members of NASN for at least the past 2 years. They must have a bachelor's degree (does not need to be in nursing) except for applicants who are pursuing a B.S.N./M.S.N. degree. Selection is based on brief essays by the applicant on the benefit of the advanced degree or course work to the applicant's school nursing practice (60%), impact on the community (25%), and educational goals (15%).
Financial Data The stipend is $1,500.
Duration 1 year.
Additional data This program was established in 1994 as the Shirley Steel Awards.
Number awarded 2 each year.
Deadline October of each year.

[676]
NATIONAL AMERICAN ARAB NURSES ASSOCIATION SCHOLARSHIPS

National American Arab Nurses Association
P.O. Box 43
Dearborn Heights, MI 48127
(313) 680-5049   E-mail: info@n-aana.org
Web: www.n-aana.org/scholarship/index.asp
Summary To provide financial assistance to nursing students who are members of the National American Arab Nurses Association (NAANA).
Eligibility This program is open to NAANA members who are studying nursing at the associate degree, bachelor's degree, master's degree, or R.N. to B.S.N. levels. Applicants must have a GPA of 3.5 or higher and a record of leadership in academic, professional, and/or student organizations. Along with their application, they must submit a 1-page essay on their career goals, leadership activities, and why they deserve the award. Financial need is not considered in the selection process. U.S. citizenship or permanent resident status is required.
Financial Data Stipends are $1,000 or $500.
Duration 1 year.
Additional data Until 2006, NAANA was named the American Arab Nurses Association.
Number awarded Varies each year.
Deadline May of each year.

[677]
NATIONAL ASSOCIATION OF SCHOOL NURSES/ AMERICAN NURSES FOUNDATION SCHOLAR AWARD

American Nurses Foundation
Attn: Nursing Research Grants Program
8515 Georgia Avenue, Suite 400
Silver Spring, MD 20910-3492
(301) 628-5227   Fax: (301) 628-5354
E-mail: anf@ana.org
Web: www.anfonline.org
Summary To provide funding to nurses interested in conducting research related to school health.
Eligibility This program is open to registered nurses who have earned a baccalaureate or higher degree and are members of the National Association of School Nurses (NASN). Applicants may be either beginning or experienced researchers, but they must be engaged in school nurse practice, education, or research. They must be planning to conduct research that is relevant to school nursing or student health (e.g., the impact of school nursing services on student health and academic outcomes, the effectiveness of health promotion and disease prevention, the cost-effectiveness of nursing services). Proposed research may be for a master's thesis or doctoral dissertation, if the project has been

approved by the principal investigator's thesis or dissertation committee.
Financial Data The grant is $3,500. Funds may not be used as a salary for the principal investigator.
Duration 1 year.
Additional data This program, established in 2010, is sponsored by the National Association of School Nurses. There is a $100 application fee.
Number awarded 1 each year.
Deadline April of each year.

[678]
NATIONAL ASSOCIATION OF SCHOOL NURSES DIRECTED RESEARCH GRANTS

National Association of School Nurses
Attn: NASN Research Committee
8484 Georgia Avenue, Suite 420
Silver Spring, MD 20910
(240) 821-1130   Toll Free: (866) 627-6767
Fax: (301) 585-1791   E-mail: nasn@nasn.org
Web: www.nasn.org/Default.aspx?tabid=371
Summary To provide funding to members of the National Association of School Nurses (NASN) who are interested in conducting research on specified school nursing issues.
Eligibility This program is open to qualified professional school nurses who have been members of the association for at least 1 year. Applicants must be 1) engaged in the practice of school nursing, the education of school nurses, or the study of school nursing as a graduate or undergraduate student; or 2) retired from school nursing. They must be interested in conducting research on 1 of several topics that are selected annually by the association as research priorities. Recently, the topics were: impact of school nursing services on student health and academic outcomes, effectiveness of health promotion and disease prevention, cost effectiveness of school health services, and predictors of successful outcomes for students needing health interventions. Selection is based on research question and purpose (5%), study aim and hypothesis (10%), background/review of literature/theoretical discussion (15%), methodology (35%), significance to school nursing (15%), qualifications of the researcher (15%), and overall quality of application (5%).
Financial Data Grants range up to $5,000 and average $2,500.
Duration 1 year.
Additional data This program, originally called the Carol Costante Research Grant, began in 1998.
Number awarded 1 to 3 each year.
Deadline February of each year.

[679]
NATIONAL ASSOCIATION OF SCHOOL NURSES RESEARCH GRANTS

National Association of School Nurses
Attn: NASN Research Committee
8484 Georgia Avenue, Suite 420
Silver Spring, MD 20910
(240) 821-1130   Toll Free: (866) 627-6767
Fax: (301) 585-1791   E-mail: nasn@nasn.org
Web: www.nasn.org/Default.aspx?tabid=371
Summary To provide funding to members of the National Association of School Nurses (NASN) who are interested in conducting research on a school nursing issue.
Eligibility This program is open to qualified professional school nurses who have been members of the association for at least 1 year. Applicants must be 1) engaged in the practice of school nursing, the education of school nurses, or the study of school nursing as a graduate or undergraduate student; or 2) retired from school nursing. They must be interested in conducting a research project on any topic that has an impact on student health and well

being. Selection is based on research question and purpose (5%), study aim and hypothesis (10%), background/review of literature/theoretical discussion (15%), methodology (35%), significance to school nursing (15%), qualifications of the researcher (15%), and overall quality of application (5%).

Financial Data Grants range up to $5,000 and average $2,500.

Duration 1 year.

Additional data This program was established in 1997 by combining 3 prior programs: the Lillian Wald Research Award, established in 1982 for research impacting the health of children; the Pauline Fenelon Research Award, established in 1987 for research in school nurse practice issues; and the Lina Rogers Award, established in 1990 for research impacting school nursing services for students.

Number awarded 1 or more each year.

Deadline February of each year.

[680]
NATIONAL STUDENT NURSES' ASSOCIATION GENERAL SCHOLARSHIPS

National Student Nurses' Association
Attn: Foundation
45 Main Street, Suite 606
Brooklyn, NY 11201
(718) 210-0705   Fax: (718) 797-1186
E-mail: nsna@nsna.org
Web: www.nsna.org

Summary To provide financial assistance to nursing or pre-nursing students.

Eligibility This program is open to students currently enrolled in state-approved schools of nursing or pre-nursing associate degree, baccalaureate, diploma, generic master's, generic doctoral, R.N. to B.S.N., R.N. to M.S.N., or L.P.N./L.V.N. to R.N. programs. Graduating high school seniors are not eligible. Support for graduate education is provided only for a first degree in nursing. Applicants must submit a 200-word description of their professional and educational goals and how this scholarship will help them achieve those goals. Selection is based on academic achievement, financial need, and involvement in student nursing organizations and community health activities. U.S. citizenship or permanent resident status is required.

Financial Data Stipends range from $1,000 to $2,500. A total of approximately $125,000 is awarded each year by the foundation for all its scholarship programs.

Duration 1 year.

Additional data This program includes the following named scholarships: the Anne Merin Memorial Scholarship, the Eileen Bowden Memorial Scholarship, the Alice Robinson Memorial Scholarship, the Jeannette Collins Memorial Scholarship, the Cleo Doster Memorial Scholarship, and the Mary Ann Tuft Scholarships. Sponsors include 3M Health Care, Bank of America, Catholic Healthcare West, Chi Eta Phi Sorority, Delmar Cengage Learning, Elsevier, HSBC Bank USA, Johnson & Johnson, Kaiser Permanente, Landau Uniforms, Pfizer, Sigma Theta Tau International, and United Healthcare. Applications must be accompanied by a $10 processing fee.

Number awarded Varies each year; recently, 63 of these scholarships were awarded.

Deadline January of each year.

[681]
NATIONAL STUDENT NURSES' ASSOCIATION SPECIALTY SCHOLARSHIPS

National Student Nurses' Association
Attn: Foundation
45 Main Street, Suite 606
Brooklyn, NY 11201
(718) 210-0705   Fax: (718) 797-1186
E-mail: nsna@nsna.org
Web: www.nsna.org

Summary To provide financial assistance to nursing students in designated specialties.

Eligibility This program is open to students currently enrolled in state-approved schools of nursing or pre-nursing associate degree, baccalaureate, diploma, generic master's, generic doctoral, R.N. to B.S.N., R.N. to M.S.N., or L.P.N./L.V.N. to R.N. programs. Graduating high school seniors are not eligible. Support for graduate education is provided only for a first degree in nursing. Applicants must designate their intended specialty, which may be anesthesia nursing, critical care, emergency, gerontology, informatics, nephrology, nurse educator, oncology, orthopedic, or perioperative. Along with their application, they must submit a 200-word description of their professional and educational goals and how this scholarship will help them achieve those goals. Selection is based on academic achievement, financial need, and involvement in student nursing organizations and community activities related to health care. U.S. citizenship or permanent resident status is required.

Financial Data Stipends range from $1,000 to $2,500. A total of approximately $125,000 is awarded each year by the foundation for all its scholarship programs.

Duration 1 year.

Additional data Funding for this program is provided in partnership with other nursing organizations, including the American Association of Nurse Anesthetists, the American Association of Critical-Care Nurses, the American Nephrology Nurses' Association, the American Organization of Nurse Executives, Decision Critical, Inc., the Emergency Nurses Association, the Infusion Nurses Society, and the Oncology Nursing Society. Applications must be accompanied by a $10 processing fee.

Number awarded Varies each year; recently 16 of these scholarships were awarded.

Deadline January of each year.

[682]
NAVY ADVANCED EDUCATION VOUCHER PROGRAM

U.S. Navy
Naval Education and Training Command
Center for Personal and Professional Development
Attn: AEV Program Office
6490 Saufley Field Road
Pensacola, FL 32509-5204
(850) 452-7271   Fax: (850) 452-1272
E-mail: rick.cusimano@navy.mil
Web: www.navycollege.navy.mil/aev/aev_home.cfm

Summary To provide financial assistance to Navy enlisted personnel who are interested in earning an undergraduate or graduate degree during off-duty hours.

Eligibility This program is open to senior enlisted Navy personnel in ranks E-7 and E-8. Applicants should be transferring to, or currently on, shore duty with sufficient time ashore to complete a bachelor's or master's degree. Personnel at rank E-7 may have no more than 16 years time in service and at E-8 no more than 18 years. The area of study must be certified by the Naval Postgraduate School as Navy-relevant.

Financial Data This program covers 100% of education costs (tuition, books, and fees). For a bachelor's degree, the maximum is $6,700 per year or a total of $20,000 per participant. For a master's degree, the maximum is $20,000 per year or a total of $40,000 per participant.

Duration Up to 36 months from the time of enrollment for a bachelor's degree; up to 24 months from the time of enrollment for a master's degree.

Additional data Recently approved majors for bachelor's degrees included human resources, construction management, information technology, emergency and disaster management, paralegal, engineering, business administration, leadership and management, nursing, strategic foreign languages, and electrical/electronic technology. Approved fields of study for master's degrees included business administration, education and training management, emergency and disaster management, engineering and technology, homeland defense and security, human resources, information technology, leadership and management, project management, and systems analysis. Recipients of this assistance incur an obligation to remain on active duty following completion of the program for a period equal to 3 times the number of months of education completed, to a maximum obligation of 36 months.

Number awarded Varies each year. Recently, 20 of these vouchers were awarded: 15 for bachelor's degrees and 5 for master's degrees.

Deadline February of each year.

[683]
NEANA SCHOLARSHIPS

American Association of Nurse Anesthetists
Attn: AANA Foundation
222 South Prospect Avenue
Park Ridge, IL 60068-4001
(847) 655-1170   Fax: (847) 692-6968
E-mail: foundation@aana.com
Web: www.aanafoundation.com

Summary To provide financial assistance to members of the American Association of Nurse Anesthetists (AANA) who are residents of the New England states and interested in obtaining further education at a program in those states.

Eligibility This program is open to members of the association who are residents of Maine, Massachusetts, New Hampshire, Rhode Island, or Vermont and/or attending a nurse anesthesia program in those states. First-year students must have completed 6 months of nurse anesthesia classes; second-year students must have completed 12 months of nurse anesthesia classes. Along with their application, they must submit a 200-word essay describing why they have chosen nurse anesthesia as a profession and their professional goals for the future. Financial need is also considered in the selection process.

Financial Data The stipend is $1,000.

Duration 1 year.

Additional data Funding for these scholarships, first awarded in 1998, is provided by the New England Assembly of Nurse Anesthetists (NEANA). The application processing fee is $25.

Number awarded 2 each year.

Deadline March of each year.

[684]
NEBRASKA STUDENT NURSE ANESTHETIST SCHOLARSHIP

Nebraska Association of Nurse Anesthetists
Attn: Foundation
625 South 14th Street, Suite A
Lincoln, NE 68508
(402) 436-2165   Fax: (402) 436-2169
Web: www.neana.org/foundation.shtml

Summary To provide financial assistance to residents of Nebraska who are completing a nurse anesthesia program.

Eligibility This program is open to residents of Nebraska who are in the final 12 months of a nurse anesthesia program.

Financial Data The stipend is $1,000.

Duration 1 year.

Additional data This scholarship was first awarded in 2003.

Number awarded 1 each year.

Deadline Deadline not specified.

[685]
NEBRASKA STUDENT NURSE ANESTHETISTS SCHOLARSHIP

American Association of Nurse Anesthetists
Attn: AANA Foundation
222 South Prospect Avenue
Park Ridge, IL 60068-4001
(847) 655-1170   Fax: (847) 692-6968
E-mail: foundation@aana.com
Web: www.aanafoundation.com

Summary To provide financial assistance to members of the American Association of Nurse Anesthetists (AANA) from any state who are completing a clinical rotation in Nebraska.

Eligibility This program is open to members of the association from any state who have completed or will complete a clinical rotation in Nebraska prior to graduation from a nurse anesthesia program. Applicants must be second-year students who have completed 12 months of nurse anesthesia classes. Along with their application, they must submit a 200-word essay describing why they have chosen nurse anesthesia as a profession and their professional goals for the future. Financial need is also considered in the selection process.

Financial Data The stipend is $1,000.

Duration 1 year.

Additional data Funding for this scholarship, first awarded in 2003, is provided by the Nebraska Association of Nurse Anesthetists. The application processing fee is $25.

Number awarded 1 each year.

Deadline March of each year.

[686]
NEF DOCTORAL SCHOLARSHIPS

Nurses Educational Funds, Inc.
Attn: Scholarship Coordinator
304 Park Avenue South, 11th Floor
New York, NY 10010
(212) 590-2443   Fax: (212) 590-2446
E-mail: info@n-e-f.org
Web: www.n-e-f.org

Summary To provide financial assistance to nurses who are interested in working on a doctoral degree.

Eligibility This program is open to registered nurses who are members of a national professional nursing organization and are enrolled in a nursing or nursing-related program at the doctoral level. Applicants must have a GPA of 3.6 or higher. They must be U.S. citizens or have declared their official intention of becoming a citizen. Along with their application, they must submit an 800-word essay on their professional goals and potential for making a contribution to the nursing profession. Selection is based on academic excellence and the essay's content and clarity.

Financial Data Stipends range from $2,500 to $10,000, depending on the availability of funds.

Duration 1 year.

Additional data The highest-ranked applicant is awarded the Isabel Hampton Robb Scholarship. There is a $20 application fee.

Number awarded Varies each year; recently, 9 of these scholarships were awarded.

Deadline February of each year.

[687]
NEF MASTER'S SCHOLARSHIPS

Nurses Educational Funds, Inc.
Attn: Scholarship Coordinator
304 Park Avenue South, 11th Floor
New York, NY 10010
(212) 590-2443   Fax: (212) 590-2446
E-mail: info@n-e-f.org
Web: www.n-e-f.org

Summary To provide financial assistance to nurses who are interested in working on a master's degree.

Eligibility This program is open to registered nurses who are members of a national professional nursing organization and enrolled full or part time in an accredited master's degree program in nursing. Applicants must have completed at least 12 credits and have a cumulative GPA of 3.6 or higher. They must be U.S. citizens or have declared their official intention of becoming a citizen. Along with their application, they must submit an 800-word essay on their professional goals and potential for making a contribution to the nursing profession. Selection is based on academic excellence and the essay's content and clarity.

Financial Data Awards range from $2,500 to $10,000, depending on the availability of funds.

Duration 1 year.

Additional data The highest-ranked applicant is awarded the Isabel McIsaac Scholarship. There is a $20 application fee.

Number awarded Varies each year; recently, 7 of these scholarships were awarded.

Deadline February of each year.

[688]
NEONATAL NURSING ACADEMIC SCHOLARSHIP AWARD

Academy of Neonatal Nursing
2270 Northpoint Parkway
Santa Rosa, CA 95407-7398
(707) 568-2168   Fax: (707) 569-0786
Web: www.academyonline.org/awards_scholarships.html

Summary To provide financial assistance to members of the Academy of Neonatal Nursing (ANN) who are working on an undergraduate or graduate degree in neonatal nursing or a related nursing major.

Eligibility This program is open to ANN members who have been in good standing for at least 2 years. Applicants must have at least 2 years of neonatal practice experience with at least 1 of those years completed in the past 18 months. They must be enrolled in a nursing academic degree program or a neonatal graduate program in which they have completed at least 2 degree-required courses with a GPA of 3.0 or higher. Only professionally-active neonatal nurses are eligible, i.e., currently engaged in a clinical, research, or educational role that contributes directly to the health care of neonates or to the nursing profession and taking 15 contact hours of continuing education a year. Along with their application, they must submit a 200-word essay on why they are pursuing their education and how attainment of this degree will benefit them in their professional role. Financial need is not considered in the selection process.

Financial Data The stipend is $1,000. Funds are paid directly to the recipient and the educational program.

Duration 1 year; recipients are not eligible for another scholarship for 5 years.

Number awarded 1 each year.

Deadline May of each year.

[689]
NEPHROLOGY NURSES CAREER MOBILITY SCHOLARSHIPS

American Nephrology Nurses' Association
Attn: ANNA National Office
200 East Holly Avenue
P.O. Box 56
Pitman, NJ 08071-0056
(856) 256-2320   Toll Free: (888) 600-2662
Fax: (856) 589-7463   E-mail: annascholarships@ajj.com
Web: www.annanurse.org

Summary To provide financial assistance to members of the American Nephrology Nurses' Association (ANNA) who are interested in working on a baccalaureate or advanced degree in nursing.

Eligibility Applicants must be current association members, have been members for at least 2 years, be actively involved in nephrology nursing-related health care services, and be accepted or enrolled in a baccalaureate or higher degree program in nursing. Along with their application, they must submit a 250-word essay on their career and educational goals that includes the expected time frame for completing their degree, the application of the award to meet expected expenses, and the impact of the completion of the degree program on their nephrology nursing practice.

Financial Data The stipend is $2,000.

Duration 1 year.

Additional data These scholarships were first awarded in 1993.

Number awarded 5 each year.

Deadline October of each year.

[690]
NEPHROLOGY NURSING CERTIFICATION COMMISSION CAREER MOBILITY SCHOLARSHIPS

American Nephrology Nurses' Association
Attn: ANNA National Office
200 East Holly Avenue
P.O. Box 56
Pitman, NJ 08071-0056
(609) 256-2320   Toll Free: (888) 600-2662
Fax: (856) 589-7463   E-mail: annascholarships@ajj.com
Web: www.annanurse.org

Summary To provide financial assistance to members of the American Nephrology Nurses' Association (ANNA) who are Certified Nephrology Nurses or Certified Dialysis Nurses and are interested in working on a baccalaureate or graduate degree in nursing to enhance their nephrology nursing practice.

Eligibility Applicants must have a current credential as a Certified Nephrology Nurse (CNN) or Certified Dialysis Nurse (CDN) administered by the Nephrology Nursing Certification Commission (NNCC), be current association members, have been members for at least 2 years, be actively involved in nephrology nursing related health care services, and be accepted or enrolled in a baccalaureate or higher degree program in nursing. Along with their application, they must submit a 250-word essay on their career and educational goals that includes the expected time frame for completing their degree, the application of the award to meet expected expenses, and the impact of the completion of the degree program on their nephrology nursing practice.

Financial Data The stipend is $2,000.

Duration 1 year.

Additional data Funds for this program, established in 1993, are supplied by the NNCC.

Number awarded 3 each year.

Deadline October of each year.

[691]
NEW ENGLAND AREA FUTURE LEADERSHIP AWARD

American Society of Safety Engineers
Attn: ASSE Foundation
1800 East Oakton Street
Des Plaines, IL 60018
(847) 768-3435   Fax: (847) 768-3434
E-mail: agabanski@asse.org
Web: www.asse.org/foundation/scholarships/scholarships.php

Summary To provide financial assistance to upper-division and graduate student members of the American Society of Safety Engineers (ASSE). especially those from the Northeast.

Eligibility This program is open to ASSE student members who are working on an undergraduate or graduate degree in occupational safety, health, and environment or a closely-related field (e.g., industrial or environmental engineering, environmental science, industrial hygiene, occupational health nursing). Undergraduates must be full-time students who have completed at least 60 semester hours with a GPA of 3.0 or higher. Graduate students must also be enrolled full time, have completed at least 9 semester hours with a GPA of 3.5 or higher, and have earned a GPA of 3.0 or higher as an undergraduate. Along with their application, they must submit 2 essays of 300 words or less: 1) why they are seeking a degree in occupational safety and health or a closely-related field, a brief description of their current activities, and how those relate to their career goals and objectives; and 2) why they should be awarded this scholarship (including career goals and financial need). Priority is given first to residents of New England, and second to residents of the ASSE Region VIII (which covers the 6 New England states plus New York, New Jersey, and Pennsylvania). U.S. citizenship is not required.

Financial Data The stipend is $1,000 per year.

Duration 1 year; recipients may reapply.

Additional data This program was established in 2008.

Number awarded 1 each year.

Deadline November of each year.

[692]
NEW ENGLAND NAVY NURSE CORPS ASSOCIATION SCHOLARSHIP

New England Navy Nurse Corps Association
c/o Maria K. Carroll, Scholarship Committee
22 William Drive
Middletown, RI 02842-5266

Summary To provide financial assistance to registered nurses (R.N.s) and nursing students working on a bachelor's or master's degree at a college or university in New England.

Eligibility This program is open to R.N.s and nursing students in the New England states. Applicants must be working on a bachelor's or master's degree in nursing and have a GPA of 2.3 or higher. They must have completed at least 1 clinical nursing course. Along with their application, they must submit a 500-word essay on why they are qualified for this scholarship, their career goals, and their potential for contribution to the profession.

Financial Data The stipend is $1,000.

Duration 1 year.

Number awarded 2 each year.

Deadline May of each year.

[693]
NEW HAMPSHIRE ASSOCIATION OF NURSE ANESTHETISTS SCHOLARSHIP

American Association of Nurse Anesthetists
Attn: AANA Foundation
222 South Prospect Avenue
Park Ridge, IL 60068-4001
(847) 655-1170   Fax: (847) 692-6968
E-mail: foundation@aana.com
Web: www.aanafoundation.com

Summary To provide financial assistance to members of the American Association of Nurse Anesthetists (AANA) who are residents of New Hampshire or working on a nurse anesthesia degree in the state.

Eligibility This program is open to members of the association who are residents of New Hampshire or attending a nurse anesthesia program in the state. First-year students must have completed 6 months of nurse anesthesia classes; second-year students must have completed 12 months of nurse anesthesia classes. Along with their application, they must submit a 200-word essay describing why they have chosen nurse anesthesia as a profession and their professional goals for the future. Financial need is also considered in the selection process.

Financial Data The stipend is $1,000.

Duration 1 year.

Additional data Funding for this program is provided by the New Hampshire Association of Nurse Anesthetists. The application processing fee is $25.

Number awarded 1 each year.

Deadline March of each year.

[694]
NEW HAMPSHIRE WORKFORCE INCENTIVE PROGRAM FORGIVABLE LOANS

New Hampshire Postsecondary Education Commission
Attn: Financial Aid Programs Coordinator
3 Barrell Court, Suite 300
Concord, NH 03301-8543
(603) 271-2555, ext. 360   Fax: (603) 271-2696
TDD: (800) 735-2964
E-mail: cynthia.capodestria@pec.state.nh.us
Web: www.nh.gov/postsecondary/financial/wip.html

Summary To provide scholarship/loans to New Hampshire residents who are interested in attending college in the state to prepare for careers in nursing and other designated professions.

Eligibility This program is open to residents of New Hampshire who wish to prepare for careers in fields designated by the commission as shortage areas. Currently, the career shortage areas are education (chemistry, general science, mathematics, physical sciences, physics, special education, and world languages), and nursing (L.P.N. through graduate). Applicants must be enrolled as a junior, senior, or graduate student at a college in New Hampshire and able to demonstrate financial need.

Financial Data Stipends are determined by the institution; recently, they averaged $1,200 per year. This is a scholarship/loan program; recipients must agree to pursue, within New Hampshire, the professional career for which they receive training. Recipients of loans for 1 year have their notes cancelled upon completion of 1 year of full-time service; repayment by service must be completed within 3 years from the date of licensure, certification, or completion of the program. Recipients of loans for more than 1 year have their notes cancelled upon completion of 2 years of full-time service; repayment by service must be completed within 5 years from the date of licensure, certification, or completion of the program. If the note is not cancelled because of service, the recipient must repay the loan within 2 years.

Duration 1 year; may be renewed.

Additional data The time for repayment of the loan, either in cash or through professional service, is extended while the recipient is 1) engaged in a course of study, at least on a half-time basis, at an institution of higher education; 2) serving on active duty as a member of the armed forces of the United States, or as a member of VISTA, the Peace Corps, or AmeriCorps, for a period up to 3 years; 3) temporarily totally disabled for a period up to 3 years; or 4) unable to secure employment because of the need to care for a disabled spouse, child, or parent for a period up to 12 months. The repayment obligation is cancelled if the recipient is unable to work because of a permanent total disability, receives relief under federal bankruptcy laws, or dies. This program went into effect in 1999.
Number awarded Varies each year; recently, 45 of these loans were awarded.
Deadline May of each year for fall semester; December of each year for spring semester.

[695]
NEW JERSEY HFMA MEMBER SCHOLARSHIP

Healthcare Financial Management Association-New Jersey Chapter
Attn: Laura A. Hess
P.O. Box 6422
Bridgewater, NJ 08807
Toll Free: (888) 652-4362   Fax: (908) 722-8775
E-mail: njhfma@aol.com
Web: www.hfmanj.org/Scholarship-Information.page
Summary To provide financial assistance to members of the New Jersey Chapter of the Healthcare Financial Management Association (HFMA) and their families who are interested in working on a degree related to health care administration at a school in any state.
Eligibility Applicants must have been a member of the chapter for at least 2 years or the spouse or dependent of a 2-year member. They must be enrolled in an accredited college, university, nursing school, or other allied health professional school in any state. Preference is given to applicants working on a degree in finance, accounting, health care administration, or a field of study related to health care. Along with their application, they must submit an essay describing their educational and professional goals and the role of this scholarship in helping achieve those. Selection is based on the essay, merit, academic achievement, civic and professional activities, course of study, and content of the application. Financial need is not considered.
Financial Data The stipend ranges up to $3,000.
Duration 1 year.
Number awarded 1 or more each year.
Deadline March of each year.

[696]
NEW JERSEY STATE NURSES ASSOCIATION RESEARCH GRANTS

New Jersey State Nurses Association
Attn: Institute for Nursing
1479 Pennington Road
Trenton, NJ 08618-2661
(609) 883-5335   Toll Free: (888) UR-NJSNA
Fax: (609) 883-5343   E-mail: institute@njsna.org
Web: www.njsna.org/displaycommon.cfm?an=5
Summary To provide funding to members of the New Jersey Nurses Association who are interested in conducting research.
Eligibility This program is open to current members of the association who have the research knowledge, skills, and resources to prepare a scientifically sound research proposal and carry out the project if it is funded. Projects may be empirical or non-empirical. Applicants must submit a proposal that includes their aims, background and significance of the research, previous

work, publications, methods, facilities, budget, and curriculum vitae. Doctoral students are encouraged to apply.
Financial Data The grant is $1,000.
Duration 1 year.
Number awarded 1 or more each year.
Deadline May of each year.

[697]
NEW MEXICO NURSE EDUCATOR LOAN-FOR-SERVICE PROGRAM

New Mexico Higher Education Department
Attn: Financial Aid Division
2048 Galisteo Street
Santa Fe, NM 87505-2100
(505) 476-8411   Toll Free: (800) 279-9777
Fax: (505) 476-8454   E-mail: Theresa.acker@state.nm.us
Web: hed.state.nm.us
Summary To provide loans-for-service to nursing education students from New Mexico who are willing to work in the state after graduation.
Eligibility This program is open to residents of New Mexico interested in working on a bachelor's, master's, or doctoral degree to prepare for a career as a nursing educator. Applicants must have been accepted by a New Mexico public postsecondary institution in a program that will enable them to enhance or gain employment in a nursing faculty position at a public college or university in the state. Along with their application, they must submit an essay explaining their need for this assistance and why they are interested in becoming a nurse educator in New Mexico. U.S. citizenship or eligible non-citizen status is required.
Financial Data The loan is $5,000 per year for enrollment in 9 credit hours and above, $3,000 per year for enrollment in 6 to 8 credit hours, or $1,500 per year for enrollment in 5 credit hours or less. This is a loan-for-service program; for every year of service as a nursing faculty member in New Mexico, a portion of the loan is forgiven. If the entire service agreement is fulfilled, 100% of the loan is eligible for forgiveness. Penalties may be assessed if the service agreement is not satisfied.
Duration 1 year; may be renewed.
Number awarded Varies each year, depending on the availability of funds.
Deadline June of each year.

[698]
NEW MEXICO NURSING LOAN-FOR-SERVICE PROGRAM

New Mexico Higher Education Department
Attn: Financial Aid Division
2048 Galisteo Street
Santa Fe, NM 87505-2100
(505) 476-8411   Toll Free: (800) 279-9777
Fax: (505) 476-8454   E-mail: Theresa.acker@state.nm.us
Web: hed.state.nm.us
Summary To provide loans-for-service to nursing students from New Mexico willing to work in underserved areas of the state after graduation.
Eligibility This program is open to residents of New Mexico interested in preparing for a career as a nurse (including a licensed practical nursing certificate, associate degree in nursing, bachelor of science in nursing, master of science in nursing, or advanced practice nurse). Applicants must be enrolled or accepted in an accredited program at a New Mexico public postsecondary institution. As a condition of the loan, they must declare an intent to practice in a designated shortage area of New Mexico for at least 1 year after completing their education. Along with their application, they must submit a brief essay on why they want to enter the field of nursing and obligate themselves to a

rural practice in New Mexico. U.S. citizenship or eligible non-citizen status is required.

Financial Data The loan depends on the financial need of the recipient, to a total of $12,000 per year. This is a loan-for-service program; for every year of service as a nurse in New Mexico, a portion of the loan is forgiven. If the entire service agreement is fulfilled, 100% of the loan is eligible for forgiveness. Penalties may be assessed if the service agreement is not satisfied.

Duration 1 year; may be renewed up to 3 additional years.

Number awarded Varies each year, depending on the availability of funds.

Deadline June of each year.

[699]
NEW MEXICO STUDENT ANESTHETIST SCHOLARSHIP

American Association of Nurse Anesthetists
Attn: AANA Foundation
222 South Prospect Avenue
Park Ridge, IL 60068-4001
(847) 655-1170　　　　　　Fax: (847) 692-6968
E-mail: foundation@aana.com
Web: www.aanafoundation.com

Summary To provide financial assistance to members of the American Association of Nurse Anesthetists (AANA), especially those from New Mexico, who are interested in obtaining further education.

Eligibility This program is open to members of the association who are either residents of New Mexico or planning to return to the state following graduation. Applicants must be currently enrolled in an accredited nurse anesthesia education program in any state. First-year students must have completed 6 months of nurse anesthesia classes; second-year students must have completed 12 months of nurse anesthesia classes. Along with their application, they must submit a 200-word essay describing why they have chosen nurse anesthesia as a profession and their professional goals for the future. Financial need is also considered in the selection process.

Financial Data The stipend is $2,000.

Duration 1 year.

Additional data Funds for this scholarship, first awarded in 2004, are provided by the New Mexico Association of Nurse Anesthetists. The application processing fee is $25.

Number awarded 1 each year.

Deadline March of each year.

[700]
NEW YORK ACADEMY OF MEDICINE STUDENT ESSAY PRIZE IN THE HISTORY OF MEDICINE AND PUBLIC HEALTH

New York Academy of Medicine
Attn: Student Essay
1216 Fifth Avenue
New York, NY 10029-5202
(212) 822-7314　　　　　　Fax: (212) 822-7338
E-mail: historyessay@nyam.org
Web: www.nyam.org/grants/studentessay.shtml

Summary To recognize and reward graduate students in health-related fields who submit outstanding essays on the history of medicine or public health.

Eligibility This competition is open to graduate students in medical, public health, pharmacy, or nursing programs in the United States. Applicants must submit an essay, approximately 2,000 to 3,000 words in length, on topics in the history of public health or medicine as they relate to urban health issues, social or environmental factors in the health of urban populations, institutional histories, or specific diseases. Selection is based on the quality and originality of the research, the significance of the topic,

and appropriateness for publication in the *Journal of Urban Health*..

Financial Data The prize is $500.

Duration The prize is awarded annually.

Additional data This prize was first awarded in 2005.

Number awarded 1 each year.

Deadline March of each year.

[701]
NEW YORK EMPIRE STATE CHALLENGE SCHOLARSHIP

Emergency Nurses Association
Attn: ENA Foundation
915 Lee Street
Des Plaines, IL 60016-6569
(847) 460-4100　　　　Toll Free: (800) 900-9659, ext. 4100
Fax: (847) 460-4004　　　　E-mail: foundation@ena.org
Web: www.ena.org

Summary To provide financial assistance to members of the Emergency Nurses Association (ENA) who are working on a master's degree.

Eligibility This program is open to emergency nurses (R.N.) who are working on a master's degree. Applicants must have been members of the association for at least 12 months and have a GPA of 3.0 or higher. They must submit a 1-page statement on their professional and educational goals and how this scholarship will help them attain those goals. Selection is based on content and clarity of the goal statement (45%), professional association involvement (35%), presentation of the application (10%), and letters of reference (10%).

Financial Data The stipend is $5,000.

Duration 1 year.

Additional data This program is funded by the New York ENA State Council.

Number awarded 1 each year.

Deadline May of each year.

[702]
NORTH CAROLINA MASTER'S NURSE SCHOLARS PROGRAM

North Carolina State Education Assistance Authority
Attn: Nurse Scholars Program
10 T.W. Alexander Drive
P.O. Box 13663
Research Triangle Park, NC 27709-3663
(919) 549-8614　　　　Toll Free: (800) 700-1775
Fax: (919) 248-4687　　　　E-mail: information@ncseaa.edu
Web: www.ncseaa.edu/MNSP.htm

Summary To provide loans-for-service to nurses in North Carolina who are interested in returning to school in the state to work on a master's degree.

Eligibility This program is open to North Carolina residents who have a B.S.N. degree and plan to work full time on a master's degree in nursing at a college, university, or hospital in the state to work as a master's level nurse or to teach in an accredited nurse education program in the state. Applicants must have a GPA of 3.2 or higher. Selection is based on academic record, teaching and leadership experience and potential, research and publishing experience and results, and desire to practice nursing on a full-time basis in North Carolina. Financial need is not considered.

Financial Data The award is $6,500 per year for full-time study or $3,250 per year for part-time study. This is a loan-for-service program. Each year of service in North Carolina after graduation as a master's-prepared nurse or a teacher in a nurse education program cancels 1 year of support. If recipients do not work as a nurse in North Carolina after graduation, they must repay the loan plus 10% interest. Recipients have up to 7 years to repay loans with service or 10 years to repay in cash.

Duration 1 year; may be renewed up to 2 additional years.

Additional data The North Carolina General Assembly created this program in 1989; the first recipients were funded for the 1990-91 academic year.

Number awarded Varies each year; recently, a total of 94 students were receiving $477,000 through this program.

Deadline May of each year.

[703]
NORTH CAROLINA NURSE EDUCATORS OF TOMORROW PROGRAM

North Carolina State Education Assistance Authority
Attn: Nurse Educators of Tomorrow Program
10 T.W. Alexander Drive
P.O. Box 13663
Research Triangle Park, NC 27709-3663
(919) 549-8614   Toll Free: (800) 700-1775
Fax: (919) 248-4687   E-mail: information@ncseaa.edu
Web: www.ncseaa.edu/NET.htm

Summary To provide loans-for-service to residents of North Carolina who are working on a graduate degree in nursing and interested in returning to the state to teach nursing after graduation.

Eligibility This program is open to North Carolina residents who are enrolled in a master's or doctoral degree program in nursing education or any other area of the nursing field that will permit them to become nursing instructors in an approved program in the state. Applicants must have completed a baccalaureate degree with a GPA of 3.2 or higher and be enrolled full time. Selection is based on academic record, leadership potential, and desire to become a nursing instructor in North Carolina. Priority is given to students at North Carolina nursing schools. U.S. citizenship is required.

Financial Data The award is $15,000 per year. This is a loan-for-service program. Recipients must teach full time as a nurse educator in North Carolina for each year of funding they receive. If they fail to complete that service requirement, they must repay all funds received with 10% interest. They have up to 7 years to repay the loan in service or 10 years to repay in cash.

Duration 1 year; renewable for 1 additional year for master's degree students or 2 years for doctoral students.

Additional data The North Carolina General Assembly created this program in 2006.

Number awarded Varies each year; recently, a total of 123 students were receiving a total of $1,785,000 in support through this program.

Deadline May of each year.

[704]
NORTH CAROLINA STATE CONTRACTUAL SCHOLARSHIP FUND PROGRAM

North Carolina State Education Assistance Authority
Attn: Grants, Training, and Outreach Department
10 T.W. Alexander Drive
P.O. Box 13663
Research Triangle Park, NC 27709-3663
(919) 549-8614   Toll Free: (800) 700-1775
Fax: (919) 248-4687   E-mail: information@ncseaa.edu
Web: www.ncseaa.edu/SCSF.htm

Summary To provide financial assistance to residents of North Carolina enrolled at private colleges and universities in the state.

Eligibility This program is open to North Carolina residents who are enrolled full or part time at approved North Carolina private colleges and universities. Applicants must normally be undergraduates, although they may have a bachelor's degree if they are enrolled in a licensure program for teachers or nurses.

Students enrolled in a program of study in theology, divinity, religious education, or any other program of study designed primarily for career preparation in a religious vocation are not eligible. Financial need is considered in the selection process.

Financial Data Stipends depend on the need of the recipient and the availability of funds. Recently, they averaged more than $2,600 per year.

Duration 1 year.

Additional data Recipients are selected by the financial aid offices of the eligible private institutions in North Carolina. This program was established in 1971.

Number awarded Varies each year; recently, a total of 16,137 students received $42,992,813 through this program.

Deadline Deadline not specified.

[705]
NORTH CAROLINA STUDENT LOAN PROGRAM FOR HEALTH, SCIENCE, AND MATHEMATICS

North Carolina State Education Assistance Authority
Attn: Health, Science, and Mathematics Program
10 T.W. Alexander Drive
P.O. Box 13663
Research Triangle Park, NC 27709-3663
(919) 549-8614   Toll Free: (800) 700-1775
Fax: (919) 248-4687   E-mail: information@ncseaa.edu
Web: www.ncseaa.edu/HSM.htm

Summary To provide forgivable loans to North Carolina residents who are interested in preparing for a career as a primary care physician, allied health professional, or science and mathematics educator.

Eligibility This program is open to North Carolina residents who have been accepted as full-time students in an accredited associate, baccalaureate, master's, or doctoral program leading to a degree in 1 of the following areas: audiology, cardiology, chiropractic medicine, clinical psychology, communications assistant, cytotechnology, dental hygiene, dentistry, mathematics education, medical social work, medical technology, nurse midwifery, nursing, nursing administration, nursing anesthetist, nursing family practitioner, nutritional sciences, occupational therapy/assistant, oncology, optometry, osteopathic medicine, pharmacy, physician assistant in primary care, physical therapy/assistant, podiatry, primary care physician, radiological technology, respiratory therapy/technician, science education, speech language pathology, or veterinary medicine. Applicants must be enrolled or planning to enroll full time at a college or university in North Carolina unless they are working on a degree in a field not offered at a North Carolina institution (i.e., chiropractic medicine, optometry, osteopathic medicine, or podiatry). Selection is based on major, academic capability, and financial need.

Financial Data Maximum loans are $3,000 per year for associate degree and certificate programs, $5,000 per year for baccalaureate degree/certificate programs, $6,500 per year for master's degree programs, or $8,500 per year for health- professional doctoral programs. The interest rate is 4% while the borrowers are attending school and 10% after they leave school. Loans (including accrued interest) are forgiven if the recipients work in North Carolina in their professional area for 1 year for each year of support received; primary care physicians and some allied health professionals must work in designated shortage areas in the state to qualify for loan forgiveness.

Duration 1 year; renewable for 1 additional year for diploma, associate, certificate, and master's degree programs, for 2 additional years for baccalaureate degree programs, or for 3 additional years for doctoral programs.

Additional data This program, formerly known as the North Carolina Medical Student Loan Program, was established in 1945.

Number awarded Varies each year; recently, a total of 390 students were receiving $2,578,178 in support through this program.
Deadline April of each year.

[706]
NORTH DAKOTA NURSING EDUCATION LOAN PROGRAM

North Dakota Board of Nursing
919 South Seventh Street, Suite 504
Bismarck, ND 58504-5881
(701) 328-9777   Fax: (701) 328-9785
Web: www.ndbon.org

Summary To provide forgivable loans to students in North Dakota who are working on an undergraduate degree, graduate degree, or continuing education program in nursing.
Eligibility This program is open to 1) students enrolled in a North Dakota board-approved or recognized undergraduate nursing education program for practical nurses or registered nurses; 2) nurses who have a current North Dakota license and have been accepted into or are currently enrolled in a graduate program that is acceptable to the Board of Nursing, and 3) nurses who are residents of North Dakota and interested in taking refresher courses. All applicants must demonstrate financial need. Along with their application, they must submit official transcripts, co-signer information, 3 letters of reference, personal financial information, a financial aid inquiry form (except for graduate students), and a student status form verifying their acceptance and expected enrollment date in the nursing program or major.
Financial Data Students in a licensed practical nurse program who plan to complete studies for an associate degree in nursing may receive up to $1,000 per year. Students in a registered nurse program who plan to complete a baccalaureate degree in nursing may receive up to $1,500 per year. Graduate students may receive up to $2,500 to complete their master's degree in nursing. Graduate students working on a doctoral degree in nursing may receive up to $5,000. Licensed practical nurses or registered nurses may receive up to the cost of a continuing education/refresher course. This is a scholarship/loan program. Recipients must agree to work as a nurse in North Dakota after graduation; the repayment rate will be $1 for each hour of employment. If employment in North Dakota is terminated before the loan is canceled, or the recipient does not work in North Dakota, or the recipient does not pass the NCLEX examination within 180 days of graduation, the loan must be repaid. The interest rate charged is approximately 9%.
Duration 2 years for students in a licensed practical nurse program; the last 2 years for students in a baccalaureate nursing degree program.
Additional data Recipients may request a deferment of payment if they proceed directly to the next level of education. There is a $15 application fee. The spouse of an applicant is not acceptable as the co-signer of the note. The co-signer should be a North Dakota resident. If the co-signer is not a North Dakota resident, the applicant must provide a letter of explanation. Proof of majority of the co-signer (18 years or older) may be required. Undergraduate recipients must be enrolled in school in a minimum of 6 credits per semester or 12 credits per year.
Number awarded 30 to 35 each year.
Deadline June of each year.

[707]
NORTH FLORIDA CHAPTER SAFETY EDUCATION SCHOLARSHIP

American Society of Safety Engineers
Attn: ASSE Foundation
1800 East Oakton Street
Des Plaines, IL 60018
(847) 768-3435   Fax: (847) 768-3434
E-mail: agabanski@asse.org
Web: www.asse.org/foundation/scholarships/scholarships.php

Summary To provide financial assistance to undergraduate and graduate student members of the American Society of Safety Engineers (ASSE) from Florida.
Eligibility This program is open to undergraduate and graduate students who are working on a degree in occupational safety, health, and environment or a closely-related field (e.g., industrial or environmental engineering, environmental science, industrial hygiene, occupational health nursing). Priority is given first to part- and full-time students who belong to the ASSE North Florida Chapter; second to full-time students at any Florida college or university; and third to full-time students at an ASAC/ABET accredited program in any state. Undergraduates must have completed at least 60 semester hours with a GPA of 3.0 or higher. Graduate students must have completed at least 9 semester hours with a GPA of 3.5 or higher and have earned a GPA of 3.0 or higher as an undergraduate. Full-time students must be ASSE student members; part-time students must be ASSE general or professional members. Along with their application, they must submit 2 essays of 300 words or less: 1) why they are seeking a degree in occupational safety and health or a closely-related field, a brief description of their current activities, and how those relate to their career goals and objectives; and 2) why they should be awarded this scholarship (including career goals and financial need). U.S. citizenship is not required.
Financial Data The stipend is $1,000 per year.
Duration 1 year; recipients may reapply.
Additional data This program is sponsored by the ASSE North Florida Chapter.
Number awarded 1 each year.
Deadline November of each year.

[708]
NOVA FOUNDATION SCHOLARSHIPS

Nurses Organization of Veterans Affairs
Attn: NOVA Foundation
47595 Watkins Island Square
Sterling, VA 20165
(703) 444-5587   Fax: (703) 444-5597
E-mail: nova@vanurse.org
Web: www.vanurse.org/scholarship.html

Summary To provide financial assistance to employees of the U.S. Department of Veterans Affairs (VA) who are working on an undergraduate or graduate degree in nursing.
Eligibility This program is open to VA employees who are enrolled or accepted for enrollment in an NLN-accredited baccalaureate, master's, post-master's, or doctoral degree program in nursing. Diploma and associate degree programs are not eligible. Selection is based on career goals, professional and civic activities, academic performance, and recommendations. U.S. citizenship is required.
Financial Data The stipend is $1,500.
Duration 1 year.
Number awarded 8 each year.
Deadline May of each year.

[709]
NSNA MOBILITY SCHOLARSHIPS

National Student Nurses' Association
Attn: Foundation
45 Main Street, Suite 606
Brooklyn, NY 11201
(718) 210-0705   Fax: (718) 797-1186
E-mail: nsna@nsna.org
Web: www.nsna.org

Summary   To provide financial assistance to nurses interested in pursuing additional education.

Eligibility   This program is open to 1) registered nurses enrolled in programs leading to a baccalaureate or master's degree in nursing or 2) licensed practical and vocational nurses enrolled in programs leading to licensure as a registered nurse. Graduating high school seniors are not eligible. Applicants must submit a 200-word description of their professional and educational goals and how this scholarship will help them achieve those goals. Selection is based on academic achievement, financial need, and involvement in student nursing organizations and community activities related to health care. U.S. citizenship or permanent resident status is required.

Financial Data   Stipends range from $1,000 to $2,500. A total of approximately $155,000 is awarded each year by the foundation for all its scholarship programs.

Duration   1 year.

Additional data   Applications must be accompanied by a $10 processing fee.

Number awarded   Varies each year. Recently, 2 of these scholarships were awarded, both sponsored by Anthony J. Jannetti, Inc.

Deadline   January of each year.

[710]
NURSE EDUCATORS OF ILLINOIS GRADUATE SCHOLARSHIPS

Nurse Educators of Illinois
Attn: Award Committee
P.O. Box 695
Morton Grove, IL 60053
(847) 983-0954   E-mail: neionline@neionline.org
Web: www.neionline.org/NEI%20Scholarship.htm

Summary   To provide financial assistance to graduate student members of Nurse Educators of Illinois who are working on a master's or doctorate in nursing.

Eligibility   This program is open to full- or part-time (half-time or more) students from Illinois who are working on a graduate degree with an emphasis on nursing, including a Ph.D., D.N.Sc., D.N.P., or NLNAC- or CCNE-accredited M.S. Applicants must have a GPA of 3.5 or higher (official transcript is required) and a record of leadership in the nursing profession. Nurse Educators of Illinois membership on an individual or program level is required.

Financial Data   The stipend is $1,000.

Duration   1 year.

Additional data   Nurse Educators of Illinois was founded in 2004 as a successor to the Illinois League for Nursing.

Number awarded   Varies each year.

Deadline   June of each year.

[711]
NURSES CHARITABLE TRUST/AORN/AMERICAN NURSES FOUNDATION SCHOLAR AWARD

American Nurses Foundation
Attn: Nursing Research Grants Program
8515 Georgia Avenue, Suite 400
Silver Spring, MD 20910-3492
(301) 628-5227   Fax: (301) 628-5354
E-mail: anf@ana.org
Web: www.anfonline.org

Summary   To provide funding to perioperative nurses interested in conducting research.

Eligibility   This program is open to registered nurses who have earned a baccalaureate or higher degree and are members of the Association of periOperative Registered Nurses (AORN). Applicants may be either beginning or experienced researchers. Proposed research may be for a master's thesis or doctoral dissertation if the project has been approved by the principal investigator's thesis or dissertation committee.

Financial Data   The grant is $10,000. Funds may not be used as a salary for the principal investigator.

Duration   1 year.

Additional data   This program was established in 2000 with funding provided by the Nurses Charitable Trust of District V of the Florida Nurses Association and by AORN. There is a $100 application fee.

Number awarded   1 each year.

Deadline   April of each year.

[712]
NURSES FOUNDATION OF WISCONSIN SCHOLARSHIP

Wisconsin Nurses Association
Attn: Nurses Foundation of Wisconsin, Inc.
6117 Monona Drive, Suite 1
Madison, WI 53716
(608) 221-0383   Fax: (608) 221-2788
E-mail: info@wisconsinnurses.org
Web: www.wisconsinnurses.org

Summary   To provide financial assistance to registered nurses in Wisconsin who are interested in continuing their education at a school in any state.

Eligibility   This program is open to registered nurses in Wisconsin who are interested in working on a bachelor's or advanced degree in nursing at a school in any state. Applicants must be members of the Wisconsin Nurses Association. They must submit a copy of their Wisconsin Certificate of Registration, a copy of their association membership card, a letter that identifies their professional goals, a summary of their financial need, and 2 letters of support. Selection is based on financial need and potential to make a contribution to nursing in Wisconsin.

Financial Data   The stipend is $1,000.

Duration   1 year.

Number awarded   Varies each year; recently, 2 of these scholarships were awarded.

Deadline   April of each year.

[713]
NURSING ECONOMIC$ FOUNDATION SCHOLARSHIP

Nursing Economic$ Foundation
c/o Jannetti Publications, Inc.
200 East Holly Avenue
P.O. Box 56
Pitman, NJ 08071-0056
(856) 256-2318   Fax: (856) 589-7463
E-mail: nefound@ajj.com
Web: www.nursingeconomics.net

Summary To provide financial assistance to students working on a master's or doctoral nursing degree with an emphasis on administration or management.
Eligibility This program is open to R.N.s who have been accepted at or are currently enrolled in an accredited, degree-granting master's or doctoral nursing program with an emphasis on administration or management. Applicants must plan to continue in the field of nursing in a leadership, administration, or management position upon completion of the degree. Along with their application, they must submit tuition information for their degree program, a curriculum vitae, transcripts, and official GRE or Miller Analogies test scores (even if their school does not require them). U.S. citizenship is required.
Financial Data The stipend is $5,000. Checks are made out jointly to the recipient and the school. Funds must be used for tuition and other school-related fees (excluding room, board, insurance, and athletic fees).
Duration 1 year; nonrenewable.
Number awarded Up to 4 each year.
Deadline May of each year.

[714]
NURSING EDUCATION ASSISTANCE LOAN PROGRAM

South Dakota Board of Nursing
4305 South Louise Avenue, Suite 201
Sioux Falls, SD 57106-3115
(605) 362-2760 Fax: (605) 362-2768
Web: doh.sd.gov/boards/nursing/loan.aspx
Summary To provide forgivable loans to South Dakota residents interested in preparing for a career as a nurse.
Eligibility This program is open to South Dakota residents who have been accepted into an approved nursing education program (for licensed practical nurses, registered nurses, or advanced practice nurses). Applicants must be planning to work on a diploma, associate degree, baccalaureate, master's degree, or doctorate. They must be able to demonstrate financial need. U.S. citizenship is required.
Financial Data The amount of each loan is determined annually by the South Dakota Board of Nursing, up to a maximum of $1,000 per full academic year. Funds may be used only for direct educational expenses (e.g., tuition, books, and fees), not for room or board. Recipients may elect to repay the loan either in full (within 5 years) or by employment in nursing in the state at the conversion rate of $1 per hour.
Duration 1 year; recipients may reapply. Loans must be repaid within 5 years (either in cash or by service as a nurse in South Dakota).
Additional data The South Dakota Legislature authorized this program in 1989. Monies to fund the program are generated by a $10 fee charged to all LPNs and RNs in South Dakota at the time of license renewal.
Number awarded Varies each year.
Deadline May of each year for students in registered nursing and advanced practice nursing programs; September of each year for students in licensed practical nursing programs.

[715]
NURSING EXCELLENCE FELLOWSHIP IN HEMOPHILIA

National Hemophilia Foundation
Attn: Manager of Healthcare Provider Programs
116 West 32nd Street, 11th Floor
New York, NY 10001
(212) 328-3745 Toll Free: (800) 42-HANDI, ext. 3745
Fax: (212) 328-3799 E-mail: mjohnson@hemophilia.org
Web: www.hemophilia.org

Summary To provide funding to registered nurses interested in conducting nursing research or clinical projects related to hemophilia.
Eligibility This program is open to registered nurses from an accredited nursing school enrolled in a graduate nursing program or practicing hemophilia nursing. Applicants must be interested in conducting a nursing research or a clinical project. Preference is given to applicants who are endorsed by a federally-funded hemophilia treatment center. Current topics of interest include, but are not limited to, the development of clinical pathways, measurable outcomes in bleeding disorders care, service utilization, epidemiology, patient and community education, rehabilitation, therapeutic modalities, psychosocial issues, women's health, liver disease, and HIV/AIDS. Selection is based on scientific merit and relevance to the research priorities of the National Hemophilia Foundation.
Financial Data The grant is $13,500 per year.
Duration 1 year.
Number awarded 1 each year.
Deadline Letters of intent must be submitted by January of each year. Completed applications are due in March.

[716]
NURSING FOUNDATION OF RHODE ISLAND RESEARCH GRANTS

Nursing Foundation of Rhode Island
Attn: Research Grant Committee
P.O. Box 41702
Providence, RI 02940
(401) 223-9680 E-mail: nfri@rinursingfoundation.org
Web: www.rinursingfoundation.org/grants.htm
Summary To provide funding to Rhode Island nurses or agencies interested in conducting research related to clinical nursing or nursing education.
Eligibility Applicants may be individuals or agencies (principal investigator must have at least a B.S.N. degree) who are interested in conducting research on 1) clinical nursing that will improve patient care or 2) nursing education that will improve curriculum and/or retention of students. Graduate students are eligible to conduct thesis or dissertation research. Preference is given to Rhode Island residents.
Financial Data Grants are a maximum of $2,500. Funds may be used for supplies, mailing and postage, analysis and searches, consultants, and computers. The purchase of equipment may not be approved if available through borrowing or rental (rental fees will be approved). Grant funds may not be used as salary for the principal investigator or secretarial assistance.
Duration Up to 1 year.
Additional data Recipients must write a final report detailing results, conclusions, and recommendations at the end of the research study.
Number awarded Varies each year; recently, 12 of these grants, with a total value of $18,732, were awarded.
Deadline April of each year.

[717]
ODONA SCHOLARSHIPS

Ohio Directors of Nursing Administration in Long Term Care
Attn: Scholarship Committee
190 East Pacemont Road
Columbus, OH 43202
Toll Free: (866) 226-3662
Web: www.odonaltc.org/pages/scholarships.asp
Summary To provide financial assistance for additional training to members of Ohio Directors of Nursing Administration in Long Term Care (ODONA).
Eligibility This program is open to ODONA members who have been working in long-term care for at least 1 year as directors of

nursing (DON) or assistant directors of nursing (ADON). Applicants must be planning to enroll in a formal educational program related to their work at a school of nursing in any state. Along with their application, they must submit a narrative of at least 100 words on why they wish to be considered for a scholarship and how it will impact their practice.

Financial Data   Stipends range from $500 to $1,500.

Duration   1 year.

Number awarded   Up to 5 each year: 1 in each of Ohio's 5 regions.

Deadline   January of each year.

[718]
OHIO ASSOCIATION OF ADVANCED PRACTICE NURSES SCHOLARSHIPS

Ohio Association of Advanced Practice Nurses
Attn: Scholarship
5818 Wilmington Pike, Suite 300
Dayton, OH 45459
Toll Free: (866) 668-3839   Fax: (866) 529-6822
E-mail: Scholarships-Awards@oaapn.org
Web: oaapn.org/scholarship.php

Summary   To provide financial assistance to students preparing to become an advanced practice nurse at a school in Ohio.

Eligibility   This program is open to students currently enrolled full or part time in a program in Ohio leading to a master's degree as an advanced practice nurse or in a post-master's certificate program. Applicants must have completed at least 12 hours of graduate work with a GPA of 3.2 or higher. Membership in the Ohio Association of Advanced Practice Nurses (OAAPN) is considered in the selection process but is not required. Service to OAAPN is also considered but is not mandatory. Along with their application, they must submit an essay on their career goals and their plans for advanced practice nursing after graduation.

Financial Data   The stipend is $1,000.

Duration   1 year.

Additional data   Recipients are expected to serve as an advanced practice nurse in Ohio for at least 1 year after graduation.

Number awarded   4 each year.

Deadline   September of each year.

[719]
OHIO NURSE EDUCATION ASSISTANCE LOAN PROGRAM FOR INSTRUCTORS

Ohio Board of Regents
Attn: State Grants and Scholarships
30 East Broad Street, 36th Floor
Columbus, OH 43215-3414
(614) 466-4818   Toll Free: (888) 833-1133
Fax: (614) 466-5866
E-mail: nealp_admin@regents.state.oh.us
Web: regents.ohio.gov/sgs/nealp/instructors.php

Summary   To provide scholarship/loans to students in Ohio who intend to prepare for a career as a nursing instructor.

Eligibility   This program is open to Ohio residents who are enrolled at least half time in an approved master's degree nurse education program in the state. Applicants must be a registered nurse with 2 years of clinical experience in nursing. Along with their application, they must submit a letter of intent stating how they intend to practice as a faculty member at a pre-licensure or post-licensure program in Ohio upon completion of their academic program. Financial need is also considered in the selection process. U.S. citizenship or permanent resident status is required.

Financial Data   The maximum award is currently $5,000 per year. This is a scholarship/loan program; up to 100% of the loan may be forgiven at the rate of 25% per year if the recipient serves

as a nurse instructor under specified conditions for up to 4 years. If the loan is not repaid with service, it must be repaid in cash with interest at the rate of 8% per year.

Duration   1 year; renewable for up to 3 additional years.

Additional data   This program is administered by the Ohio Board of Regents with assistance from the Ohio Board of Nursing.

Number awarded   Varies each year.

Deadline   July of each year.

[720]
OKLAHOMA NURSING STUDENT ASSISTANCE PROGRAM

Physician Manpower Training Commission
Attn: Nursing Program Coordinator
5500 North Western Avenue, Suite 201
Oklahoma City, OK 73118
(405) 843-5667   Fax: (405) 843-5792
E-mail: michelle.cecil@pmtc.state.ok.us
Web: www.pmtc.state.ok.us/nsap.htm

Summary   To provide scholarship/loans to nursing students from Oklahoma who are interested in practicing in rural communities in the state.

Eligibility   This program is open to residents of Oklahoma who have been admitted to an accredited program of nursing in any state at the L.P.N., A.D.N., B.S.N., or M.S.N. level. Applicants must be interested in practicing nursing in Oklahoma communities, especially rural communities. They may apply either for direct funding from the state or with matching support from a health institution in the state, such as a hospital, nursing home, or other health care entity. Along with their application, they must submit ACT scores, high school and/or college GPA, and documentation of financial need. U.S. citizenship is required.

Financial Data   The minimum scholarship/loan provided by the state for all levels is $500 per year. The maximum is $1,750 per year for L.P.N. students, $2,000 per year for A.D.N. students, or $2,500 per year for B.S.N. or M.S.N. students. The loan is forgiven if the nurse fulfills a work obligation at an approved health institution in Oklahoma of 1 year for each year of financial assistance received; participants in the matching program must work for their sponsor. Nurses who decide not to fulfill their work obligation are required to repay the principal amount plus 12% interest and a possible penalty of up to 98% of the principal.

Duration   Funding is available for completion of an L.P.N. program, for 2 years for an A.D.N. program, or the final 2 years of a B.S.N. or M.S.N. program.

Additional data   This program was established in 1982.

Number awarded   Between 250 and 300 of these awards are granted each year. Since the program began, more than 5,250 nursing students have received support.

Deadline   June of each year.

[721]
ONCOLOGY NURSING SOCIETY FOUNDATION/ REHABILITATION NURSING FOUNDATION GRANT

Association of Rehabilitation Nurses
Attn: Rehabilitation Nursing Foundation
4700 West Lake Avenue
Glenview, IL 60025-1485
(847) 375-4710   Toll Free: (800) 229-7530
Fax: (877) 734-9384   E-mail: info@rehabnurse.org
Web: www.rehabnurse.org/research/researchgrants.html

Summary   To provide funding to graduate nursing students and professionals interested in conducting research involving rehabilitation nursing in patients with cancer.

Eligibility   The principal investigator for the research project must be a registered nurse who is active in rehabilitation or who has demonstrated interest in and significant contributions to rehabilitation nursing. Membership in the Association of Rehabilitation Nurses (ARN) is not required. Graduate students may apply. The proposed research project should advance rehabilitation nursing in patients with cancer.

Financial Data The grant is $10,000.

Duration The project must be completed within 2 years.

Additional data This program is cosponsored by the Oncology Nursing Society Foundation and the Rehabilitation Nursing Foundation of the ARN.

Number awarded 1 each year.

Deadline January of each year.

[722]
ONF-SMITH EDUCATION SCHOLARSHIP

Oregon Nurses Association
Attn: Oregon Nurses Foundation
18765 S.W. Boones Ferry Road, Suite 200
Tualatin, OR 97062-8498
(503) 293-0011   Fax: (503) 293-0013
E-mail: tangedal@oregonrn.org
Web: www.oregonrn.org

Summary To provide financial assistance to residents of any state who are working on an undergraduate or graduate degree in nursing at a school in Oregon.

Eligibility This program is open to students from any state who are currently enrolled in an accredited bachelor's or graduate program in nursing in Oregon and have a GPA of 3.0 or higher. Applicants who are already registered nurses must be a member of the Oregon Nurses Association; applicants who are not yet registered nurses must be a member of an Oregon affiliate of the National Student Nurses Association. Selection is based on leadership abilities and experiences (35%); experiences with other cultures, minority groups, and underserved populations (30%); career plans in nursing (30%); and reasons for needing this funding (5%).

Financial Data The stipend is $1,000. Funds are paid directly to the recipient's school.

Duration 1 year.

Number awarded 1 or more each year.

Deadline February of each year.

[723]
ONS FOUNDATION MASTER'S AND POST-MASTER'S NURSE PRACTITIONER CERTIFICATE SCHOLARSHIPS

Oncology Nursing Society
Attn: ONS Foundation
125 Enterprise Drive
Pittsburgh, PA 15275-1214
(412) 859-6100   Toll Free: (866) 257-4ONS
Fax: (412) 859-6163   E-mail: foundation@ons.org
Web: www.ons.org/Awards/FoundationAwards/Masters

Summary To provide financial assistance to registered nurses interested in working on a master's or post-master's degree in advanced practice oncology nursing.

Eligibility Applicants must 1) be registered nurses with a demonstrated interest in and commitment to oncology nursing; 2) have a previous bachelor's or master's degree in nursing; 3) be enrolled in or applying to an academic master's degree or post-master's nurse practitioner certificate program in an NLN- or CCNE-accredited school of nursing; and 4) never have received this award from this sponsor. Along with their application, they must submit 1) an essay of 250 words or less on their role in caring for persons with cancer, and 2) a statement of their professional goals and the relationship of those goals to the advancement of oncology nursing. Financial need is not considered in the selection process.

Financial Data The stipend is $3,000.

Duration 1 year.

Additional data This program is supported by Novartis Oncology, Genentech BioOncology, Oncology Hematology Care, Inc., and the Oncology Nursing Certification Corporation. Upon completion of their degree, recipients must submit a summary of the educational activities in which they participated. Applications must be accompanied by a $5 fee.

Number awarded Varies each year; recently, 19 of these scholarships were awarded.

Deadline January of each year.

[724]
OSANA SCHOLARSHIPS

American Association of Nurse Anesthetists
Attn: AANA Foundation
222 South Prospect Avenue
Park Ridge, IL 60068-4001
(847) 655-1170   Fax: (847) 692-6968
E-mail: foundation@aana.com
Web: www.aanafoundation.com

Summary To provide financial assistance to members of the American Association of Nurse Anesthetists (AANA) from any state who are interested in obtaining further education at a program in Ohio.

Eligibility This program is open to members of the association from any state who are currently enrolled in an accredited nurse anesthesia education program in Ohio. Applicants must be in the final 12 months of their program. Along with their application, they must submit a 200-word essay describing why they have chosen nurse anesthesia as a profession and their professional goals for the future. Financial need is also considered in the selection process.

Financial Data The stipend is $1,000.

Duration 1 year.

Additional data Funding for this scholarship, first awarded in 1995, is provided by the Ohio State Association of Nurse Anesthetists (OSANA). The application processing fee is $25.

Number awarded 2 each year.

Deadline March of each year.

[725]
PALMER CARRIER CRNA SCHOLARSHIP

American Association of Nurse Anesthetists
Attn: AANA Foundation
222 South Prospect Avenue
Park Ridge, IL 60068-4001
(847) 655-1170   Fax: (847) 692-6968
E-mail: foundation@aana.com
Web: www.aanafoundation.com

Summary To provide financial assistance to members of the American Association of Nurse Anesthetists (AANA) who are interested in working on a doctoral degree.

Eligibility This program is open to members of the association who are certified or recertified CRNAs and working on a doctoral degree in an accredited nurse anesthesia education program. Applicants must have a long-term goal to remain in a leadership capacity in education and/or research upon completion of graduate study, be actively involved at the state or national level in the profession of nurse anesthesia, and demonstrate a commitment to furthering the profession of nurse anesthesia. Along with their application, they must submit a 300-word essay describing their current involvement in nurse anesthesia education, practice, or research; how funding will enhance their educational and professional goals; their research or capstone project; how the degree sought will influence their career; and their long-term goals for participating in a leadership capacity.

Financial Data The stipend is $5,000.

Duration 1 year.

Additional data This scholarship was first awarded in 2002. The application processing fee is $25.

Number awarded 1 each year.

Deadline April of each year.

[726]
PALMER CARRIER STUDENT SCHOLARSHIP

American Association of Nurse Anesthetists
Attn: AANA Foundation
222 South Prospect Avenue
Park Ridge, IL 60068-4001
(847) 655-1170   Fax: (847) 692-6968
E-mail: foundation@aana.com
Web: www.aanafoundation.com

Summary To provide financial assistance to members of the American Association of Nurse Anesthetists (AANA) who are interested in obtaining further education.

Eligibility This program is open to members of the association who are currently enrolled in an accredited nurse anesthesia education program. First-year students must have completed 6 months of nurse anesthesia classes; second-year students must have completed 12 months of nurse anesthesia classes. Along with their application, they must submit a 200-word essay describing why they have chosen nurse anesthesia as a profession and their professional goals for the future. Financial need is also considered in the selection process. Preference is given to second-year students in Illinois.

Financial Data The stipend is $3,000.

Duration 1 year.

Additional data This scholarship was first awarded in 2002. The application processing fee is $25.

Number awarded 1 each year.

Deadline March of each year.

[727]
PAMELA STINSON KIDD MEMORIAL DOCTORAL SCHOLARSHIP

Emergency Nurses Association
Attn: ENA Foundation
915 Lee Street
Des Plaines, IL 60016-6569
(847) 460-4100   Toll Free: (800) 900-9659, ext. 4100
Fax: (847) 460-4004   E-mail: foundation@ena.org
Web: www.ena.org

Summary To provide financial assistance for doctoral study to nurses who are members of the Emergency Nurses Association (ENA).

Eligibility This program is open to nurses (R.N.) who are working on a doctoral degree in nursing. Applicants must have been members of the association for at least 12 months and have a GPA of 3.0 or higher. Their dissertation must be related to emergency nursing. Along with their application, they must submit 1) a 100-word statement on their professional and educational goals and how this scholarship will help them attain those goals; and 2) a 100-word explanation of how this scholarship will further the practice of emergency nursing. Selection is based on content and clarity of the goal statement (45%), professional association involvement (35%), presentation of the application (10%), and letters of reference (10%).

Financial Data The stipend is $10,000.

Duration 1 year; nonrenewable.

Number awarded 1 each year.

Deadline May of each year.

[728]
PATRICIA SMITH CHRISTENSEN SCHOLARSHIP

Sigma Theta Tau International
Attn: Research Services
550 West North Street
Indianapolis, IN 46202-3191
(317) 634-8171   Toll Free: (888) 634-7575
Fax: (317) 634-8188   E-mail: research@stti.iupui.edu
Web: www.nursingsociety.org

Summary To provide financial assistance to graduate nursing students working on a degree in the area of maternal-child or pediatric nursing.

Eligibility This program is open to registered nurses who are enrolled in a master's or doctoral degree program in nursing. If other qualifications are equal, preference is given to Canadian residents and to members of Sigma Theta Tau International. Applicants must submit a letter outlining their reasons for pursuing advanced nursing education in the area of maternal-child or pediatric nursing and providing details about their current program and future career plans. Selection is based on demonstrated potential for advanced study and research.

Financial Data The stipend is $1,000.

Duration 1 year.

Number awarded 1 every other year.

Deadline March of odd-numbered years.

[729]
PATSY QUINT OCCUPATIONAL HEALTH NURSES ENDOWED SCHOLARSHIP

Kansas State Nurses Association
Attn: Kansas Nurses Foundation
1109 S.W. Topeka Boulevard
Topeka, KS 66612-1602
(785) 233-8638   Fax: (785) 233-5222
E-mail: ksna@ksna.net
Web: www.nursingworld.org/SNAS/KS/Knf.htm

Summary To provide financial assistance to nurses in Kansas interested in working on a degree in occupational health at a school in the state.

Eligibility This program is open to residents of Kansas who are either 1) R.N.s currently in occupational health and working on a baccalaureate degree, or 2) occupational health nurses working on a master's or doctoral degree with an emphasis on occupational health. Applicants must have a GPA of 3.0 or higher. Along with their application, they must submit a personal narrative on their anticipated role in nursing in Kansas.

Financial Data The stipend is $500.

Duration 1 year.

Number awarded 1 each year.

Deadline June of each year.

[730]
PAULINE THOMPSON CLINICAL NURSING RESEARCH AWARD

Pennsylvania State Nurses Association
Attn: Nursing Foundation of Pennsylvania
2578 Interstate Drive, Suite 101
Harrisburg, PA 17110
(717) 692-0542   Toll Free: (888) 707-PSNA
Fax: (717) 692-4540   E-mail: nfp@panurses.org
Web: www.panurses.org/2008/section.cfm?SID=21&ID=4

Summary To provide funding to members of the Pennsylvania State Nurses Association who are interested in conducting a clinical research project.

Eligibility This program is open to members of the Pennsylvania State Nurses Association who are interested in conducting research focusing on a clinical topic that directly affects patient/client care. Applicants must have previous experience or education related to the research process or be working in consultation with a nurse who has a background or experience in the research process. They may have obtained no more than $5,000 in research funds from any other source for this specific project. The research may be conducted as part of the requirements for a master's or doctoral degree in nursing at an institution in Pennsylvania.

Financial Data The grant is $2,000.

Duration 1 year.

Additional data The recipient must attend the foundation's annual banquet to receive the award. The recipient will be the guest of the foundation at the banquet and financial support for travel and overnight accommodations will be provided if necessary. In addition, the recipient must submit a report annually or at the completion of the research project (whichever comes first).

Number awarded 1 or more each year.

Deadline May of each year.

[731]
PENNSYLVANIA ASSOCIATION OF SCHOOL NURSES AND PRACTITIONERS CERTIFIED SCHOOL NURSE SCHOLARSHIP

Pennsylvania Association of School Nurses and Practitioners
c/o Michelle Ficca, Scholarship Chair
Bloomsburg University of Pennsylvania
3136 MCHS
Bloomsburg, PA 17815
(570) 389-4000   E-mail: pasnapweb@pasnap.org
Web: www.pasnap.org/education/scholarships.html

Summary To provide financial assistance to students in Pennsylvania preparing for a career as a school nurse.

Eligibility This program is open to 1) nursing and nurse practitioner students in Pennsylvania intending to practice school nursing and enrolled or accepted in a B.S.N. or school nurse certification program; and 2) certified school nurses working on a graduate degree in nursing in Pennsylvania. Applicants must submit a 1-page letter outlining their goals in school nursing, a copy of their acceptance letter or official transcript, a current resume, and a copy of their current nursing license. Selection is based on a random drawing from all qualified applications; financial need is not considered.

Financial Data The stipend is $1,000. Funds are paid directly to the financial aid office in the recipient's institution.

Duration 1 year.

Number awarded 2 each year.

Deadline March of each year.

[732]
PENS ACADEMIC EDUCATION SCHOLARSHIPS

Pediatric Endocrinology Nursing Society
Attn: President-Elect
7794 Grow Drive
Pensacola, FL 32514
(850) 484-5223   Toll Free: (877) 936-7367
Fax: (850) 484-8762   E-mail: pens@peutzamc.com
Web: www.pens.org/scholarships.html

Summary To provide financial assistance for further education to members of the Pediatric Endocrinology Nursing Society (PENS).

Eligibility This program is open to R.N.s currently employed in pediatric endocrine nursing who have been members of PENS for at least 3 years. Applicants must be working on a degree in nursing; preference is given to those working on a B.S.N. degree and to first-time applicants. Along with their application, they must submit a copy of their R.N. license card, curriculum vitae or resume, statement of fees from the college or university, transcript of grades or (if beginning course work) a letter of acceptance, a list of professional organizations to which they belong,

information on PENS activities in which they have participated, a list of volunteer or community service, and documentation of financial need.

Financial Data The stipend is $1,000 per year.

Duration 1 year. Members are eligible for 2 scholarships in a 5-year period.

Number awarded Varies each year.

Deadline March or August of each year.

[733]
PETER GILI SCHOLARSHIP AWARD

ExceptionalNurse.com
Attn: Scholarship Committee
13019 Coastal Circle
Palm Beach Gardens, FL 33410
(561) 627-9872   Fax: (561) 776-9254
TDD: (561) 776-9442   E-mail: ExceptionalNurse@aol.com
Web: www.ExceptionalNurse.com/scholarship.php

Summary To provide financial assistance to nursing students who have a disability.

Eligibility This program is open to students with a documented disability or medical challenge who have applied to, or have already been admitted to, a college or university nursing program on a full-time basis. Applicants must submit an essay on how they plan to contribute to the nursing profession and how their disability will influence their practice as a nurse. Selection is based on the essay, transcripts of high school and/or college courses completed, activities and honors received, 3 letters of recommendation, and financial need.

Financial Data The stipend is $500.

Duration 1 year; nonrenewable.

Number awarded 1 each year.

Deadline May of each year.

[734]
PFIZER COMMUNITY INNOVATIONS GRANT PROGRAM

Nurse Practitioner Healthcare Foundation
Attn: Scholarship Selection Committee
2647 134th Avenue N.E.
Bellevue, WA 98005-1813
(425) 861-0911   Fax: (425) 861-0907
Web: www.nphealthcarefoundation.org

Summary To provide funding to nurse practitioners and graduate nurse practitioner students interested in conducting an educational project related to community innovation.

Eligibility This program is open to professional nurse practitioners and students currently enrolled in a nationally-accredited graduate nurse practitioner program. Applicants must be interested in conducting an educational project designed to foster innovation at the local community level in the areas of service, education, or research. Selection is based on the quality of the project, the target community, and the anticipated value of the project to the community. U.S. citizenship or permanent resident status is required.

Financial Data The initial grant is $2,500, paid at the time of the award. Upon completion of the project, an additional $500 is awarded to support project dissemination (e.g., travel expenses for presenting at a national meeting, editing a paper for publication, preparing a poster).

Duration The project must be completed within 2 years.

Additional data This program is sponsored by Pfizer.

Number awarded 8 each year.

Deadline November of each year.

[735]
PHILLIPS/LAIRD SCHOLARSHIP

Minnesota Nurses Association
Attn: Minnesota Nurses Association Foundation
1625 Energy Park Drive, Suite 200
St. Paul, MN 55108
(651) 414-2822   Toll Free: (800) 536-4662, ext. 122
Fax: (651) 695-7000   E-mail: linda.owens@mnnurses.org
Web: www.mnnurses.org

Summary To provide financial assistance to members of the Minnesota Nurses Association (MNA) who are interested in working on a baccalaureate or graduate degree in nursing.

Eligibility This program is open to MNA members who have a current R.N. licensure and have been accepted into an approved program of study leading to a baccalaureate or graduate academic degree in nursing. Applicants must submit a brief description of their career goals following their graduation. Selection is based on that statement, professional activities, demonstrated leadership ability, scholarship in nursing, MNA activities, and community involvement. Preference is given to nurses who live or work in the "former" MNA District 13 (e.g., Owatonna, Waseca, Northfield, Faribault, Rice County).

Financial Data The stipend is $2,000 per year.

Duration 1 year; may be renewed.

Number awarded 1 each year.

Deadline May of each year.

[736]
PHYSIO-CONTROL AACN SMALL PROJECTS GRANTS

American Association of Critical-Care Nurses
Attn: Research Department
101 Columbia
Aliso Viejo, CA 92656-4109
(949) 362-2000, ext. 551
Toll Free: (800) 809-CARE, ext. 551
Fax: (949) 362-2020   E-mail: research@aacn.org
Web: www.aacn.org

Summary To provide funding to investigators, including students, who wish to conduct research on acute myocardial infarction or resuscitation.

Eligibility This program is open to investigators interested in conducting a research project focusing on aspects of acute myocardial infarction, resuscitation, or sudden cardiac death. Applicants must be proposing to conduct research related to patient education, competency-based education, staff development, CQI projects, outcomes evaluation, or small clinical research studies. Funds may be awarded for new projects, projects in progress, or projects required for an academic degree. Collaborative projects are encouraged and may involve interdisciplinary teams, multiple nursing units, home health, subacute and transitional care, other institutions, or community agencies.

Financial Data The maximum grant is $1,500. Funds may be used to cover direct project expenses, such as printed materials, small equipment, supplies (including computer software), and assistive personnel. They may not be used for salaries or institutional overhead.

Additional data Funds for these grants are provided by Physio-Control, Inc.

Number awarded 1 each year.

Deadline September of each year.

[737]
PHYSIO-CONTROL ACADEMIC SCHOLARSHIP

American Association of Occupational Health Nurses, Inc.
Attn: AAOHN Foundation
7794 Grow Drive
Pensacola, FL 32514
(850) 474-6963   Toll Free: (800) 241-8014
Fax: (850) 484-8762   E-mail: aaohn@aaohn.org
Web: www.aaohn.org/scholarships/academic-study.html

Summary To provide financial assistance to registered nurses who are working on a bachelor's or graduate degree to prepare for a career in occupational and environmental health.

Eligibility This program is open to registered nurses who are enrolled in a baccalaureate or graduate degree program. Applicants must demonstrate an interest in, and commitment to, occupational and environmental health. Along with their application, they must submit a 500-word narrative on their professional goals as they relate to the academic activity and the field of occupational and environmental health. Selection is based on that essay (50%), impact of education on applicant's career (20%), and 2 letters of recommendation (30%).

Financial Data The stipend is $3,000.

Duration 1 year; may be renewed up to 2 additional years.

Additional data Funding for this program is provided by Physio-Control, Inc.

Number awarded 1 each year.

Deadline January of each year.

[738]
PHYSIO-CONTROL SCHOLARSHIP

Emergency Nurses Association
Attn: ENA Foundation
915 Lee Street
Des Plaines, IL 60016-6569
(847) 460-4100   Toll Free: (800) 900-9659, ext. 4100
Fax: (847) 460-4004   E-mail: foundation@ena.org
Web: www.ena.org

Summary To provide financial assistance to members of the Emergency Nurses Association (ENA) who are working on a master's degree.

Eligibility This program is open to emergency nurses (R.N.) who are working on a master's degree. Applicants must have been members of the association for at least 12 months and have a GPA of 3.0 or higher. They must submit a 1-page statement on their professional and educational goals and how this scholarship will help them attain those goals. Selection is based on content and clarity of the goal statement (45%), professional association involvement (35%), presentation of the application (10%), and letters of reference (10%).

Financial Data The stipend is $3,000.

Duration 1 year.

Additional data This program is funded by Physio-Control, Inc.

Number awarded 2 each year.

Deadline May of each year.

[739]
POUDRE VALLEY HEALTH SYSTEM NIGHTINGALE SCHOLARSHIP

Colorado Nurses Foundation
7400 East Arapahoe Road, Suite 211
Centennial, CO 80112
(303) 694-4728   Fax: (303) 694-4869
E-mail: mail@cnfound.org
Web: www.cnfound.org/scholarships.html

Summary To provide financial assistance to undergraduate and graduate nursing students in Colorado who are willing to work in designated communities following graduation.

Eligibility This program is open to Colorado residents who are enrolled in an approved nursing program in the state. Applicants may be 1) second-year students in an associate degree program; 2) junior or senior level B.S.N. undergraduate students; 3) R.N.s enrolled in a baccalaureate or higher degree program in a school of nursing; 4) R.N.s with a master's degree in nursing, currently practicing in Colorado and enrolled in a doctoral program; or 5) students in the second or third year of a Doctorate Nursing Practice (D.N.P.) program. They must be willing to work in Fort Collins, Loveland, or Estes Park, Colorado following graduation. Undergraduates must have a GPA of 3.25 or higher and graduate students must have a GPA of 3.5 or higher. Selection is based on professional philosophy and goals, dedication to the improvement of patient care in Colorado, demonstrated commitment to nursing, critical thinking skills, potential for leadership, involvement in community and professional organizations, recommendations, GPA, and financial need.

Financial Data The stipend is $1,000.

Duration 1 year.

Number awarded 2 each year.

Deadline October of each year.

[740]
PREDOCTORAL RESEARCH TRAINING FELLOWSHIPS IN EPILEPSY

Epilepsy Foundation
Attn: Research Department
8301 Professional Place
Landover, MD 20785-2237
(301) 459-3700   Toll Free: (800) EFA-1000
Fax: (301) 577-2684   TDD: (800) 332-2070
E-mail: grants@efa.org
Web: www.epilepsyfoundation.org/research/grants.cfm

Summary To provide funding to doctoral candidates in nursing and other designated fields for dissertation research on a topic related to epilepsy.

Eligibility This program is open to full-time graduate students working on a Ph.D. in biochemistry, genetics, neuroscience, nursing, pharmacology, pharmacy, physiology, or psychology. Applicants must be conducting dissertation research on a topic relevant to epilepsy under the guidance of a mentor with expertise in the area of epilepsy investigation. Applications from women, members of minority groups, and people with disabilities are especially encouraged. Selection is based on the relevance of the proposed work to epilepsy, the applicant's qualifications, the mentor's qualifications, the scientific quality of the proposed dissertation research, the quality of the training environment for research related to epilepsy, and the adequacy of the facility.

Financial Data The grant is $20,000, consisting of $19,000 for a stipend and $1,000 to support travel to attend the annual meeting of the American Epilepsy Society.

Duration 1 year.

Additional data Support for this program, which began in 1998, is provided by many individuals, families, and corporations, especially the American Epilepsy Society, Abbott Laboratories, Ortho-McNeil Pharmaceutical, and Pfizer Inc.

Number awarded Varies each year.

Deadline August of each year.

[741]
PREVENTIVE CARDIOVASCULAR NURSES ASSOCIATION/AMERICAN NURSES FOUNDATION SCHOLAR AWARD

American Nurses Foundation
Attn: Nursing Research Grants Program
8515 Georgia Avenue, Suite 400
Silver Spring, MD 20910-3492
(301) 628-5227   Fax: (301) 628-5354
E-mail: anf@ana.org
Web: www.anfonline.org

Summary To provide funding to nurses interested in conducting research related to cardiovascular disease.

Eligibility This program is open to registered nurses who have earned a baccalaureate or higher degree. Applicants may be either beginning or experienced researchers. They must be planning to conduct research that is related to the prevention of cardiovascular disease. Proposed research may be for a master's thesis or doctoral dissertation, if the project has been approved by the principal investigator's thesis or dissertation committee.

Financial Data The grant is $5,000. Funds may not be used as a salary for the principal investigator.

Duration 1 year.

Additional data This program, established in 2010, is sponsored by the Preventive Cardiovascular Nurses Association. There is a $100 application fee.

Number awarded 1 each year.

Deadline April of each year.

[742]
PROCTER & GAMBLE ENDOWED SCHOLARSHIP IN GASTROENTEROLOGY

Nurse Practitioner Healthcare Foundation
Attn: Scholarship Selection Committee
2647 134th Avenue N.E.
Bellevue, WA 98005-1813
(425) 861-0911   Fax: (425) 861-0907
Web: www.nphealthcarefoundation.org

Summary To provide financial assistance to students preparing for a career as a nurse practitioner with an emphasis on gastroenterology.

Eligibility This program is open to students currently enrolled in a nationally-accredited nurse practitioner program at the master's, post-master's, or doctoral level. Applicants must have clinical and/or research interests in the field of gastroenterology. They must describe what they plan to do in their chosen area to enhance their ability to make an innovative or unique contribution to the overall care of patients with potential or ongoing gastroenterological problems. U.S. citizenship or permanent resident status is required.

Financial Data The stipend is $1,000.

Duration 1 year; nonrenewable.

Additional data This program, established in 2006, is sponsored by the Procter & Gamble Company.

Number awarded 1 each year.

Deadline December of each year.

[743]
PROCTER & GAMBLE ENDOWED SCHOLARSHIP IN SERVICE

Nurse Practitioner Healthcare Foundation
Attn: Scholarship Selection Committee
2647 134th Avenue N.E.
Bellevue, WA 98005-1813
(425) 861-0911   Fax: (425) 861-0907
Web: www.nphealthcarefoundation.org

Summary   To provide financial assistance to students preparing for a career as a nurse practitioner.
Eligibility   This program is open to students currently enrolled in a nationally-accredited nurse practitioner program at the master's, post-master's, or doctoral level. Applicants must have made a significant, positive leadership contribution on campus, in the community, or in patient care while working on an advanced degree. They must describe how they will use this scholarship to advance their skills as a nurse practitioner leader, including past and current leadership experience and potential opportunities to enact the leadership role to influence the profession and their care of patients as a nurse practitioner. U.S. citizenship or permanent resident status is required.
Financial Data   The stipend is $1,000.
Duration   1 year; nonrenewable.
Additional data   This program, established in 2006, is sponsored by the Procter & Gamble Company.
Number awarded   1 each year.
Deadline   December of each year.

[744]
PROMISE OF NURSING REGIONAL FACULTY FELLOWSHIP PROGRAM

National Student Nurses' Association
Attn: Foundation
45 Main Street, Suite 606
Brooklyn, NY 11201
(718) 210-0705   Fax: (718) 797-1186
E-mail: nsna@nsna.org
Web: www.nsna.org

Summary   To provide financial assistance to registered nurses enrolled in a graduate program in selected areas to prepare for a career as a nurse educator.
Eligibility   This program is open to registered nurses who have a baccalaureate degree. Applicants must be currently enrolled in state-approved graduate schools of nursing in the Dallas/Fort Worth area of Texas, the Houston/Galveston area of Texas (Austin, Brazoria, Chamber, Colorado, Fort Bend, Galveston, Harris, Liberty, Matagorda, Montgomery, Walker, Waller, and Wharton counties), central Florida, southern Florida, southern California (Los Angeles, Orange, Riverside, San Bernardino, Santa Barbara, and Ventura counties), or the states of Georgia, Louisiana, Massachusetts, Mississippi, New Jersey, Oregon, Pennsylvania, or Washington. They must be able to document a commitment to nurse-educator role preparation and plan to serve in a nurse-educator role upon completion of their program. Along with their application, they must submit a 200-word description of their education, research, and career goals and how this fellowship will help them achieve those goals. Financial need is also considered in the selection process. U.S. citizenship or permanent resident status is required.
Financial Data   Stipends range from $1,000 to $7,500.
Duration   1 year.
Additional data   This program is supported by fundraising events sponsored by Johnson & Johnson. Applications must be accompanied by a $10 processing fee.
Number awarded   Varies each year.
Deadline   March of each year.

[745]
PROMISE OF NURSING SCHOLARSHIPS

National Student Nurses' Association
Attn: Foundation
45 Main Street, Suite 606
Brooklyn, NY 11201
(718) 210-0705   Fax: (718) 797-1186
E-mail: nsna@nsna.org
Web: www.nsna.org

Summary   To provide financial assistance to nursing or pre-nursing students at schools in selected geographic locations.
Eligibility   This program is open to students currently enrolled in state-approved schools of nursing or pre-nursing associate degree, baccalaureate, diploma, generic master's, generic doctoral, R.N. to B.S.N., R.N. to M.S.N., or L.P.N./L.V.N. to R.N. programs. Graduating high school seniors are not eligible. Support for graduate education is provided only for a first degree in nursing. Applicants must be attending school in the Dallas/Fort Worth area of Texas, the Houston/Galveston area of Texas (Austin, Brazoria, Chamber, Colorado, Fort Bend, Galveston, Harris, Liberty, Matagorda, Montgomery, Walker, Waller, and Wharton counties), central Florida, southern Florida, southern California (Los Angeles, Orange, Riverside, San Bernardino, Santa Barbara, and Ventura counties), or the states of Georgia (graduate students only), Louisiana, Maryland, Massachusetts, Mississippi, New Jersey (graduate students only), Oregon, Pennsylvania, Tennessee, or Washington. Selection is based on academic achievement, financial need, and involvement in student nursing organizations and community health activities.
Financial Data   Stipends range from $1,000 to $2,500.
Duration   1 year.
Additional data   This program, offered for the first time in 2003, is supported by fundraising events sponsored by Johnson & Johnson. Applications must be accompanied by a $10 processing fee.
Number awarded   Varies each year. Recently, 57 of these scholarships were awarded: 2 in Dallas/Fort Worth, Texas; 1 in Houston/Galveston, Texas; 2 in central Florida; 9 in southern California; 9 in Maryland; 11 in Massachusetts; 4 in New Jersey; 5 in Pennsylvania; 3 in Tennessee; and 11 in Washington.
Deadline   January of each year.

[746]
RED AND LOLA FEHR SCHOLARSHIP

Colorado Nurses Foundation
7400 East Arapahoe Road, Suite 211
Centennial, CO 80112
(303) 694-4728   Fax: (303) 694-4869
E-mail: mail@cnfound.org
Web: www.cnfound.org/scholarships.html

Summary   To provide financial assistance to residents of Colorado who are working on a graduate degree in nursing at a college or university in the state to prepare for a career as a nursing faculty member.
Eligibility   This program is open to Colorado residents who have been accepted as a student in an approved nursing program in the state. Applicants must be working on a graduate degree to prepare for a career as a nursing faculty member. They must have a GPA of 3.5 or higher. Selection is based on professional philosophy and goals, dedication to the improvement of patient care in Colorado, demonstrated commitment to nursing, critical thinking skills, potential for leadership, involvement in community and professional organizations, recommendations, GPA, and financial need.
Financial Data   The stipend is $1,000.
Duration   1 year.
Number awarded   2 each year.
Deadline   October of each year.

[747]
RENATTA S. LOQUIST SCHOLARSHIP FOR GRADUATE NURSING EDUCATION

South Carolina Nurses Foundation, Inc.
Attn: Palmetto Gold Committee
1821 Gadsden Street
Columbia, SC 29201
(803) 252-4781   Fax: (803) 779-3870
E-mail: info@scpalmettogold.org
Web: www.scpalmettogold.org

Summary To provide fellowship/loans to students from any state working on a graduate nursing degree in South Carolina and planning to become a nursing educator in the state.

Eligibility This program is open to residents of any state who are accepted to or enrolled in a graduate nursing program at a university in South Carolina. Applicants must be willing to commit to teaching in a South Carolina state-approved nursing program for at least 3 years after completion of their graduate degree. They must apply through their school of nursing.

Financial Data The stipend is $2,000. This is a fellowship/loan program; recipients who do not fulfill their commitment to teach nursing in South Carolina must repay all funds received.

Duration 1 year.

Additional data This program, which began in 2007, operates through the Palmetto Gold Project of the South Carolina Nurses Foundation, with funding from the BlueCross BlueShield of South Carolina Foundation.

Number awarded 1 each year.

Deadline Nominations must be submitted by October of each year.

[748]
RICE MEMORIAL SCHOLARSHIP

Ohio Nurses Association
Attn: Ohio Nurses Foundation
4000 East Main Street
Columbus, OH 43213-2983
(614) 237-5414   Fax: (614) 237-6074
E-mail: gharsheymeade@ohnurses.org
Web: www.ohnurses.org

Summary To provide financial assistance to registered nurses in Ohio who are cancer survivors or have a relative with cancer and are working on a nursing degree at a school in the state.

Eligibility This program is open to Ohio residents who have a valid Ohio nursing license and plan to continue practicing in the state. Applicants must be a cancer survivor or have a close relative who has been diagnosed with cancer. They must have a GPA of 3.5 or higher and be planning to enroll in a nursing degree program at a school in Ohio. Along with their application, they must submit a 250-word personal statement on how the cancer experience has shaped their life and practice in Ohio. Selection is based on that statement, college academic records, school activities, and community services. Membership in the Ohio Nurses Association is considered in the selection process.

Financial Data The stipend is $500 per year.

Duration 1 year; recipients may reapply if they complete 9 credit hours during the academic year.

Number awarded 1 or more each year.

Deadline January of each year.

[749]
RITA K. CHOW AND YAYE TOGASKI-BREITENBACH AMERICAN NURSES FOUNDATION SCHOLAR AWARD

American Nurses Foundation
Attn: Nursing Research Grants Program
8515 Georgia Avenue, Suite 400
Silver Spring, MD 20910-3492
(301) 628-5227   Fax: (301) 628-5354
E-mail: anf@ana.org
Web: www.anfonline.org

Summary To provide funding to nurses interested in conducting research.

Eligibility This program is open to registered nurses who have earned a baccalaureate or higher degree. Applicants must be beginning researchers who have had no more than 3 research-based publications in refereed journals and have received, as a principal investigator, no more than $15,000 in extramural funding in any 1 research area. Proposed research may be for a master's thesis or doctoral dissertation, if the project has been approved by the principal investigator's thesis or dissertation committee. There are no restrictions on the research topic.

Financial Data The grant is $3,500. Funds may not be used as a salary for the principal investigator.

Duration 1 year.

Additional data There is a $100 application fee.

Number awarded 1 each year.

Deadline April of each year.

[750]
RNF NEW INVESTIGATOR RESEARCH GRANTS

Association of Rehabilitation Nurses
Attn: Rehabilitation Nursing Foundation
4700 West Lake Avenue
Glenview, IL 60025-1485
(847) 375-4710   Toll Free: (800) 229-7530
Fax: (877) 734-9384   E-mail: info@rehabnurse.org
Web: www.rehabnurse.org/research/researchgrants.html

Summary To encourage nurses who are novice researchers to conduct research on topics related to rehabilitation nursing.

Eligibility This award is open to rehabilitation nurses who are interested in conducting research or graduate nursing students working on theses or dissertations. Applicants must not have conducted research at the doctoral level, must have a rehabilitation focus, and must not have had previous research funding of more than $5,000. Quantitative and qualitative research projects will be accepted for review. Membership in the association is not required.

Financial Data The grant is $10,000.

Duration The project must be completed within 2 years.

Number awarded 1 each year.

Deadline January of each year.

[751]
RNF RESEARCH FELLOW GRANTS

Association of Rehabilitation Nurses
Attn: Rehabilitation Nursing Foundation
4700 West Lake Avenue
Glenview, IL 60025-1485
(847) 375-4710   Toll Free: (800) 229-7530
Fax: (877) 734-9384   E-mail: info@rehabnurse.org
Web: www.rehabnurse.org/research/researchgrants.html

Summary To provide funding to graduate students and professionals interested in conducting research on topics related to rehabilitation nursing.

Eligibility The principal investigator for the research project must be a registered nurse who is active in rehabilitation or who has demonstrated interest in and significant contributions to rehabilitation nursing. Membership in the association is not required. Graduate students may apply. Research proposals that address the clinical, educational, or administrative dimensions of rehabilitation nursing are requested. Quantitative and qualitative research projects will be accepted for review.

Financial Data   The grant is $10,000.

Duration   The project must be completed within 2 years.

Number awarded   2 each year.

Deadline   January of each year.

[752]
ROBERT AND CHRISTINE GISNESS ADVANCE PRACTICE SCHOLARSHIP

Emergency Nurses Association
Attn: ENA Foundation
915 Lee Street
Des Plaines, IL 60016-6569
(847) 460-4100   Toll Free: (800) 900-9659, ext. 4100
Fax: (847) 460-4004   E-mail: foundation@ena.org
Web: www.ena.org

Summary   To provide financial assistance to members of the Emergency Nurses Association (ENA) who are working on a master's degree.

Eligibility   This program is open to emergency nurses (R.N.) who are working on a master's degree. Applicants must have been members of the association for at least 12 months and have a GPA of 3.0 or higher. They must submit a 1-page statement on their professional and educational goals and how this scholarship will help them attain those goals. Selection is based on content and clarity of the goal statement (45%), professional association involvement (35%), presentation of the application (10%), and letters of reference (10%).

Financial Data   The stipend is $3,000.

Duration   1 year.

Number awarded   1 each year.

Deadline   May of each year.

[753]
ROBERT TOMAN MEMORIAL SCHOLARSHIP

Emergency Nurses Association
Attn: ENA Foundation
915 Lee Street
Des Plaines, IL 60016-6569
(847) 460-4100   Toll Free: (800) 900-9659, ext. 4100
Fax: (847) 460-4004   E-mail: foundation@ena.org
Web: www.ena.org

Summary   To provide financial assistance to members of the Emergency Nurses Association (ENA) who are working on a master's degree.

Eligibility   This program is open to emergency nurses (R.N.) who are working on a master's degree. Applicants must have been members of the association for at least 12 months and have a GPA of 3.0 or higher. They must submit a 1-page statement on their professional and educational goals and how this scholarship will help them attain those goals. Selection is based on content and clarity of the goal statement (45%), professional association involvement (35%), presentation of the application (10%), and letters of reference (10%).

Financial Data   The stipend is $5,000.

Duration   1 year.

Additional data   This program is funded by the California ENA State Council.

Number awarded   1 each year.

Deadline   May of each year.

[754]
ROBERTA D. THIRY ENDOWED SCHOLARSHIP

Kansas State Nurses Association
Attn: Kansas Nurses Foundation
1109 S.W. Topeka Boulevard
Topeka, KS 66612-1602
(785) 233-8638   Fax: (785) 233-5222
E-mail: ksna@ksna.net
Web: www.nursingworld.org/SNAS/KS/Knf.htm

Summary   To provide financial assistance to residents of Kansas who are working on a bachelor's or higher degree in nursing.

Eligibility   This program is open to R.N.s and other students in Kansas who are working on a nursing degree. Applicants must have a GPA of 3.0 or higher. Along with their application, they must submit a personal narrative describing their anticipated role in nursing in the state of Kansas. Preference is given to full-time students. First priority is given to R.N.s admitted to the B.S.N. completion program at Kansas Wesleyan University. If no applicants qualify for that first priority, second priority is given students enrolled in the third or fourth year of the B.S.N. program at Kansas Wesleyan University. If no applicants qualify for that second priority, third priority is given to students enrolled in master's or doctoral programs, especially residents of Dickinson, Ellsworth, Lincoln, Mitchell, Ottawa, and Saline counties. If no applicants qualify for that third priority, fourth priority is given to students enrolled in other Kansas B.S.N. or graduate nursing programs.

Financial Data   The stipend is $500.

Duration   1 year.

Number awarded   1 each year.

Deadline   June of each year.

[755]
ROBERTA PIERCE SCOFIELD DOCTORAL SCHOLARSHIP

Oncology Nursing Society
Attn: ONS Foundation
125 Enterprise Drive
Pittsburgh, PA 15275-1214
(412) 859-6100   Toll Free: (866) 257-4ONS
Fax: (412) 859-6163   E-mail: foundation@ons.org
Web: www.ons.org/Awards/FoundationAwards/Doctoral

Summary   To provide financial assistance to registered nurses interested in working on a doctoral degree in oncology nursing.

Eligibility   This program is open to registered nurses who have an interest in and commitment to oncology nursing. Applicants must be enrolled in or applying to a doctoral nursing degree program or related program. If they do not have a master's degree, they must have completed the first 2 years of a doctoral program. Along with their application, they must submit brief essays on their role in caring for persons with cancer; their research area of interest and plans for a dissertation; their professional goals and how those goals relate to the advancement of oncology nursing; and how the doctoral program will assist them in achieving their goals.

Financial Data   The stipend is $5,000.

Duration   1 year; nonrenewable.

Additional data   At the end of each year of scholarship participation, recipients must submit a summary of their educational activities. Applications must be accompanied by a $5 fee.

Number awarded   1 each year.

Deadline   January of each year.

[756]
ROBIN GAINES MEMORIAL SCHOLARSHIP

New England Regional Black Nurses Association, Inc.
P.O. Box 190690
Boston, MA 02119
(617) 524-1951
Web: www.nerbna.org/org/scholarships.html

Summary To provide financial assistance to registered nurses (R.N.s) from New England who are working on a master's degree and have contributed to the African American community.
Eligibility The program is open to residents of the New England states who are R.N.s and currently working on a master's degree (nursing, advanced nursing practice, or public health) at a school in any state. Applicants must have at least 1 full year of school remaining. Along with their application, they must submit a 3-page essay that covers their career aspirations in the nursing profession; how they have contributed to the African American or other communities of color in such areas as work, volunteering, church, or community outreach; an experience that has enhanced their personal and/or professional growth; and any financial hardships that may hinder them from completing their education.
Financial Data A stipend is awarded (amount not specified).
Duration 1 year.
Number awarded 1 or more each year.
Deadline March of each year.

[757]
ROSE DHEIN SCHOLARSHIP

Minnesota Nurses Association
Attn: Minnesota Nurses Association Foundation
1625 Energy Park Drive, Suite 200
St. Paul, MN 55108
(651) 414-2822   Toll Free: (800) 536-4662, ext. 122
Fax: (651) 695-7000   E-mail: linda.owens@mnnurses.org
Web: www.mnnurses.org

Summary To provide financial assistance to members of the Minnesota Nurses Association (MNA) who are interested in working on a graduate degree in nursing in order to become a teacher.
Eligibility This program is open to MNA members who have a current R.N. licensure and have been accepted into an approved program of study leading to a graduate academic degree in nursing. Applicants must be preparing for a career as a teacher of nursing. Along with their application, they must submit a brief description of their career goals following their graduate education, particularly related to teaching nursing. Selection is based on that statement, evidence of activity in professional organizations, scholarship, and community service.
Financial Data The stipend is $3,000 per year.
Duration 1 year; may be renewed.
Number awarded 1 or more each year.
Deadline May of each year.

[758]
ROSE FEATHERSTONE MEMORIAL SCHOLARSHIP

American Association of Nurse Anesthetists
Attn: AANA Foundation
222 South Prospect Avenue
Park Ridge, IL 60068-4001
(847) 655-1170   Fax: (847) 692-6968
E-mail: foundation@aana.com
Web: www.aanafoundation.com

Summary To provide financial assistance to members of the American Association of Nurse Anesthetists (AANA), especially residents of Idaho, who are interested in obtaining further education.
Eligibility This program is open to members of the association who are currently enrolled in an accredited nurse anesthesia education program. Preference is given to residents of Idaho. First-year students must have completed 6 months of nurse anesthesia classes; second-year students must have completed 12 months of nurse anesthesia classes. Along with their application, they must submit a 200-word essay describing why they have chosen nurse anesthesia as a profession and their professional goals for

the future. Financial need is also considered in the selection process.
Financial Data The stipend is $3,000.
Duration 1 year.
Additional data This scholarship, first awarded in 2004, is supported by the Idaho Association of Nurse Anesthetists. The application processing fee is $25.
Number awarded 1 each year.
Deadline March of each year.

[759]
ROSEMARY BERKEL CRISP RESEARCH AWARD

Sigma Theta Tau International
Attn: Research Services
550 West North Street
Indianapolis, IN 46202-3191
(317) 634-8171   Toll Free: (888) 634-7575
Fax: (317) 634-8188   E-mail: research@stti.iupui.edu
Web: www.nursingsociety.org

Summary To provide funding for clinically-oriented nursing research to members of Sigma Theta Tau International.
Eligibility This program is open to registered nurses actively involved in an aspect of health care delivery, education, or research in a clinical setting. Applicants must be members of the fraternity who have a master's or doctoral degree or are enrolled in a doctoral program. They must be interested in conducting research in the areas of women's health, oncology, or pediatrics. Selection is based on the quality of the proposed research, the future potential of the applicant, appropriateness of the research budget, and feasibility of the time frame. Preference is given to applicants residing in Arkansas, Illinois, Kentucky, Missouri, or Tennessee.
Financial Data The maximum grant is $5,000.
Duration 1 year.
Number awarded 1 each year.
Deadline November of each year.

[760]
ROSEMARY SMITH, R.N. MEMORIAL SCHOLARSHIP

Massachusetts Nurses Association
Attn: Massachusetts Nurses Foundation
340 Turnpike Street
Canton, MA 02021
(781) 830-5745   Toll Free: (800) 882-2056, ext. 745
Fax: (781) 821-4445   E-mail: cmessia@mnarn.org
Web: www.massnurses.org/about-man/mns/scholarships

Summary To provide financial assistance to members of the Massachusetts Nurses Association (MNA) who are working on an undergraduate or graduate degree in nursing, labor studies, or public health policy.
Eligibility This program is open to MNA members who are registered nurses or other health care professionals. First preference is given to members of MNA's Unit 7. Applicants must be enrolled in a bachelor's or master's degree program in nursing, labor studies, or public health policy. Along with their application, they must submit a 500-word essay on their career goals, how education will enhance those goals, and their contribution to their profession. Selection is based on the essay, professional development activities, community work, and 2 professional references. Minorities are specifically encouraged to apply.
Financial Data A stipend is awarded (amount not specified).
Duration 1 year.
Additional data Unit 7 is a bargaining unit that represents registered nurses, public health nurses, nurse practitioners, nursing instructors, community psychiatric mental health nurses, community mental health nursing advisers, health care facility inspectors,

psychologists, physical therapists, occupational therapists, and audiologists.

Number awarded   1 each year.

Deadline   May of each year.

[761]
ROY ANDERSON MEMORIAL SCHOLARSHIP

Colorado Nurses Foundation
7400 East Arapahoe Road, Suite 211
Centennial, CO 80112
(303) 694-4728   Fax: (303) 694-4869
E-mail: mail@cnfound.org
Web: www.cnfound.org/scholarships.html

Summary   To provide financial assistance to residents of Colorado who are working on a bachelor's or higher degree in nursing at a college or university in the state.

Eligibility   This program is open to Colorado residents who have been accepted as a student in an approved nursing program in the state. Applicants must be working on a bachelor's or higher degree. Undergraduates must have a GPA of 3.25 or higher and graduate students must have a GPA of 3.5 or higher. Selection is based on professional philosophy and goals, dedication to the improvement of patient care in Colorado, demonstrated commitment to nursing, critical thinking skills, potential for leadership, involvement in community and professional organizations, recommendations, GPA, and financial need.

Financial Data   The stipend is $5,000.

Duration   1 year.

Number awarded   2 each year.

Deadline   October of each year.

[762]
RUTH M. WRIGHT, CRNA MEMORIAL SCHOLARSHIP

American Association of Nurse Anesthetists
Attn: AANA Foundation
222 South Prospect Avenue
Park Ridge, IL 60068-4001
(847) 655-1170   Fax: (847) 692-6968
E-mail: foundation@aana.com
Web: www.aanafoundation.com

Summary   To provide financial assistance to members of the American Association of Nurse Anesthetists (AANA) who are pursuing further education at a program in any state.

Eligibility   This program is open to members of the association who are attending a nurse anesthesia program in any state. Applicants must have completed at least 6 months of school and have a GPA of 3.0 or higher. They must be able to demonstrate a commitment to nurse anesthesia professional organizations through service to AANA, a state organization, a student nurse anesthetist organization, or a similar organization. Along with their application, they must submit a 200-word essay describing why they have chosen nurse anesthesia as a profession and their professional goals for the future. Financial need is also considered in the selection process.

Financial Data   The stipend is $3,000.

Duration   1 year.

Additional data   This program began in 2008. The application processing fee is $25.

Number awarded   3 each year.

Deadline   March of each year.

[763]
RUTH MUSKRAT BRONSON FELLOWSHIP

American Indian Graduate Center
Attn: Executive Director
4520 Montgomery Boulevard, N.E., Suite 1-B
Albuquerque, NM 87109-1291
(505) 881-4584   Toll Free: (800) 628-1920
Fax: (505) 884-0427   E-mail: aigc@aigc.com
Web: www.aigc.com/02scholarships/scholarships.htm

Summary   To provide financial assistance to Native American students interested in working on a graduate degree in nursing or other health-related field.

Eligibility   This program is open to enrolled members of U.S. federally-recognized American Indian tribes and Alaska Native groups and students who can document one-fourth degree federally-recognized Indian blood. Applicants must be enrolled full time at a graduate school in the United States. First priority is given to nursing students; second priority is given to students in other health-related fields. Along with their application, they must submit a 500-word essay on their extracurricular activities as they relate to American Indian programs at their institution, volunteer and community work as related to American Indian communities, tribal and community involvement, and making positive changes in the American Indian community with their college education. Financial need is also considered in the selection process.

Financial Data   Stipends range from $1,000 to $5,000 per academic year, depending on the availability of funds and the recipient's unmet financial need.

Duration   1 year; may be renewed.

Additional data   The application fee is $15. Since this a supplemental program, students must apply in a timely manner for federal financial aid and campus-based aid at the college they are attending to be considered for this program. Failure to apply will disqualify an applicant.

Number awarded   1 or 2 each year.

Deadline   May of each year.

[764]
SANOFI-PASTEUR AMERICAN NURSES FOUNDATION SCHOLAR AWARD

American Nurses Foundation
Attn: Nursing Research Grants Program
8515 Georgia Avenue, Suite 400
Silver Spring, MD 20910-3492
(301) 628-5227   Fax: (301) 628-5354
E-mail: anf@ana.org
Web: www.anfonline.org

Summary   To provide funding to nurses interested in conducting research on adolescent health.

Eligibility   This program is open to registered nurses who have earned a baccalaureate or higher degree. Applicants may be either beginning or experienced researchers. They must be interested in conducting research on adolescent health; projects involving adolescent immunizations are limited to those that include all of the recommended adolescent immunizations. Proposed research may be for a master's thesis or doctoral dissertation, if the project has been approved by the principal investigator's thesis or dissertation committee.

Financial Data   The grant is $8,500. Funds may not be used as a salary for the principal investigator.

Duration   1 year.

Additional data   This program is sponsored by sanofi-pasteur. There is a $100 application fee.

Number awarded   1 each year.

Deadline   April of each year.

[765]
SANOFI-PASTEUR HEALTH THROUGH IMMUNIZATION AWARDS

Nurse Practitioner Healthcare Foundation
Attn: Scholarship Selection Committee
2647 134th Avenue N.E.
Bellevue, WA 98005-1813
(425) 861-0911   Fax: (425) 861-0907
Web: www.nphealthcarefoundation.org

Summary To provide funding to nurse practitioners and graduate nurse practitioner students interested in conducting a research or educational project related to immunization.

Eligibility This program is open to professional nurse practitioners and students currently enrolled in a nationally-accredited graduate nurse practitioner program. Applicants must be interested in conducting a research or educational project in the area of immunizations. The target audience may be patients, the general public, or health care professionals. U.S. citizenship or permanent resident status is required.

Financial Data The initial grant is $2,500, paid at the time of the award. Upon completion of the project, an additional $1,000 is awarded to support project dissemination (e.g., travel expenses for presenting at a national meeting, editing a paper for publication, preparing a poster).

Duration The project must be completed within 2 years.

Additional data This program is sponsored by sanofi-pasteur.

Number awarded 3 each year.

Deadline November of each year.

[766]
SARAH COLVIN SOCIAL JUSTICE SCHOLARSHIP

Minnesota Nurses Association
Attn: Minnesota Nurses Association Foundation
1625 Energy Park Drive, Suite 200
St. Paul, MN 55108
(651) 414-2822   Toll Free: (800) 536-4662, ext. 122
Fax: (651) 695-7000   E-mail: linda.owens@mnnurses.org
Web: www.mnnurses.org

Summary To provide financial assistance to members of the Minnesota Nurses Association (MNA) who are interested in working on a baccalaureate or graduate degree in nursing and have an interest in social justice.

Eligibility This program is open to MNA members who have a current R.N. licensure and have been accepted into an approved program of study leading to a baccalaureate or graduate academic degree in nursing. Applicants must be able to document evidence of advocating for individuals and groups harmed by inequities, environmental exploitation, discrimination, and oppression. Examples of social justice issues may include (but are not limited to) working with the mentally ill, impoverished, abused, or elderly. Selection is based on a statement of career goals, professional activities, demonstrated leadership ability, scholarship in nursing, MNA activities, and community involvement.

Financial Data The stipend is $2,000 per year.

Duration 1 year; may be renewed.

Number awarded 1 each year.

Deadline May of each year.

[767]
SAYRE MEMORIAL FUND AMERICAN NURSES FOUNDATION SCHOLAR AWARD

American Nurses Foundation
Attn: Nursing Research Grants Program
8515 Georgia Avenue, Suite 400
Silver Spring, MD 20910-3492
(301) 628-5227   Fax: (301) 628-5354
E-mail: anf@ana.org
Web: www.anfonline.org

Summary To provide funding to nurses interested in conducting research.

Eligibility This program is open to registered nurses who have earned a baccalaureate or higher degree. Applicants must be beginning researchers who have had no more than 3 research-based publications in refereed journals and have received, as a principal investigator, no more than $15,000 in extramural funding in any 1 research area. They must be interested in conducting research that relates to the interaction between clinical practice and the role of those occupying leadership/management positions. Preference is given to studies examining that relationship in a community or managed care setting (as opposed to acute care). Proposed research may be for a master's thesis or doctoral dissertation, if the project has been approved by the principal investigator's thesis or dissertation committee.

Financial Data The grant is $3,500. Funds may not be used as a salary for the principal investigator.

Duration 1 year.

Additional data There is a $100 application fee.

Number awarded 1 each year.

Deadline April of each year.

[768]
SCHOLARSHIP FOR RNS MAJORING IN NURSING

Ohio Nurses Association
Attn: Ohio Nurses Foundation
4000 East Main Street
Columbus, OH 43213-2983
(614) 237-5414   Fax: (614) 237-6074
E-mail: gharsheymeade@ohnurses.org
Web: www.ohnurses.org

Summary To provide financial assistance to registered nurses in Ohio who are working on a nursing degree at a school in any state.

Eligibility This program is open to Ohio residents who have a valid Ohio nursing license. Applicants must have a GPA of 2.5 or higher as an undergraduate or 3.5 or higher if working on a graduate degree. They must be planning to enroll full time in a nursing degree program at a school in any state. Along with their application, they must submit a 100-word personal statement on how they will advance the profession of nursing in Ohio. Selection is based on that statement, college academic records, school activities, and community services.

Financial Data The stipend is $1,000 per year.

Duration 1 year; recipients may reapply for 1 additional year if they maintain a cumulative GPA of 2.5 or higher.

Number awarded 1 or more each year.

Deadline January of each year.

[769]
SCHOOL NURSE ORGANIZATION OF WASHINGTON SCHOLARSHIPS

School Nurse Organization of Washington
Attn: Professional Development Chair
P.O. 141309
Spokane Valley, WA 99214-1309
Web: www.schoolnurseorganizationofwashington.org/?ID=39

Summary To provide financial assistance to members of the School Nurse Organization of Washington (SNOW) who are interested in additional training.

Eligibility This program is open to SNOW members who are interested in working on a B.S.N., master's degree, or education staff associate certification in school nursing. Applicants must submit a 1-page essay on why they selected school nursing as a clinical specialty. Selection is based on the essay, academic achievement, professional involvement, and financial need.

Financial Data The stipend is $500.

Duration 1 year.

Additional data This program includes the Carol Hoffman Scholarship, the Martha Meyers Scholarship, and the Lifetime Members Scholarship.

Number awarded 3 each year.

Deadline February of each year.

[770]
SCHWEITZER FELLOWSHIPS

The Albert Schweitzer Fellowship
Attn: National Program Director
330 Brookline Avenue
Boston, MA 02215
(617) 667-3115   Fax: (617) 667-7989
E-mail: info@schweitzerfellowship.org
Web: www.schweitzerfellowship.org/features/us

Summary To provide health professional graduate students with an opportunity to offer direct service to underserved communities.

Eligibility This program is open to medical, nursing, pharmacy public health, social work, and other health professional students at schools in the areas where the program currently operates: Baltimore, Boston, Chicago, Greater Philadelphia, Houston/Galveston, Los Angeles, New Hampshire/Vermont, New Orleans, North Carolina, Pittsburgh, or San Francisco Bay area. Applicants must be interested in working with an existing community agency to carry out a health-related service project full time during the summer or part time during the academic year.

Financial Data The stipend in most programs is $2,000.

Duration Participants are expected to perform 200 hours of community service work.

Additional data This program began in Boston (including Worcester) in 1992, North Carolina in 1994, New Hampshire/Vermont in 1996, Chicago (including DuPage County) in 1996, Pittsburgh in 1997, Baltimore in 1999, Greater Philadelphia (Bucks, Chester, Delaware, Montgomery, and Philadelphia counties in Pennsylvania; Burlington, Camden, Gloucester, Mercer, and Salem counties in New Jersey; New Castle County in Delaware) in 2007, San Francisco Bay area (Alameda, Contra Costa, San Francisco, San Mateo, and Santa Clara counties) in 2007, Los Angeles in 2008, New Orleans in 2008, and Houston/Galveston in 2009. For the addresses of those programs and a description of available service opportunities at each, contact the headquarters in Boston.

Number awarded Varies each year.

Deadline Each program selects its own deadline, but this is generally in January.

[771]
SCOTT DOMINGUEZ-CRATERS OF THE MOON CHAPTER SCHOLARSHIP

American Society of Safety Engineers
Attn: ASSE Foundation
1800 East Oakton Street
Des Plaines, IL 60018
(847) 768-3435   Fax: (847) 768-3434
E-mail: agabanski@asse.org
Web: www.asse.org/foundation/scholarships/scholarships.php

Summary To provide financial assistance to undergraduate and graduate student members of the American Society of Safety Engineers (ASSE) from designated western states.

Eligibility This program is open to undergraduate and graduate students who are working on a degree in occupational safety, health, and environment or a closely-related field (e.g., industrial or environmental engineering, environmental science, industrial hygiene, occupational health nursing). First priority is given to residents within the service area of Craters of the Moon Chapter in Idaho; second priority is given to residents of other states in ASSE Region II (Arizona, Colorado, Montana, Nevada, New Mexico, Utah, and Wyoming). Special consideration is also given to 1) employees of a sponsoring organization or their dependents; 2) students who are serving their country through active duty in the armed forces or are honorably discharged; 3) former members of the Boy Scouts, Girl Scouts, FFA, or 4-H; 4) recipients of awards from service organizations; and 5) students who have provided volunteer service to an ASSE chapter in a leadership role. Undergraduates must have completed at least 60 semester hours with a GPA of 3.0 or higher. Graduate students must have completed at least 9 semester hours with a GPA of 3.5 or higher and have earned a GPA of 3.0 or higher as an undergraduate. Full-time students must be ASSE student members; part-time students must be ASSE general or professional members. Along with their application, they must submit 2 essays of 300 words or less: 1) why they are seeking a degree in occupational safety and health or a closely-related field, a brief description of their current activities, and how those relate to their career goals and objectives; and 2) why they should be awarded this scholarship (including career goals and financial need). U.S. citizenship is not required.

Financial Data The stipend is $1,000 per year.

Duration 1 year; recipients may reapply.

Additional data This program is sponsored by the ASSE Craters of the Moon Chapter.

Number awarded 1 each year.

Deadline November of each year.

[772]
SENATOR PATRICIA K. MCGEE NURSING FACULTY SCHOLARSHIP PROGRAM

New York State Higher Education Services Corporation
Attn: Student Information
99 Washington Avenue
Albany, NY 12255
(518) 473-1574   Toll Free: (888) NYS-HESC
Fax: (518) 473-3749   TDD: (800) 445-5234
E-mail: webmail@hesc.com
Web: www.hesc.com

Summary To provide scholarship/loans to nurses in New York who are interested in working on a graduate degree and agree to teach nursing in the state following graduation.

Eligibility This program is open to registered nurses professionally licensed to work in New York who have been residents of the state for at least 1 year. Applicants must be interested in enrolling in a master's or doctoral degree in nursing at a school in the state. They must agree to a service contract to practice as nursing faculty or adjunct clinical faculty in New York for 4 years within 3 years of completing their graduate degree. U.S. citizenship or eligible non-citizen status is required.

Financial Data The maximum stipend is $20,000 per year or the average SUNY cost of attendance, whichever is less. Funds are paid directly to the schools the recipients attend. If they fail to honor the service contract in any way, the award converts to a loan and must be repaid with interest.

Duration This program is available for up to 3 years of study.

Number awarded Varies each year.

Deadline April of each year.

[773]
SGNA RESEARCH GRANTS

Society of Gastroenterology Nurses and Associates, Inc.
Attn: Research Committee
401 North Michigan Avenue
Chicago, IL 60611-4267
(312) 321-5165   Toll Free: (800) 245-SGNA
Fax: (312) 673-6694   E-mail: sgna@smithbucklin.com
Web: www.sgna.org/Education/scholarships.cfm

Summary To provide funding to scholars and students interested in conducting a research project related to gastroenterology nursing.

Eligibility This program is open to investigators interested in conducting a research project that is timely and significant to gastroenterology nursing. Research may be done individually or as a collaborative effort. Students enrolled in an academic degree program may be included among the investigators. Preference is given to proposals that address a research priority of the sponsor: conscious sedation, expanded role of the GI practitioner, infection control, safety, patient education, or nursing intervention related to GI disease processes.

Financial Data The amount of the grant depends on the nature of the project and the availability of funds.

Duration Data collection must be completed within 1 year.

Additional data Recipients must agree to prepare a manuscript presenting the results of the research for publication in *Gastroenterology Nursing* within 6 months of completing the project.

Number awarded Varies each year.

Deadline February, July, or October of each year.

[774]
SGNA RN ADVANCING EDUCATION SCHOLARSHIP

Society of Gastroenterology Nurses and Associates, Inc.
Attn: Awards Committee
401 North Michigan Avenue
Chicago, IL 60611-4267
(312) 321-5165   Toll Free: (800) 245-SGNA
Fax: (312) 673-6694   E-mail: sgna@smithbucklin.com
Web: www.sgna.org/Education/scholarships.cfm

Summary To provide financial assistance to registered nurses (R.N.s) working in gastroenterology who are interested in enrolling in an advanced degree program.

Eligibility This program is open to R.N.s working in gastroenterology who are members of the Society of Gastroenterology Nurses and Associates (SGNA). Applicants must be enrolled in an accredited advanced degree program working on a B.S.N., M.S.N., or Ph.D. degree with a GPA of 3.0 or higher. Along with their application, they must submit a 500-word essay on a challenging situation they see in the health care environment today and how they, as an R.N. with an advanced degree, would best address and meet that challenge. Financial need is not considered in the selection process.

Financial Data The stipend is $2,500 for full-time students or $1,000 for part-time students. Funds are issued as reimbursement after the recipient has completed the proposed course work with a GPA of 3.0 or higher.

Duration 1 year.

Number awarded 1 or more each year.

Deadline July of each year.

[775]
SHARON A. SMITH SCHOLARSHIP

Massachusetts Organization of Nurse Executives
Attn: Scholarship Selection Committee
101 Cambridge Street, Suite 110
Burlington, MA 01803
(781) 272-3500   Fax: (781) 272-3505
E-mail: info@massone.org
Web: www.massone.org

Summary To provide financial assistance to members of the Massachusetts Organization of Nurse Executives (MONE) and their families who are studying nursing in college or graduate school.

Eligibility This program is open to MONE members and their immediate family (spouse, children, siblings, nieces, and nephews). Applicants must be enrolled in an accredited nursing program (B.S.N., M.S.N., or advanced practice). Along with their application, they must submit a 500-word essay on why they are working on a nursing or advanced degree and what they hope to accomplish, documentation of financial need, and the names of 2 references.

Financial Data The amount of the stipend varies each year, depending on the availability of funds.

Duration 1 year.

Number awarded Varies each year.

Deadline April of each year.

[776]
SHIP ISLAND–MRS. J.O. JONES MEMORIAL SCHOLARSHIP

United Daughters of the Confederacy
Attn: Education Director
328 North Boulevard
Richmond, VA 23220-4057
(804) 355-1636   Fax: (804) 353-1396
E-mail: hqudc@rcn.com
Web: www.hqudc.org/scholarships/scholarships.html

Summary To provide financial assistance for graduate nursing education to lineal descendants of Confederate veterans.

Eligibility Eligible to apply for these scholarships are lineal descendants of worthy Confederates or collateral descendants who are members of the Children of the Confederacy or the United Daughters of the Confederacy. Applicants must intend to study nursing at the graduate level and must submit certified proof of the Confederate record of 1 ancestor, with the company and regiment in which he served. They must have a GPA of 3.0 or higher.

Financial Data The amount of this scholarship depends on the availability of funds.

Duration 1 year; may be renewed up to 2 additional years.

Additional data Members of the same family may not hold scholarships simultaneously, and only 1 application per family will be accepted within any 1 year. All requests for applications must be accompanied by a self-addressed stamped envelope.

Number awarded 1 each year.

Deadline April of each year.

[777]
SIGMA THETA TAU INTERNATIONAL/AMERICAN NURSES FOUNDATION GRANT

Sigma Theta Tau International
Attn: Research Services
550 West North Street
Indianapolis, IN 46202-3191
(317) 634-8171   Toll Free: (888) 634-7575
Fax: (317) 634-8188   E-mail: research@stti.iupui.edu
Web: www.nursingsociety.org

204 FINANCIAL AID PROGRAMS

Summary To provide funding to beginning or experienced nurses who are interested in conducting research on a clinical topic.

Eligibility This program is open to registered nurses with a current license who have a master's or doctoral degree or are enrolled in a doctoral program. Applicants must be interested in conducting a research project on a clinical nursing topic. They may be beginning nurse researchers or experienced nurse researchers entering a new field of study. All other qualifications being equal, preference is given to Sigma Theta Tau members. Selection is based on the quality of the proposed research, the future promise of the applicant, and the research budget.

Financial Data The maximum grant is $7,500.

Duration 1 year.

Additional data This program is sponsored jointly by Sigma Theta Tau International (STTI) and American Nurses Foundation (ANF). ANF handles the selection process in odd-numbered years and STTI handles the selection process in even-numbered years. Applications are also available from the American Nurses Foundation (in odd-numbered years).

Number awarded 1 each year.

Deadline April of each year.

[778]
SIGMA THETA TAU INTERNATIONAL/ASSOCIATION OF NURSES IN AIDS CARE GRANT

Sigma Theta Tau International
Attn: Research Services
550 West North Street
Indianapolis, IN 46202-3191
(317) 634-8171   Toll Free: (888) 634-7575
Fax: (317) 634-8188   E-mail: research@stti.iupui.edu
Web: www.nursingsociety.org

Summary To provide funding to nurses or nursing graduate students who are interested in conducting research related to AIDS.

Eligibility This program is open to registered nurses who have a master's degree and/or are enrolled in a doctoral program. Applicants must be interested in conducting clinically oriented HIV/AIDS research, including studies focused on HIV prevention, symptom management, and promotion of self-care and adherence. Proposals for pilot and/or developmental research may be submitted. Membership in either Sigma Theta Tau International or the Association of Nurses in AIDS Care is required; preference is given to applicants who are members of both organizations.

Financial Data The maximum grant is $2,500.

Duration 1 year.

Additional data This program is sponsored jointly by Sigma Theta Tau International and the Association of Nurses in AIDS Care.

Number awarded 1 each year.

Deadline March of each year.

[779]
SIGMA THETA TAU INTERNATIONAL/HOSPICE AND PALLIATIVE NURSES FOUNDATION END OF LIFE NURSING CARE RESEARCH GRANT

Sigma Theta Tau International
Attn: Research Services
550 West North Street
Indianapolis, IN 46202-3191
(317) 634-8171   Toll Free: (888) 634-7575
Fax: (317) 634-8188   E-mail: research@stti.iupui.edu
Web: www.nursingsociety.org

Summary To provide funding to nurses and graduate nursing students who are interested in conducting research on end of life nursing care.

Eligibility This program is open to registered nurses who have a master's or doctoral degree or are enrolled in a doctoral pro-

gram. Applicants must be interested in conducting a research project, including pilot and/or developmental research, on end of life nursing care. Preference is given to members of Sigma Theta Tau International and/or the Hospice and Palliative Nurses Association.

Financial Data The maximum grant is $10,000.

Duration 1 year.

Additional data This program is sponsored jointly by Sigma Theta Tau International and the Hospice and Palliative Nurses Foundation.

Number awarded 1 each year.

Deadline March of each year.

[780]
SIGMA THETA TAU INTERNATIONAL/MIDWEST NURSING RESEARCH SOCIETY RESEARCH GRANT

Sigma Theta Tau International
Attn: Research Services
550 West North Street
Indianapolis, IN 46202-3191
(317) 634-8171   Toll Free: (888) 634-7575
Fax: (317) 634-8188   E-mail: research@stti.iupui.edu
Web: www.nursingsociety.org

Summary To provide funding to nurses and graduate nursing students from midwestern states interested in conducting research.

Eligibility This program is open to registered nurses who have a master's degree and/or are enrolled in a doctoral program. Applicants must be interested in conducting a research project, including pilot and/or developmental research. They must be members of both Sigma Theta Tau International and the Midwest Nursing Research Society (MNRS). All research topics and designs are eligible; multidisciplinary, historical, and international research is encouraged.

Financial Data The maximum grant is $2,500.

Duration 1 year.

Additional data This program is sponsored jointly by Sigma Theta Tau International and the MNRS.

Number awarded 1 each year.

Deadline March of each year.

[781]
SIGMA THETA TAU INTERNATIONAL/NATIONAL LEAGUE FOR NURSING GRANT

Sigma Theta Tau International
Attn: Research Services
550 West North Street
Indianapolis, IN 46202-3191
(317) 634-8171   Toll Free: (888) 634-7575
Fax: (317) 634-8188   E-mail: research@stti.iupui.edu
Web: www.nursingsociety.org

Summary To provide funding to nurses and graduate nursing students who are interested in conducting research involving the use of technology.

Eligibility This program is open to registered nurses who have a master's or doctoral degree or are enrolled in a doctoral program. Applicants must be interested in conducting a research project that will advance the science of nursing education through the use of technology in the dissemination of knowledge. Preference is given to members of Sigma Theta Tau International and/or the National League for Nursing.

Financial Data The maximum grant is $5,000.

Duration 1 year.

Additional data This program is sponsored jointly by Sigma Theta Tau International and the National League for Nursing.

Number awarded 1 each year.

Deadline May of each year.

[782]
SIGMA THETA TAU INTERNATIONAL SMALL RESEARCH GRANTS

Sigma Theta Tau International
Attn: Research Services
550 West North Street
Indianapolis, IN 46202-3191
(317) 634-8171   Toll Free: (888) 634-7575
Fax: (317) 634-8188   E-mail: research@stti.iupui.edu
Web: www.nursingsociety.org

Summary To provide funding to nurses and graduate nursing students who are interested in conducting research.

Eligibility This program is open to registered nurses with a current license who have a master's or doctoral degree or are enrolled in a doctoral program. Applicants must be interested in conducting a research project on any topic. Applications from novice researchers who have received no other national research funds are encouraged and receive special consideration. All other qualifications being equal, preference is given to Sigma Theta Tau members. Selection is based on the quality of the proposed research, the future promise of the applicant, and the applicant's research budget.

Financial Data The maximum grant is $5,000.

Duration 1 year.

Number awarded 10 to 15 each year.

Deadline November of each year.

[783]
SIGMA THETA TAU INTERNATIONAL/SOUTHERN NURSING RESEARCH SOCIETY RESEARCH GRANT

Sigma Theta Tau International
Attn: Research Services
550 West North Street
Indianapolis, IN 46202-3191
(317) 634-8171   Toll Free: (888) 634-7575
Fax: (317) 634-8188   E-mail: research@stti.iupui.edu
Web: www.nursingsociety.org

Summary To provide funding to nurses and graduate nursing students from southern states interested in conducting research.

Eligibility This program is open to registered nurses who have a master's degree and/or are enrolled in a doctoral program. Applicants must be interested in conducting a research project, including pilot and/or developmental research. They must be members of both Sigma Theta Tau International and the Southern Nursing Research Society (SNRS). All research topics and designs are eligible; multidisciplinary, historical, and international research is encouraged.

Financial Data The maximum grant is $4,500.

Duration 1 year.

Additional data This program is sponsored jointly by Sigma Theta Tau International and the SNRS.

Number awarded 1 each year.

Deadline March of each year.

[784]
SIGMA THETA TAU INTERNATIONAL/WESTERN INSTITUTE OF NURSING RESEARCH GRANT

Sigma Theta Tau International
Attn: Research Services
550 West North Street
Indianapolis, IN 46202-3191
(317) 634-8171   Toll Free: (888) 634-7575
Fax: (317) 634-8188   E-mail: research@stti.iupui.edu
Web: www.nursingsociety.org

Summary To provide funding to nurses and graduate nursing students from western states interested in conducting research.

Eligibility This program is open to registered nurses who have a master's degree and/or are enrolled in a doctoral program.

Applicants must be interested in conducting a research project, including pilot and/or developmental research. They must be members of Sigma Theta Tau International and/or the Western Institute of Nursing.

Financial Data The maximum grant is $2,500.

Duration 1 year.

Additional data This program is sponsored jointly by Sigma Theta Tau International and the Western Institute of Nursing.

Number awarded 1 each year.

Deadline November of each year.

[785]
SISTER TERESA HARRIS SCHOLARSHIP

New Jersey State Nurses Association
Attn: Institute for Nursing
1479 Pennington Road
Trenton, NJ 08618-2661
(609) 883-5335   Toll Free: (888) UR-NJSNA
Fax: (609) 883-5343   E-mail: institute@njsna.org
Web: www.njsna.org/displaycommon.cfm?an=5

Summary To provide financial assistance to New Jersey residents who are applying to or enrolled in a master's program for advanced practice nursing at a school in the state.

Eligibility Applicants must be New Jersey residents who are registered nurses applying to or currently enrolled in a master's degree program for advanced practice nursing located in the state. They must be members of the New Jersey State Nurses Association. Selection is based on financial need, GPA, and leadership potential.

Financial Data The stipend is $1,000.

Duration 1 year.

Number awarded 1 each year.

Deadline January of each year.

[786]
SOCIETY OF PEDIATRIC NURSES EDUCATIONAL SCHOLARSHIP

Society of Pediatric Nurses
7794 Grow Drive
Pensacola, FL 32514
(850) 494-9467   Toll Free: (800) 723-2902
Fax: (850) 484-8762   E-mail: spn@dancyamc.com
Web: www.pedsnurses.org/awards-amp-scholarships.html

Summary To provide financial assistance to members of the Society of Pediatric Nurses (SPN) who are working on a bachelor's or graduate degree.

Eligibility This program is open to SPN members who are currently enrolled or accepted in a B.S.N. completion program or graduate program that will advance the health care of children. Students must be nominated by a current SPN member or chapter. Along with their application, they must submit a letter of recommendation from an SPN member that addresses their interest in and/or commitment to the care of children and their families, and a letter of recommendation from a faculty member who can evaluate their potential to meet professional goals.

Financial Data The stipend is $500.

Duration 1 year.

Number awarded 1 or more each year.

Deadline November of each year.

[787]
SOHN GRADUATE SCHOLARSHIPS

Society of Otorhinolaryngology and Head-Neck Nurses, Inc.
Attn: Ear, Nose and Throat Nursing Foundation
202 Julia Street
New Smyrna Beach, FL 32168
(386) 428-1695   Fax: (386) 423-7566
E-mail: info@sohnnurse.com
Web: www.sohnnurse.com/awards.html

Summary To provide financial assistance to members of the Society of Otorhinolaryngology and Head-Neck Nurses (SOHN) who are working on a graduate degree in nursing.

Eligibility This program is open to members of the society who are able to demonstrate progress toward a master's degree in nursing. Applicants must have a GPA of 3.0 or higher. Along with their application, they must submit a copy of their current registration in a graduate nursing program, a copy of recent transcripts, a statement of current financial assistance received and required, 3 letters of recommendation, and a narrative of 750 to 1,000 words describing their past or current SOHN involvement, future SOHN goals, and desire for advancing their degree in nursing.

Financial Data Stipends range from $1,000 to $1,500.

Duration 1 year.

Number awarded 1 each year.

Deadline June of each year.

[788]
SOUTH CAROLINA NURSES CARE SCHOLARSHIPS

South Carolina Nurses Foundation, Inc.
Attn: Awards Committee Chair
1821 Gadsden Street
Columbia, SC 29201
(803) 252-4781   Fax: (803) 779-3870
E-mail: brownk1@aol.com
Web: www.scnursesfoundation.org/index_files/Page316.htm

Summary To provide financial assistance to students enrolled in an undergraduate or graduate degree nursing program in South Carolina.

Eligibility This program is open to students currently enrolled in an undergraduate or graduate nursing degree program in South Carolina. Applicants must submit documentation of financial need and brief statements of their career goals, both upon graduation and in 5 years.

Financial Data The stipend is $1,500.

Duration 1 year.

Additional data This program was established in 2002 and is funded by the sale of "Nurses Care" specialty license plates.

Number awarded 4 each year: 2 to undergraduates and 2 to graduate students.

Deadline May of each year.

[789]
SOUTH DAKOTA NURSES FOUNDATION SCHOLARSHIP

South Dakota Nurses Association
Attn: South Dakota Nurses Foundation
P.O. Box 1015
Pierre, SD 57501-1015
(605) 945-4265   Fax: (888) 425-3032
E-mail: sdnurse@midco.net
Web: www.sdnursesassociation.org

Summary To provide financial assistance to members of the South Dakota Nurses Association (SDNA) who are interested in working on a graduate degree at a school in any state.

Eligibility This program is open to residents of South Dakota who are registered nurses and have been members of SDNA for at least 1 year. Applicants must be working on a master's or doc-

toral degree in nursing or a related field at a school in any state with the intention of practicing nursing in a South Dakota high need area or teaching in a South Dakota baccalaureate or higher degree nursing education program. They must have a GPA of 3.0 or higher. Along with their application, they must submit a personal statement on their career goals, personal qualities that affect their nursing practice, and how those career goals and personal qualities correspond to the purposes of the scholarship. Selection is based on leadership, compassion, involvement in professional organizations, professional activities, and community service.

Financial Data The stipend is $1,000.

Duration 1 year.

Additional data This scholarship was first offered in 2007.

Number awarded 1 each year.

Deadline July of each year.

[790]
SOUTHERN NURSING RESEARCH SOCIETY/ AMERICAN NURSES FOUNDATION SCHOLAR AWARD

American Nurses Foundation
Attn: Nursing Research Grants Program
8515 Georgia Avenue, Suite 400
Silver Spring, MD 20910-3492
(301) 628-5227   Fax: (301) 628-5354
E-mail: anf@ana.org
Web: www.anfonline.org

Summary To provide funding to members of the Southern Nursing Research Society (SNRS) who are interested in conducting research.

Eligibility This program is open to registered nurses who have earned a baccalaureate or higher degree. Applicants may be either beginning or experienced researchers. Proposed research may be for a master's thesis or doctoral dissertation if the project has been approved by the principal investigator's thesis or dissertation committee. There are no restrictions on the research topic, but applicants must be current SNRS members.

Financial Data Grants are $4,000 or $3,500. Funds may not be used as a salary for the principal investigator.

Duration 1 year.

Additional data Funding for this program is provided by the Southern Nursing Research Society. There is a $100 application fee.

Number awarded 2 each year: 1 at $4,000 and 1 at $3,500.

Deadline April of each year.

[791]
SOUTHERN NURSING RESEARCH SOCIETY DISSERTATION AWARD

Southern Nursing Research Society
10200 West 44th Avenue, Suite 304
Wheat Ridge, CO 80033
Toll Free: (877) 314-SNRS
E-mail: snrs@resourcecenter.com
Web: snrs.org/research/dissertationgrants.html

Summary To provide dissertation research funding to doctoral candidates who are members of the Southern Nursing Research Society (SNRS).

Eligibility This program is open to students currently enrolled in doctoral study at a school or college of nursing in the southern states. Applicants must be members of the SNRS whose dissertation topic has been approved. They must submit evidence that their proposed research topic meets the requirements for the dissertation and that it can be supported at the proposed institution or facility. Selection is based on significance to nursing, scientific merit, innovation, appropriateness of methodology to the research question, qualifications of the applicant to conduct the study, adequacy of human subjects and/or animal protection, and appropriateness of the environment, budget, and time frame.

Financial Data   The grant is $3,000.

Duration   1 year.

Additional data   The application fee is $25.

Number awarded   1 each year.

Deadline   February of each year.

[792]
SOUTHERN NURSING RESEARCH SOCIETY SMALL GRANT AWARD

Southern Nursing Research Society
10200 West 44th Avenue, Suite 304
Wheat Ridge, CO 80033
Toll Free: (877) 314-SNRS
E-mail: snrs@resourcecenter.com
Web: snrs.org/research/smallgrants.html

Summary   To provide research funding to student and professional members of the Southern Nursing Research Society (SNRS).

Eligibility   This program is open to SNRS members who are new investigators interested in initiating or building a program of research that advances nursing science and practice. Applicants may not have received more than $30,000 in research funding during the past 2 years. Students are eligible, although they may not be conducting research for course credit. Selection is based on significance to nursing, scientific merit, innovation, appropriateness of methodology to the research question, qualifications of the applicant to conduct the study, adequacy of human subjects and/or animal protection, and appropriateness of the environment, budget, and time frame.

Financial Data   The amount of the grant depends on the nature of the proposal.

Duration   1 year.

Additional data   The application fee is $50 or $25 for students.

Number awarded   1 each year.

Deadline   September of each year.

[793]
ST. FRANCIS SCHOOL OF NURSING ALUMNI OF PITTSBURGH, PA SCHOLARSHIP FUND

Pittsburgh Foundation
Attn: Scholarship Coordinator
Five PPG Place, Suite 250
Pittsburgh, PA 15222-5414
(412) 394-2649   Fax: (412) 391-7259
E-mail: turnerd@pghfdn.org
Web: www.pittsburghfoundation.org

Summary   To provide financial assistance to students working on an undergraduate or graduate degree in nursing.

Eligibility   This program is open to 1) students working on their first academic degree or diploma that leads to professional licensure as a registered nurse, and 2) licensed registered nurses working on an advanced degree in nursing. Applicants must have a GPA of 3.0 or higher and be able to demonstrate financial need. Along with their application, they must submit brief essays on their prior work experience, prior education, financial obligations, extracurricular activities and volunteer work, past achievements related to nursing, and career goals. U.S. citizenship is required.

Financial Data   A stipend is awarded (amount not specified).

Duration   1 year.

Additional data   This scholarship was first awarded in 2007.

Number awarded   1 or more each year.

Deadline   December of each year.

[794]
STEPHANIE CARROLL SCHOLARSHIP

National Association Directors of Nursing Administration in Long Term Care
Attn: Education/Scholarship Committee
11353 Reed Hartman Highway, Suite 210
Cincinnati, OH 45241
(513) 791-3679   Toll Free: (800) 222-0539
Fax: (513) 791-3699   E-mail: info@nadona.org
Web: www.nadona.org/wysiwyg.php?wID=6

Summary   To provide financial assistance to nursing undergraduate and graduate students who plan to practice in long-term care or geriatrics.

Eligibility   This program is open to students entering or continuing in an accredited undergraduate or graduate nursing program. Applicants must indicate an intent to practice in long-term care or geriatrics for at least 2 years after graduation. Along with their application, they must submit an essay of at least 100 words on why they have chosen nursing as a career, why they are seeking this degree and how it will impact their nursing practice, and their commitment to the nursing profession, including their goals for their nursing career after graduation. Financial need is considered in the selection process.

Financial Data   The stipend is $5,000.

Duration   1 year.

Number awarded   At least 1 each year.

Deadline   June of each year.

[795]
STRYKER STRATEGIC SPONSOR SCHOLARSHIP

Emergency Nurses Association
Attn: ENA Foundation
915 Lee Street
Des Plaines, IL 60016-6569
(847) 460-4100   Toll Free: (800) 900-9659, ext. 4100
Fax: (847) 460-4004   E-mail: foundation@ena.org
Web: www.ena.org

Summary   To provide financial assistance to members of the Emergency Nurses Association (ENA) who are working on a master's degree.

Eligibility   This program is open to emergency nurses (R.N.s) who are working on a master's degree. Applicants must have been members of the association for at least 12 months and have a GPA of 3.0 or higher. They must submit a 1-page statement on their professional and educational goals and how this scholarship will help them attain those goals. Selection is based on content and clarity of the goal statement (45%), professional association involvement (35%), presentation of the application (10%), and letters of reference (10%).

Financial Data   The stipend is $5,000.

Duration   1 year.

Additional data   This program is funded by Stryker, an ENA Strategic Sponsor.

Number awarded   1 each year.

Deadline   May of each year.

[796]
SUSAN STEIN SCHOLARSHIP

American College of Nurse-Midwives
Attn: ACNM Foundation, Inc.
8403 Colesville Road, Suite 1550
Silver Spring, MD 20910-6374
(240) 485-1850   Fax: (240) 485-1818
Web: www.midwife.org/foundation_award.cfm

Summary   To provide financial assistance for midwifery education to student members of the American College of Nurse-Midwives (ACNM) who have had a personal experience with breast cancer.

Eligibility This program is open to ACNM members who are currently enrolled in an accredited basic midwife education program and have successfully completed 1 academic or clinical semester/quarter or clinical module. Applicants must have had or currently have a personal experience with breast cancer, either their own or a family member's. Along with their application, they must submit a 300-word essay on the effect of breast cancer on their identity as a midwife. Selection is based primarily on the quality of the application, although leadership potential, financial need, academic achievement, and personal goals may also be considered.
Financial Data The stipend is $3,000.
Duration 1 year.
Additional data This program was established in 2010.
Number awarded 1 each year.
Deadline May of each year.

[797]
TANA EDUCATION DISTRICT #6 SCHOLARSHIP

American Association of Nurse Anesthetists
Attn: AANA Foundation
222 South Prospect Avenue
Park Ridge, IL 60068-4001
(847) 655-1170   Fax: (847) 692-6968
E-mail: foundation@aana.com
Web: www.aanafoundation.com

Summary To provide financial assistance to members of the American Association of Nurse Anesthetists from Texas who are interested in obtaining further education at a school in the state.
Eligibility This program is open to members of the association who are registered nurses licensed to practice in Texas and currently enrolled in an accredited nurse anesthesia education program in the state. First-year students must have completed 6 months of nurse anesthesia classes; second-year students must have completed 12 months of nurse anesthesia classes. Along with their application, they must submit a 200-word essay describing why they have chosen nurse anesthesia as a profession and their professional goals for the future. Financial need is also considered in the selection process.
Financial Data The stipend is $1,000.
Duration 1 year.
Additional data Funding for this scholarship, first awarded in 2000, is provided by the Texas Association of Nurse Anesthetists (TANA) Education District #6. The application processing fee is $25.
Number awarded 1 each year.
Deadline March of each year.

[798]
TCNS RESEARCH AWARD

Transcultural Nursing Society
c/o Lisa A. Dobson, Business Manager
Madonna University
36600 Schoolcraft Road
Livonia, MI 48150-1176
Toll Free: (888) 432-5470   Fax: (734) 432-5463
E-mail: ldobson@tcns.org
Web: www.tcns.org/Foundationawards.html

Summary To provide funding for doctoral or postdoctoral research to members of the Transcultural Nursing Society (TCNS).
Eligibility This program is open to doctoral students in nursing and nurses who have received a doctoral degree within the past 3 years. Applicants must have been a member of the society for 2 out of the past 5 years. They must be interested in conducting a research project related to transcultural nursing.
Financial Data The grant is $3,000.

Number awarded 1 each year.
Deadline October of each year.

[799]
TENNESSEE GRADUATE NURSING LOAN FORGIVENESS PROGRAM

Tennessee Student Assistance Corporation
Parkway Towers
404 James Robertson Parkway, Suite 1510
Nashville, TN 37243-0820
(615) 741-1346   Toll Free: (800) 342-1663
Fax: (615) 741-6101   E-mail: TSAC.Aidinfo@tn.gov
Web: www.tn.gov/collegepays/mon_college/nurse_lf.html

Summary To provide forgivable loans to nurses in Tennessee who are interested in working on an advanced degree at a school in the state to prepare for a career as a nursing teacher or administrator.
Eligibility This program is open to residents of Tennessee who have a license as a registered nurse. Applicants must be interested in working on a master's or post-master's degree in nursing education at an eligible institution in Tennessee. They must agree to enter a faculty or administrative position in a Tennessee nursing education program following completion of their degree program. U.S. citizenship is required.
Financial Data The maximum loan is $7,000 per year of full-time enrollment or $3,500 per year of part-time enrollment. Funds are disbursed directly to the educational institution. For each year of full- or part-time employment in a teaching or administrative capacity in a Tennessee nursing education program, 25% of the amount borrowed is forgiven. If recipients fail to fulfill that service obligation, they must repay all funds received in cash with 9% interest.
Duration 1 year of full-time enrollment or equivalent part-time enrollment; may be renewed for up to 3 additional full-time or equivalent years, provided the recipient maintains satisfactory academic progress.
Number awarded Varies each year.
Deadline February of each year.

[800]
TENNESSEE NURSES FOUNDATION MEMORIAL EDUCATIONAL SCHOLARSHIP PROGRAM

Tennessee Nurses Association
Attn: Tennessee Nurses Foundation
545 Mainstream Drive, Suite 405
Nashville, TN 37228-1296
(615) 254-0350   Toll Free: (800) 467-1350
Fax: (615) 254-0303   E-mail: tnf@tnaonline.org
Web: www.tnaonline.org/tnf-initiatives.html

Summary To provide financial assistance to members of the Tennessee Nurses Association (TNA) who are working on a degree at a school in any state.
Eligibility This program is open to Tennessee residents who have been a continuous member of the TNA for at least 1 year. Applicants must be working on a baccalaureate, master's, or doctoral degree at an accredited institution of higher education in any state. Selection is based on available funds, financial need, leadership potential, and sustained association involvement.
Financial Data The stipend depends on the need of the recipient and the availability of funds.
Duration 1 year.
Additional data Recipients must maintain membership in the Tennessee Nurses' Association throughout the educational period.
Number awarded Varies each year.
Deadline February or August of each year.

[801]
TENNESSEE RURAL HEALTH LOAN FORGIVENESS PROGRAM

Tennessee Student Assistance Corporation
Parkway Towers
404 James Robertson Parkway, Suite 1510
Nashville, TN 37243-0820
(615) 741-1346   Toll Free: (800) 342-1663
Fax: (615) 741-6101   E-mail: TSAC.Aidinfo@tn.gov
Web: www.tn.gov/collegepays/mon_college/ruralhealth.html

Summary To provide forgivable loans to residents of Tennessee who are working on a degree at a school in the state to prepare for a career as a physician, dentist, physician assistant, or nurse practitioner and practice in an underserved area of the state.

Eligibility This program is open to students currently enrolled full time at a postsecondary educational institution in Tennessee that has a school of medicine that offers an M.D. degree, a school of osteopathic medicine that offers a D.O. degree, a school of dentistry that offers a D.D.S. or D.M.D. degree, a physician assistant program, or a master's or doctoral degree as a nurse practitioner. Applicants must have been residents of Tennessee for at least 1 year. They must agree to practice their profession in a health resource shortage area following completion of their program of study for 1 year per year of support received.

Financial Data The maximum loan is $12,000 per year or the cost of tuition, mandatory fees, books, and equipment, whichever is less. Funds are disbursed directly to the educational institution. If recipients fail to fulfill their service agreement, they must repay all funds received in cash with 9% interest.

Duration 1 year; may be renewed up to 4 additional years or until completion of the program.

Additional data This program was established in 2008.

Number awarded 50 each year.

Deadline August of each year.

[802]
TEXAS OUTSTANDING RURAL SCHOLAR RECOGNITION PROGRAM

Office of Rural Community Affairs
Attn: Rural Health Unit
1700 North Congress Street, Suite 220
P.O. Box 12877
Austin, TX 78711-2877
(512) 936-6701   Toll Free: (800) 544-2042
Fax: (512) 936-6776   E-mail: agrant@orca.state.tx.us
Web: www.orca.state.tx.us/index.php/Home/Grants

Summary To provide scholarship/loans to outstanding Texas students who are interested in preparing for a career in health care in rural areas.

Eligibility This program is open to Texas residents who are either high school seniors in the top quarter of their graduating class or college students who have earned a GPA of 3.0 or higher. Applicants must be enrolled or intend to enroll in an eligible academic institution in Texas to become a health care professional and arrange to be sponsored by an organization in 1 of the 177 rural counties in the state. Eligible health care professions include medicine (with a residency in family practice, emergency medicine, general internal medicine, general pediatrics, general surgery, or general obstetrics and gynecology), dentistry, optometry, nursing, pharmacy, chiropractic, behavioral health, and allied health (rehabilitative services, radiology technician, medical laboratory technician, health systems management, and dietary and nutritional services). Eligible sponsoring organizations include local hospitals, rural health clinics, and community organizations. Funds are awarded on a competitive basis. Selection is based on academic achievements, essay content, sponsor's financial commitment, community statement of need, and overall quality of the nominee.

Financial Data The amount of the forgivable loan award is based on the cost of attendance at the recipient's academic institution. Sponsoring communities pledge to cover half the student's educational expenses; the state covers the other half. Students must pledge to provide 1 year of work in the sponsoring community for each year of support they receive while in college.

Duration 1 year; may be renewed.

Number awarded Varies each year.

Deadline May of each year for fall semester; September of each year for spring semester; January of each year for summer semesters.

[803]
TEXAS PROFESSIONAL NURSING SCHOLARSHIPS

Texas Higher Education Coordinating Board
Attn: Grants and Special Programs
1200 East Anderson Lane
P.O. Box 12788, Capitol Station
Austin, TX 78711-2788
(512) 427-6340   Toll Free: (800) 242-3062
Fax: (512) 427-6127   E-mail: grantinfo@thecb.state.tx.us
Web: www.collegeforalltexans.com

Summary To provide financial assistance to Texas students who are interested in preparing for a career as a professional nurse.

Eligibility This program is open to undergraduate or graduate students who are residents of Texas and enrolled at least half time in a program leading to licensure as a professional nurse at a college or university in the state. Applicants must be able to demonstrate financial need.

Financial Data The stipend depends on the need of the recipient, to a maximum of $2,500.

Duration 1 academic year.

Additional data Some of these funds are targeted to students from rural communities and some to graduate students.

Number awarded Varies each year; recently, 944 of these scholarships were awarded.

Deadline Applicants should contact the financial aid director at the professional nursing school in which they plan to enroll for appropriate deadline dates.

[804]
TEXAS SAFETY FOUNDATION SCHOLARSHIP

American Society of Safety Engineers
Attn: ASSE Foundation
1800 East Oakton Street
Des Plaines, IL 60018
(847) 768-3435   Fax: (847) 768-3434
E-mail: agabanski@asse.org
Web: www.asse.org/foundation/scholarships/scholarships.php

Summary To provide financial assistance to upper-division and graduate student members of the American Society of Safety Engineers (ASSE), especially those from Texas.

Eligibility This program is open to ASSE student members who are working on an undergraduate or graduate degree in occupational safety, health, and environment or a closely-related field (e.g., industrial or environmental engineering, environmental science, industrial hygiene, occupational health nursing). Priority is given to residents of Texas or students attending a university in the state. Undergraduates must be full-time students who have completed at least 60 semester hours with a GPA of 3.0 or higher. Graduate students must also be enrolled full time, have completed at least 9 semester hours with a GPA of 3.5 or higher, and have earned a GPA of 3.0 or higher as an undergraduate. Along with their application, they must submit 2 essays of 300 words or less: 1) why they are seeking a degree in occupational safety and health or a closely-related field, a brief description of their current activities, and how those relate to their career goals and objectives; and 2) why they should be awarded this scholarship (including career goals and financial need). U.S. citizenship is not required.

Financial Data　The stipend is $2,500 per year.

Duration　1 year; recipients may reapply.

Additional data　This program, established in 2008, is supported by the Texas Safety Foundation.

Number awarded　1 each year.

Deadline　November of each year.

[805]
TEXAS WAIVER PROGRAM FOR REGISTERED NURSES ENROLLED IN POSTGRADUATE NURSING DEGREE PROGRAMS

Texas Higher Education Coordinating Board
Attn: Grants and Special Programs
1200 East Anderson Lane
P.O. Box 12788, Capitol Station
Austin, TX 78711-2788
(512) 427-6340　　　　　　　　Toll Free: (800) 242-3062
Fax: (512) 427-6127　　　　E-mail: grantinfo@thecb.state.tx.us
Web: www.collegeforalltexans.com

Summary　To provide a partial tuition exemption to registered nurses working on a graduate degree at a public college or university in Texas.

Eligibility　This program is open to registered nurses who are authorized to practice professional nursing in Texas. Applicants must enroll in a program designed to lead to a master's degree or other higher degree in nursing and intend to teach in a program in Texas designed to prepare students for licensure as registered nurses. Non-immigrant aliens are eligible if they are authorized to practice professional nursing in Texas and have a BCIS status that will allow them to remain in Texas and work.

Financial Data　This program provides a waiver of nonresident tuition.

Duration　1 year.

Number awarded　Varies each year; recently, 3 of these waivers were granted.

Deadline　Deadline not specified.

[806]
THE GREAT 100 SCHOLARSHIP PROGRAM

The Great 100, Inc.
P.O. Box 4875
Greensboro, NC 27404-4875
Toll Free: (800) 729-1975　　　E-mail: mperdue@hprhs.com
Web: www.great100.org/Scholarship/index.asp

Summary　To provide financial assistance to undergraduate and graduate students in North Carolina who are interested in working on a degree in nursing.

Eligibility　This program is open to students working on an associate degree in nursing, a diploma in nursing, a bachelor's degree in nursing, a master's degree in nursing, or a Ph.D. in a field related to nursing. Each year, the sponsor selects schools in North Carolina that offer nursing degrees and invites them to nominate students for these awards. The letters of nomination must indicate how the student promotes and advances the profession of nursing in a positive way in the practice setting and/or in the community, and actively seeks ways to support nurses and other health care providers; demonstrate integrity, honesty, and accountability, and functions within scope of practice; displays commitment to patients, families, and colleagues; demonstrates caring and assists others to grow and develop; and radiates energy and enthusiasm, and contributes/makes a difference to overall outcomes in the practice setting. Schools make the final selection of recipients.

Financial Data　The stipend is $1,000.

Duration　1 year.

Additional data　This program was established in 1989.

Number awarded　Varies each year. Recently, 20 of these scholarships were awarded: 6 to A.D.N./Diploma students, 6 to B.S.N. students, 6 to M.S.N. students, and 2 to Ph.D. students.

Deadline　March of each year.

[807]
THOMAS J. BURNS MEMORIAL SCHOLARSHIP

American Association of Nurse Anesthetists
Attn: AANA Foundation
222 South Prospect Avenue
Park Ridge, IL 60068-4001
(847) 655-1170　　　　　　　　　　Fax: (847) 692-6968
E-mail: foundation@aana.com
Web: www.aanafoundation.com

Summary　To provide financial assistance to members of the American Association of Nurse Anesthetists (AANA) from any state pursuing further education at a program in Wisconsin.

Eligibility　This program is open to members of the association who are residents of any state attending a nurse anesthesia program in Wisconsin. First-year students must have completed 6 months of nurse anesthesia classes; second-year students must have completed 12 months of nurse anesthesia classes. Along with their application, they must submit a 200-word essay describing why they have chosen nurse anesthesia as a profession and their professional goals for the future. Financial need is also considered in the selection process.

Financial Data　The stipend is $3,000.

Duration　1 year.

Additional data　The application processing fee is $25.

Number awarded　1 each year.

Deadline　March of each year.

[808]
THOMPSON SCHOLARSHIP FOR WOMEN IN SAFETY

American Society of Safety Engineers
Attn: ASSE Foundation
1800 East Oakton Street
Des Plaines, IL 60018
(847) 768-3435　　　　　　　　　　Fax: (847) 768-3434
E-mail: agabanski@asse.org
Web: www.asse.org/foundation/scholarships/scholarships.php

Summary　To provide financial assistance to graduate students, especially women, working on a degree in safety-related fields (including occupational health nursing).

Eligibility　This program is open to students working on a graduate degree in safety engineering, safety management, occupational health nursing, occupational medicine, risk management, ergonomics, industrial hygiene, fire safety, environmental safety, environmental health, or another safety-related field. Priority is given to women. Applicants must be full-time students who have completed at least 9 semester hours with a GPA of 3.5 or higher. Their undergraduate GPA must have been 3.0 or higher. Along with their application, they must submit 2 essays of 300 words or less: 1) why they are seeking a degree in occupational safety and health or a closely-related field, a brief description of their current activities, and how those relate to their career goals and objectives; and 2) why they should be awarded this scholarship (including career goals and financial need). U.S. citizenship is not required.

Financial Data　The stipend is $1,000 per year.

Duration　1 year; recipients may reapply.

Number awarded　1 each year.

Deadline　November of each year.

[809]
TRANSCULTURAL NURSING SOCIETY SCHOLARSHIP AWARD

Transcultural Nursing Society
c/o Lisa A. Dobson, Business Manager
Madonna University
36600 Schoolcraft Road
Livonia, MI 48150-1176
Toll Free: (888) 432-5470   Fax: (734) 432-5463
E-mail: ldobson@tcns.org
Web: www.tcns.org/Foundationawards.html

Summary To provide financial assistance to members of the Transcultural Nursing Society from any country who are working on a graduate degree in nursing.

Eligibility This program is open to members of the society from any country who are already enrolled part or full time in a graduate degree course of study. Applicants must have a focus on transcultural, cross cultural, or international nursing. Along with their application, they must submit 1) a brief description of graduate courses to be completed that are relevant to transcultural nursing; 2) a statement indicating why they are pursuing a focus on transcultural nursing; and 3) a statement of career goals.

Financial Data The stipend is $1,000.

Duration 1 year.

Number awarded 1 or more each year.

Deadline October of each year.

[810]
TUFTS HEALTH PLAN FOUNDATION NURSE SCHOLARS PROGRAM

Massachusetts Hospital Association
Attn: Massachusetts Hospital Research and Educational
  Association
5 New England Executive Park
Burlington, MA 01803-5096
(781) 262-6006   E-mail: knelson@mhalink.org
Web: www.patientsfirstma.org/workforce.cfm

Summary To provide loans-for-service to residents of Massachusetts and Rhode Island who are working on a graduate degree in nursing and planning to teach nursing in those states.

Eligibility This program is open to residents of Massachusetts and Rhode Island who have completed at least 1 year in a master's or doctoral nursing program at designated schools in those states. Applicants must be committed to teaching nursing in Massachusetts or Rhode Island after completing their degree program. Underrepresented minorities are particularly encouraged to apply. They must be U.S. citizens, permanent residents, refugees, or qualified immigrants. Selection is based on evidence of commitment to a career in nursing education in Massachusetts and Rhode Island and to mentoring, recruiting, and retaining future nurses and nurse colleagues; commitment to and quality of nursing education professional development plan; potential to contribute to the advancement of nursing education; and leadership potential.

Financial Data The stipend is $10,000. Funds may be used for tuition, fees, and other personal expenses directly related to education. Recipients must sign a letter of commitment to provide a 1-year payback in a teaching role in an academic setting in Massachusetts or Rhode Island. Failure to complete the payback commitment will require that funding be repaid to the program by the recipient.

Duration 1 year; nonrenewable.

Additional data This program was established in 2007 by the Tufts Health Plan Foundation. For a list of the designated colleges and universities, contact the Massachusetts Hospital Association.

Number awarded 1 or more each year.

Deadline March of each year.

[811]
TYLENOL SCHOLARSHIPS

McNeil Consumer and Specialty Pharmaceuticals
c/o International Scholarship and Tuition Services, Inc.
200 Crutchfield Avenue
Nashville, TN 37210
(615) 320-3149   Toll Free: (866) 851-4275
Fax: (615) 320-3151   E-mail: contactus@applyists.com
Web: www.tylenol.com

Summary To provide financial assistance for college or graduate school to students intending to prepare for a career in nursing or another health-related field.

Eligibility This program is open to students who have completed at least 1 year of an undergraduate or graduate course of study at an accredited 2-year or 4-year college, university, or vocational/technical school. Applicants must be working on a degree in health education, medicine, nursing, pharmacy, or public health. Along with their application, they must submit 1) a 500-word essay on the experiences or persons that have contributed to their plans to prepare for a career in a health-related field, and 2) a 100-word summary of their professional plans. Selection is based on the essays, academic record, community involvement, and college GPA.

Financial Data Stipends are $10,000 or $5,000.

Duration 1 year.

Additional data This program is sponsored by McNeil Consumer and Specialty Pharmaceuticals, maker of Tylenol products, and administered by International Scholarship and Tuition Services (formerly Scholarship Program Administrators, Inc.).

Number awarded 40 each year: 10 at $10,000 and 30 at $5,000.

Deadline May of each year.

[812]
UNITED HEALTH FOUNDATION LATINO HEALTH SCHOLARS PROGRAM

Hispanic College Fund
Attn: Scholarship Processing
1301 K Street, N.W., Suite 450-A West
Washington, DC 20005
(202) 296-5400   Toll Free: (800) 644-4223
Fax: (202) 296-3774   E-mail: hcf-info@hispanicfund.org
Web: scholarships.hispanicfund.org/applications

Summary To provide financial assistance to Hispanic American undergraduate and graduate students who are interested in preparing for a career in the health field.

Eligibility This program is open to U.S. citizens and permanent residents of Hispanic background (at least 1 grandparent must be 100% Hispanic) who are high school seniors or graduates. Applicants must be enrolled or planning to enroll full time at an accredited 2- or 4-year college, university, or vocational/technical school to work on an undergraduate or graduate degree in a health-related field. They must have a GPA of 3.0 or higher, be able to demonstrate financial need, and be able to demonstrate a commitment to working in underserved communities, including community health centers. Relevant fields of study include medicine, nursing, mental health, pharmacy, public health, allied health, and health sciences.

Financial Data Stipends range from $2,500 to $5,000 per year, depending on the need of the recipient. Funds are paid directly to the student's college or university to help cover tuition and fees.

Duration 1 year; recipients may reapply.

Additional data This program is sponsored by MasterCard. All applications must be submitted online; no paper applications are available.

Number awarded Varies each year; recently, a total of $42,500 was available for this program.

Deadline March of each year.

[813]
UNITED HOSPICE FOUNDATION SCHOLARSHIP PROGRAM

United Hospice Foundation
Attn: Executive Director
1626 Jeurgens Court
Norcross, GA 30093
(678) 533-6462   Toll Free: (800) 956-5354
Fax: (678) 533-6463
E-mail: fpoole@unitedhospicefoundation.org
Web: www.unitedhospicefoundation.org/scholarships.html

Summary To provide financial assistance to residents of designated southeastern states who are working on a degree in nursing, pharmacy, or therapy to prepare for a career working in hospice or long-term care.

Eligibility This program is open to residents of Florida, Georgia, North Carolina, or South Carolina who are enrolled at an educational institution in any state. Applicants must be accepted or enrolled in 1) a nursing program and working on a diploma, associate, bachelor's, or master's degree as a registered nurse (R.N.) or licensed practical nurse (L.P.N.); 2) a school of pharmacy and working on a Pharm.D. degree; or 3) a school of rehabilitation working on a degree in physical therapy, occupational therapy, or speech therapy. They must be able to demonstrate financial need and a strong commitment to hospice nursing, long-term care, and/or pain management.

Financial Data The stipend is $1,000 per year.

Duration 1 year; recipients may reapply, provided they maintain a "B" average.

Additional data This program includes the following named awards: the Neil L. Pruitt, Sr. Scholarship, the Dorothy Shell Scholarship, the Coy Williamson Scholarship, and the Robin W. Bryson Scholarship.

Number awarded 1 or more each year.

Deadline June of each year.

[814]
UPS FOUNDATION ACADEMIC SCHOLARSHIPS

American Association of Occupational Health Nurses, Inc.
Attn: AAOHN Foundation
7794 Grow Drive
Pensacola, FL 32514
(850) 474-6963   Toll Free: (800) 241-8014
Fax: (850) 484-8762   E-mail: aaohn@aaohn.org
Web: www.aaohn.org/scholarships/academic-study.html

Summary To provide financial assistance to registered nurses who are working on a bachelor's or graduate degree to prepare for a career in occupational and environmental health.

Eligibility This program is open to registered nurses who are enrolled in a baccalaureate or graduate degree program. Applicants must demonstrate an interest in, and commitment to, occupational and environmental health. Along with their application, they must submit a 500-word narrative on their professional goals as they relate to the academic activity and the field of occupational and environmental health. Selection is based on that essay (50%), impact of education on applicant's career (20%), and 2 letters of recommendation (30%).

Financial Data The stipend is $2,500.

Duration 1 year; may be renewed up to 2 additional years.

Additional data Funding for this program is provided by the UPS Foundation.

Number awarded 2 each year.

Deadline January of each year.

[815]
UTAH NURSES FOUNDATION GRANT-IN-AID SCHOLARSHIPS

Utah Nurses Association
Attn: Utah Nurses Foundation
4505 South Wasatch Boulevard, Suite 135
Salt Lake City, UT 84124
(801) 272-4510   Fax: (801) 272-4322
E-mail: una@xmission.com
Web: www.utahnursesassociation.com

Summary To provide scholarship/loans to Utah residents who are interested in working on a nursing degree at a school in the state.

Eligibility This program is open to Utah residents who have completed at least 1 semester of core nursing courses in an accredited registered nursing program (undergraduate or graduate) in the state. Undergraduate students must be involved in their school's chapter of the National Student Nurse Association. Registered nurses completing a baccalaureate or advanced nursing degree must be members of the Utah Nurses Association. Applicants must have a GPA of 3.0 or higher and be able to demonstration financial need. Along with their application, they must submit a narrative statement describing their anticipated role in nursing in Utah upon completion of the nursing program. Preference is given to applicants engaged in full-time study. Selection is based on the following priorities: 1) R.N.s working on a B.S.N.; 2) graduate and postgraduate nursing students; 3) students in formal nursing programs (advanced practice nurses); and 4) undergraduate nursing students. U.S. citizenship is required.

Financial Data A stipend is awarded (amount not specified). Funds may be used only for tuition and books. Recipients must agree to work for a Utah health care facility or Utah educational institution as a full-time employee for at least 1 year (2 years if part time). If they fail to complete their educational program or work requirement, they must repay all funds received.

Duration 1 year; may be renewed 1 additional year.

Additional data Recipients must agree to join the Utah Nurses Association within 6 months of graduation.

Deadline May or September of each year.

[816]
VERMONT ASSOCIATION OF NURSE ANESTHETISTS STUDENT SCHOLARSHIP

American Association of Nurse Anesthetists
Attn: AANA Foundation
222 South Prospect Avenue
Park Ridge, IL 60068-4001
(847) 655-1170   Fax: (847) 692-6968
E-mail: foundation@aana.com
Web: www.aanafoundation.com

Summary To provide financial assistance to members of the American Association of Nurse Anesthetists (AANA), especially residents of Vermont, who are interested in obtaining further education.

Eligibility This program is open to members of the association who are currently enrolled in an accredited nurse anesthesia education program. Preference is given to residents of Vermont. If no student from Vermont applies, the second choice is for a student enrolled at a school in New England. First-year students must have completed 6 months of nurse anesthesia classes; second-year students must have completed 12 months of nurse anesthesia classes. Along with their application, they must submit a 200-word essay describing why they have chosen nurse anesthesia as a profession and their professional goals for the future. Financial need is also considered in the selection process.

Financial Data The stipend is $2,000.

Duration 1 year.

Additional data This scholarship, first awarded in 2009, is supported by the Vermont Association of Nurse Anesthetists. The application processing fee is $25.

Number awarded 1 each year.

Deadline March of each year.

[817]
VIRGINIA ASSOCIATION OF NURSE ANESTHETISTS SCHOLARSHIP

American Association of Nurse Anesthetists
Attn: AANA Foundation
222 South Prospect Avenue
Park Ridge, IL 60068-4001
(847) 655-1170   Fax: (847) 692-6968
E-mail: foundation@aana.com
Web: www.aanafoundation.com

Summary To provide financial assistance to members of the American Association of Nurse Anesthetists (AANA) from Virginia who are interested in obtaining further education at a school in the state.

Eligibility This program is open to members of the association from Virginia who are currently enrolled in an accredited nurse anesthesia education program in the state. First-year students must have completed 6 months of nurse anesthesia classes; second-year students must have completed 12 months of nurse anesthesia classes. Along with their application, they must submit a 200-word essay describing why they have chosen nurse anesthesia as a profession and their professional goals for the future. Financial need is also considered in the selection process.

Financial Data The stipend is $1,000.

Duration 1 year.

Additional data Funds for this scholarship, first awarded in 2005, are provided by the Virginia Association of Nurse Anesthetists. The application processing fee is $25.

Number awarded 1 each year.

Deadline March of each year.

[818]
VIRGINIA C. PHILLIPS GRADUATE SCHOLARSHIP AWARD

South Carolina Nurses Foundation, Inc.
Attn: Virginia C. Phillips Scholarship Fund
1821 Gadsden Street
Columbia, SC 29201
(803) 252-4781   Fax: (803) 779-3870
E-mail: brownk1@aol.com
Web: www.scnursesfoundation.org

Summary To provide financial assistance to residents of South Carolina who are enrolled in a graduate program in nursing or public health in any state.

Eligibility This program is open to South Carolina residents who have successfully completed at least 12 hours of graduate course work in a program in nursing or public health. Applicants must be a current member of a professional organization and have already made some contribution to the field of public/community health nursing. Along with their application, they must submit a 1- to 2-page statement that describes their past contributions to public/community health nursing and their future career goals in nursing. Financial need is not considered in the selection process.

Financial Data The stipend is $1,500.

Duration 1 year.

Additional data This program, which began in 1980, is operated in partnership with the South Carolina Department of Health and Environmental Control (SCDHEC).

Number awarded 1 each year.

Deadline July of each year.

[819]
VIRGINIA HENDERSON CLINICAL RESEARCH GRANT

Sigma Theta Tau International
Attn: Research Services
550 West North Street
Indianapolis, IN 46202-3191
(317) 634-8171   Toll Free: (888) 634-7575
Fax: (317) 634-8188   E-mail: research@stti.iupui.edu
Web: www.nursingsociety.org

Summary To provide funding for clinically-oriented nursing research to members of Sigma Theta Tau International.

Eligibility This program is open to registered nurses actively involved in some aspect of health care delivery, education, or research in a clinical setting. Applicants must be members of the fraternity who have a master's or doctoral degree in nursing or are enrolled in a doctoral program. Selection is based on the quality of the proposed research, future potential of the applicant, appropriateness of the research budget, and feasibility of the time frame.

Financial Data The maximum grant is $5,000.

Duration 1 year.

Number awarded 1 every other year.

Deadline November of odd-numbered years.

[820]
VIRGINIA KELLEY AMERICAN NURSES FOUNDATION SCHOLAR AWARD

American Nurses Foundation
Attn: Nursing Research Grants Program
8515 Georgia Avenue, Suite 400
Silver Spring, MD 20910-3492
(301) 628-5227   Fax: (301) 628-5354
E-mail: anf@ana.org
Web: www.anfonline.org

Summary To provide funding to nurses or graduate nursing students interested in conducting research on women's health.

Eligibility This program is open to registered nurses who have earned a baccalaureate or higher degree. Applicants must be beginning researchers who have had no more than 3 research-based publications in refereed journals and have received, as a principal investigator, no more than $15,000 in extramural funding in any 1 research area. They must be interested in conducting research on women's health. Proposed research may be for a master's thesis or doctoral dissertation if the project has been approved by the principal investigator's thesis or dissertation committee.

Financial Data The grant is $3,500. Funds may not be used as a salary for the principal investigator.

Duration 1 year.

Additional data There is a $100 application fee.

Number awarded 1 each year.

Deadline April of each year.

[821]
VIRGINIA PAULSON MEMORIAL SCHOLARSHIP

Colorado Nurses Foundation
7400 East Arapahoe Road, Suite 211
Centennial, CO 80112
(303) 694-4728   Fax: (303) 694-4869
E-mail: mail@cnfound.org
Web: www.cnfound.org/scholarships.html

Summary To provide financial assistance to undergraduate and graduate nursing students in Colorado who are members of the Colorado Nurses Association (CNA) or Colorado Student Nurses Association (CSNA).

Eligibility This program is open to Colorado residents who have been accepted as a student in an approved nursing program in the state. Applicants may be 1) second-year students in an associate degree program; 2) junior or senior level B.S.N. undergraduate students; 3) R.N.s enrolled in a baccalaureate or higher degree program in a school of nursing; 4) R.N.s with a master's degree in nursing, currently practicing in Colorado and enrolled in a doctoral program; or 5) students in the second or third year of a Doctorate Nursing Practice (D.N.P.) program. They must be current members of CNA or CSNA. Undergraduates must have a GPA of 3.25 or higher and graduate students must have a GPA of 3.5 or higher. Selection is based on professional philosophy and goals, dedication to the improvement of patient care in Colorado, demonstrated commitment to nursing, critical thinking skills, potential for leadership, involvement in community and professional organizations, recommendations, GPA, and financial need.

Financial Data The stipend is $1,000.

Duration 1 year.

Number awarded 1 each year.

Deadline October of each year.

[822]
VIRGINIA S. CLELAND AMERICAN NURSES FOUNDATION SCHOLAR AWARD

American Nurses Foundation
Attn: Nursing Research Grants Program
8515 Georgia Avenue, Suite 400
Silver Spring, MD 20910-3492
(301) 628-5227   Fax: (301) 628-5354
E-mail: anf@ana.org
Web: www.anfonline.org

Summary To provide funding to nurses and graduate nursing students interested in conducting research on health policy.

Eligibility This program is open to registered nurses who have earned a baccalaureate or higher degree. Applicants may be either beginning or experienced researchers. They must be interested in conducting research on nursing health policy. Proposed research may be for a master's thesis or doctoral dissertation if the project has been approved by the principal investigator's thesis or dissertation committee.

Financial Data The grant is $3,500. Funds may not be used as a salary for the principal investigator.

Duration 1 year.

Additional data There is a $100 application fee.

Number awarded 1 each year.

Deadline April of each year.

[823]
VIRGINIA STONE AMERICAN NURSES FOUNDATION SCHOLAR AWARD

American Nurses Foundation
Attn: Nursing Research Grants Program
8515 Georgia Avenue, Suite 400
Silver Spring, MD 20910-3492
(301) 628-5227   Fax: (301) 628-5354
E-mail: anf@ana.org
Web: www.anfonline.org

Summary To provide funding to nurses and graduate nursing students interested in conducting research on clinical gerontological issues.

Eligibility This program is open to registered nurses who have earned a baccalaureate or higher degree. Applicants must be experienced researchers who have had more than 3 research-based publications in refereed journals and have received, as a principal investigator, more than $15,000 in extramural funding in any 1 research area. They must be interested in conducting research that relates to clinical gerontological nursing issues. The proposed research may be for a master's thesis or doctoral dissertation, if the project has been approved by the principal investigator's thesis or dissertation committee.

Financial Data The grants are $20,000 or $10,000. Funds may not be used as a salary for the principal investigator.

Duration 1 year.

Additional data There is a $100 application fee.

Number awarded 2 each year: 1 at $20,000 and 1 at $10,000.

Deadline April of each year.

[824]
WASHINGTON STATE HEALTH PROFESSIONAL SCHOLARSHIP PROGRAM

Washington Higher Education Coordinating Board
917 Lakeridge Way
P.O. Box 43430
Olympia, WA 98504-3430
(360) 596-4817   Toll Free: (888) 535-0747
Fax: (360) 664-9273   TDD: (360) 753-7809
E-mail: health@hecb.wa.gov
Web: www.hecb.wa.gov

Summary To provide scholarship/loans for primary care health professional education to students who agree to work in designated areas of Washington after graduation.

Eligibility Applicants must be enrolled or accepted for enrollment in an accredited program leading to eligibility for licensure in Washington State as a physician, osteopathic physician and surgeon, pharmacist, licensed midwife or certified nurse-midwife, physician assistant, nurse practitioner, nurse faculty, dentist, dental hygienist, registered nurse, or practical nurse. They must be U.S. citizens, but Washington residency is not required. Selection is based on prior experience in a rural or shortage area, academic and humanitarian achievements, letters of recommendation, academic standing, and commitment and experience in serving the medically underserved or shortage areas. Preference is given to applicants with community sponsorship and support. The community sponsor may be a rural hospital, a rural health care facility, a community clinic, or a local health care provider that can provide training or employment opportunities. Support should be a financial commitment that may include educational and living stipends, matching funds, or employment and training opportunities.

Financial Data The stipend is intended to cover eligible expenses: tuition, books, equipment, fees, and room and board. This is a scholarship/loan program. Recipients who fail to complete the course of study are required to repay the amount received, plus a penalty and interest. Scholars who fail to serve in a designated rural, underserved urban, or other health professional shortage areas in Washington are required to repay the scholarship, with penalty plus interest.

Duration Up to 5 years.

Additional data This program is jointly administered with the Washington State Department of Health.

Number awarded Varies each year.

Deadline April of each year.

[825]
WASHINGTON STATE NURSES FOUNDATION SCHOLARSHIPS

Washington State Nurses Association
Attn: Washington State Nurses Foundation
575 Andover Park West, Suite 101
Seattle, WA 98188-9961
(206) 575-7979   Fax: (206) 575-1908
E-mail: wsnf@wsna.org
Web: www.wsna.org/WSNF/Scholarship

Summary To provide financial assistance to students in Washington preparing for a career as a registered nurse in the state.

Eligibility This program is open to nursing students who are residents of Washington or attending a college or university in the state. Applicants must have a GPA of 3.0 or higher in a program leading to an associate, baccalaureate, or graduate degree. They must submit essays on the following topics: 1) their participation in school and volunteer activities, including offices and positions of leadership; 2) honors and awards they have received and the relevance of those to nursing; 3) special or unusual life experiences or activities that have made an impact on their nursing career or that assisted them to decide on nursing as a profession; 4) their long- and short-term goals for their nursing career; 5) what they anticipate their role in the Washington State Nurses Association (WSNA) will be, why it is important to them, and (if they are already an R.N.) their involvement in the organization and reasons for participation; and 6) their past work experience (both paid and volunteer) and why this may or may not impact their career in nursing. Undergraduate students must have completed at least 12 nursing credits in the R.N. program. Applicants who are already R.N.s must be members of the WSNA. Financial need is not considered in the selection process.

Financial Data The stipend is $1,000.

Duration 1 year.

Number awarded Varies each year; recently, 5 of these scholarships were awarded.

Deadline February of each year.

[826]
WATSON MIDWIVES OF COLOR SCHOLARSHIP

American College of Nurse-Midwives
Attn: ACNM Foundation, Inc.
8403 Colesville Road, Suite 1550
Silver Spring, MD 20910-6374
(240) 485-1850   Fax: (240) 485-1818
Web: www.midwife.org/foundation_award.cfm

Summary To provide financial assistance for midwifery education to students of color who belong to the American College of Nurse-Midwives (ACNM).

Eligibility This program is open to ACNM members of color who are currently enrolled in an accredited basic midwife education program and have successfully completed 1 academic or clinical semester/quarter or clinical module. Applicants must submit a 150-word essay on their 5-year midwifery career plans and a 100-word essay on their intended future participation in the local, regional, and/or national activities of the ACNM. Selection is based on leadership potential, financial need, academic history, and potential for future professional contribution to the organization.

Financial Data The stipend is $3,000.

Duration 1 year.

Number awarded Varies each year; recently, 3 of these scholarships were awarded.

Deadline March of each year.

[827]
WATSON PHARMA CAREER MOBILITY SCHOLARSHIP

American Nephrology Nurses' Association
Attn: ANNA National Office
200 East Holly Avenue
P.O. Box 56
Pitman, NJ 08071-0056
(856) 256-2320   Toll Free: (888) 600-2662
Fax: (856) 589-7463   E-mail: annascholarships@ajj.com
Web: www.annanurse.org

Summary To provide financial assistance to members of the American Nephrology Nurses' Association (ANNA) who are interested in working on a baccalaureate or advanced degree in nursing.

Eligibility Applicants must be current association members, have been members for at least 2 years, be actively involved in nephrology nursing related health care services, and be accepted or enrolled in a baccalaureate or higher degree program in nurs-

ing. Along with their application, they must submit a 250-word essay on their career and educational goals that includes the expected time frame for completing their degree, the application of the award to meet expected expenses, and the impact of the completion of the degree program on their nephrology nursing practice.

Financial Data The stipend is $2,500.

Duration 1 year.

Additional data This scholarship, first awarded in 2003, is sponsored by Watson Pharma, Inc.

Number awarded 1 each year.

Deadline October of each year.

[828]
WEST TEXAS ANESTHESIA SEMINARS SCHOLARSHIP

American Association of Nurse Anesthetists
Attn: AANA Foundation
222 South Prospect Avenue
Park Ridge, IL 60068-4001
(847) 655-1170   Fax: (847) 692-6968
E-mail: foundation@aana.com
Web: www.aanafoundation.com

Summary To provide financial assistance to members of the American Association of Nurse Anesthetists from Texas who are interested in obtaining further education.

Eligibility This program is open to members of the association who are registered nurses licensed to practice in Texas and currently enrolled in an accredited nurse anesthesia education program in the state. Applicants must be second-year students who have completed 12 months of nurse anesthesia classes. Along with their application, they must submit a 200-word essay describing why they have chosen nurse anesthesia as a profession and their professional goals for the future. Financial need is also considered in the selection process.

Financial Data The stipend is $1,000.

Duration 1 year.

Additional data Funding for this scholarship, first awarded in 2002, is provided by the Texas Association of Nurse Anesthetists (TANA) Education District #4, sponsor of the West Texas Anesthesia Seminars. The application processing fee is $25.

Number awarded 1 each year.

Deadline March of each year.

[829]
WESTERN INSTITUTE OF NURSING/AMERICAN NURSES FOUNDATION SCHOLAR AWARD

American Nurses Foundation
Attn: Nursing Research Grants Program
8515 Georgia Avenue, Suite 400
Silver Spring, MD 20910-3492
(301) 628-5227   Fax: (301) 628-5354
E-mail: anf@ana.org
Web: www.anfonline.org

Summary To provide funding to members of the Western Institute of Nursing (WIN) who are interested in conducting research.

Eligibility This program is open to registered nurses who have earned a baccalaureate or higher degree. Applicants may be either beginning or experienced researchers. Proposed research may be for a master's thesis or doctoral dissertation if the project has been approved by the principal investigator's thesis or dissertation committee. There are no restrictions on the research topic, but applicants must be current WIN members.

Financial Data The grant is $3,500. Funds may not be used as a salary for the principal investigator.

Duration 1 year.

Additional data Funding for this program is provided by the WIN. There is a $100 application fee.

Number awarded 1 each year.
Deadline April of each year.

[830]
WESTERN INSTITUTE OF NURSING DISSERTATION GRANT

Western Institute of Nursing
c/o OHSU School of Nursing
3455 S.W. Veterans Hospital Road
Portland, OR 97239-2941
(503) 494-0869   Fax: (503) 494-3691
E-mail: win@ohsu.edu
Web: www.ohsu.edu/son/win/students/dissertationgrant.shtml

Summary To provide funding for dissertation research to doctoral candidates in nursing who are members of both the Western Institute of Nursing (WIN) and the Council for the Advancement of Nursing Science (CANS).

Eligibility This program is open to nursing doctoral candidates who are members of both WIN and CANS. Applicants must submit a research proposal that conforms to standard NIH guidelines. Their chair or adviser must verify that 1) the proposed work is acceptable to meet dissertation requirements, and 2) the student has the ability and resources to complete the proposed work.

Financial Data The grant covers research expenses, to a maximum of $5,000.

Duration 1 year.

Additional data This program is supported by WIN in conjunction with CANS.

Number awarded 1 each year.

Deadline October of each year.

[831]
WILLIAM C. RAY, CIH, CSP ARIZONA SCHOLARSHIP

American Society of Safety Engineers
Attn: ASSE Foundation
1800 East Oakton Street
Des Plaines, IL 60018
(847) 768-3435   Fax: (847) 768-3434
E-mail: agabanski@asse.org
Web: www.asse.org/foundation/scholarships/scholarships.php

Summary To provide financial assistance to upper-division and graduate student members of the American Society of Safety Engineers (ASSE).

Eligibility This program is open to ASSE student members who are working on an undergraduate or graduate degree in occupational safety, health, and environment or a closely-related field (e.g., industrial or environmental engineering, environmental science, industrial hygiene, occupational health nursing). Undergraduates must be full-time students who have completed at least 60 semester hours with a GPA of 3.0 or higher. Graduate students must also be enrolled full time, have completed at least 9 semester hours with a GPA of 3.5 or higher, and have earned a GPA of 3.0 or higher as an undergraduate. Along with their application, they must submit 2 essays of 300 words or less: 1) why they are seeking a degree in occupational safety and health or a closely-related field, a brief description of their current activities, and how those relate to their career goals and objectives; and 2) why they should be awarded this scholarship (including career goals and financial need). U.S. citizenship is not required.

Financial Data The stipend is $2,000 per year.

Duration 1 year; recipients may reapply.

Number awarded 1 each year.

Deadline November of each year.

[832]
WISCONSIN ORGANIZATION OF NURSE EXECUTIVES ADVANCED DEGREE EDUCATIONAL STIPEND PROGRAM

Wisconsin Organization of Nurse Executives, Inc.
c/o Kathryn Olson, Professional Development Committee
Saint Joseph's Hospital, Patient Care Services
611 St. Joseph Avenue
Marshfield, WI 54449
(715) 387-7592   Fax: (715) 387-7616
E-mail: kathryn.olson@ministryhealth.org
Web: www.w-one.org

Summary To provide financial assistance to nurses in Wisconsin who are interested in working on an advanced degree in nursing leadership at a school in any state.

Eligibility This program is open to Wisconsin nurses working on a master's (M.S.N.) or doctoral (Ph.D. or D.N.P.) degree substantially related to nursing leadership. Applicants must have a GPA of 3.0 or higher. Along with their application, they must submit a letter identifying their professional goals and how they plan to attain them, the way they plan to affect nursing and patient care in Wisconsin, areas of interest, memberships in professional and community organizations and any related activities, the topic of their planned research or project, and how they perceive their role as a nursing leader in the future.

Financial Data The stipend is $1,000.

Duration 1 year; nonrenewable.

Number awarded 1 or more each year.

Deadline July of each year.

[833]
WISCONSIN ORGANIZATION OF NURSE EXECUTIVES NURSING ADMINISTRATION RESEARCH GRANT

Wisconsin Organization of Nurse Executives, Inc.
c/o Kathryn Olson, Professional Development Committee
Saint Joseph's Hospital, Patient Care Services
611 St. Joseph Avenue
Marshfield, WI 54449
(715) 387-7592   Fax: (715) 387-7616
E-mail: kathryn.olson@ministryhealth.org
Web: www.w-one.org

Summary To provide funding to professional and student nurses in Wisconsin who are interested in conducting research related to nursing leadership.

Eligibility This program is open to residents of Wisconsin who have a nursing license and are interested in conducing research related to nursing leadership. Applicants must submit a 5-page description of their proposed research; students must include a letter of reference from their major professor. They may not have received funding for research from the sponsoring organization in the 3 previous years. Along with their application, they must submit a letter identifying their professional goals and how they plan to attain them, the way they plan to affect nursing and patient care in Wisconsin, areas of interest, memberships in professional and community organizations and any related activities, the topic of their planned research or project, and how they perceive their role as a nursing leader in the future.

Financial Data The grant is $1,000.

Duration Funds must be spent within 1 year.

Number awarded 1 or more each year.

Deadline September of each year.

[834]
WOCN SOCIETY ADVANCED EDUCATION SCHOLARSHIP PROGRAM

Wound, Ostomy and Continence Nurses Society
Attn: Scholarship Committee
15000 Commerce Parkway, Suite C
Mt. Laurel, NJ 08054
Toll Free: (888) 224-WOCN   E-mail: info@wocn.org
Web: www.wocn.org/Education/Scholarships

Summary   To provide financial assistance to members of the Would, Ostomy and Continence Nurses (WOCN) Society interested in working on an undergraduate or graduate degree.

Eligibility   This program is open to active members of the society who have a current, unrestricted R.N. license and are working on a baccalaureate, master's, or doctoral degree or N.P. certificate. Applicants must provide evidence of current or previous employment as a wound, ostomy, and/or continence nurse during the last 3 years, proof of WOCNCB certification, and proof of current enrollment or acceptance into an accredited nursing program or other accredited college or university program for non-nursing degrees. Selection is based on merit, compliance with the eligibility requirements, and financial need.

Financial Data   The stipend is $2,000.

Duration   1 year.

Number awarded   Varies each year; recently, 3 of these scholarships were awarded.

Deadline   April or October of each year.

[835]
WVSNA/BERNICE L. VANCE SCHOLARSHIP

West Virginia Nurses Association
Attn: Scholarship Board of Trustees
405 Capitol Street, Suite 600
P.O. Box 1946
Charleston, WV 25327
(304) 342-1169   Toll Free: (800) 400-1226
Fax: (304) 414-3369   E-mail: centraloffice@wvnurses.org
Web: www.wvnurses.org/scholarship.html

Summary   To provide financial assistance to nurses in West Virginia who are enrolled in an accredited nursing program in any state and a member of the West Virginia Nurses Association (WVNA) or the West Virginia Student Nurses Association (WVSNA).

Eligibility   This program is open to native West Virginians who have been employed as a nurse in the state for at least 1 year, are enrolled in an accredited nursing program in any state, and are a member of either the WVSNA or WVNA. Applicants must submit the names of at least 2 personal references, a copy of their transcript, documentation of financial need, a self-evaluation form, an evaluation from a faculty adviser, and an evaluation from a clinical adviser.

Financial Data   A stipend is awarded (amount not specified).

Duration   1 year; recipients may reapply.

Number awarded   Varies each year.

Deadline   June of each year.

Sponsoring Organization Index

The Sponsoring Organization Index makes it easy to identify agencies that offer financial aid specifically to undergraduate and graduate nursing students. In this index, the sponsoring organizations are listed alphabetically, word by word. In addition, we've used an alphabetical code (within parentheses) to help you identify the focus of the funding offered by the organizations: U = Undergraduates; G = Graduate Students. For example, if the name of a sponsoring organization is followed by (U) 241, a program sponsored by that organization is described in the Undergraduate section, in entry 241. If that sponsoring organization's name is followed by another entry number—for example, (G) 701—the same or a different program sponsored by that organization is described in the Graduate Students section, in entry 701. Remember: the numbers cited here refer to program entry numbers, not to page numbers in the book.

A

Abbott Laboratories, (U) 101, (G) 526, 740

Academy of Medical-Surgical Nurses, (U) 226, (G) 645

Academy of Neonatal Nursing, (U) 112, 260, (G) 536-537, 688

African-American/Caribbean Education Association, Inc., (U) 231

AfterCollege, (U) 3, (G) 412

Alabama State Nurses Association, (U) 7, 35, (G) 414

Alabama-West Florida United Methodist Foundation, Inc., (U) 219

Alaska Community Foundation, (U) 84

The Albert Schweitzer Fellowship, (G) 770

Alpha Tau Delta, (U) 235, (G) 420

Alpharma Pharmaceuticals, LLC, (G) 419

American Academy of Nurse Practitioners, (G) 410, 421, 423, 498, 552, 659

American Academy of Nursing, (G) 468

American Assembly for Men in Nursing, (U) 14, (G) 424

American Association for the History of Nursing, (G) 407

American Association of Colleges of Nursing, (G) 590

American Association of Critical-Care Nurses, (U) 15, (G) 402-406, 425, 524, 736

American Association of Nurse Anesthetists, (U) 254, (G) 408-409, 415, 431, 492, 494-496, 515, 538, 540-541, 559, 567, 588, 595-596, 604, 608, 621, 626, 640, 649-651, 681, 683, 685, 693, 699, 724-726, 762, 797, 807, 817, 828

American Association of Occupational Health Nurses, Inc., (U) 2, 374, (G) 411, 814

American Cancer Society, (G) 503, 554

American College of Emergency Physicians. New Hampshire Chapter, (U) 265

American College of Nurse Practitioners, (G) 426

American College of Nurse-Midwives, (U) 46, 353, 391, (G) 427, 462, 796, 826

American Indian Graduate Center, (G) 763

American Legion. Americanism and Children & Youth Division, (G) 517

American Legion. Arizona Auxiliary, (U) 24-25

American Legion. Arkansas Auxiliary, (U) 27

American Legion. California Auxiliary, (U) 54

American Legion. Colorado Auxiliary, (U) 71

American Legion. Connecticut Auxiliary, (U) 77

American Legion. Georgia Auxiliary, (U) 124

American Legion. Idaho Auxiliary, (U) 149

American Legion. Illinois Auxiliary, (U) 153

American Legion. Indiana Auxiliary, (U) 157

American Legion. Iowa Auxiliary, (U) 163

American Legion. Maryland Auxiliary, (U) 213

American Legion. Massachusetts Department, (U) 172

American Legion. Michigan Auxiliary, (U) 229

American Legion. Minnesota Auxiliary, (U) 233

American Legion. Missouri Department, (U) 223

American Legion. New Jersey Auxiliary, (U) 269

American Legion. New Mexico Auxiliary, (U) 270

American Legion. North Carolina Department, (U) 70

American Legion. Ohio Auxiliary, (U) 296

American Legion. Oregon Auxiliary, (U) 304

American Legion. South Dakota Auxiliary, (U) 199

American Legion. Virginia Auxiliary, (U) 379

American Legion. Wisconsin Auxiliary, (U) 395

American Nephrology Nurses' Association, (U) 9, 18, 167, 261-262, 392, (G) 416, 433, 460, 581, 689-690, 827

American Nurses Association of California, (U) 369, (G) 469

American Nurses Association of Maine, (U) 16

American Nurses Credentialing Center, (G) 625

American Nurses Foundation, (G) 428, 435, 484, 506, 508, 519, 550, 563, 584, 593, 598, 616, 627, 630, 677, 711, 741, 749, 767, 820, 822-823

American Psychiatric Nurses Association, (G) 429

American Radio Relay League, (U) 394

American Society of PeriAnesthesia Nurses, (U) 37, (G) 451

Residency Index

Some programs listed in this book are restricted to residents of a particular state or region. Others are open to applicants wherever they may live. The Residency Index will help you pinpoint programs available only to residents in your area as well as programs that have no residency restrictions at all (these are listed under the term "United States"). To use this index, look up the geographic areas that apply to you (always check the listings under "United States"), jot down the entry numbers listed after the applicant category that applies to you (Undergraduates or Graduate Students), and use those numbers to find the program descriptions in the directory. To help you in your search, we've provided some "see also" references in each index entry. Remember: the numbers cited here refer to program entry numbers, not to page numbers in the book.

A

Alabama: **Undergraduates,** 7, 35, 198, 219; **Graduate Students,** 414-415. See also Southern states; United States

Alaska: **Undergraduates,** 66, 84, 327; **Graduate Students,** 452, 476. See also United States

Arizona: **Undergraduates,** 24-26, 130, 339; **Graduate Students,** 440-441, 551, 771. See also United States; Western states

Arkansas: **Undergraduates,** 27, 198; **Graduate Students,** 442, 505, 632, 759. See also Southern states; United States

C

California: **Undergraduates,** 11, 54, 105, 334, 369; **Graduate Students,** 418, 454-455, 469. See also United States; Western states

Colorado: **Undergraduates,** 44, 64, 71-73, 91, 130, 145, 192, 321, 331, 339, 380, 382; **Graduate Students,** 459, 473, 481-483, 502, 551, 564, 610, 739, 746, 761, 771, 821. See also United States; Western states

Connecticut: **Undergraduates,** 41, 53, 76-78, 185, 263; **Graduate Students,** 467, 485-487, 509, 511, 691. See also New England states; Northeastern states; United States

D

Delaware: **Undergraduates,** 86, 204; **Graduate Students,** 515. See also Northeastern states; Southeastern states; Southern states; United States

F

Florida: **Undergraduates,** 4, 62, 67, 89, 98, 107, 110, 128, 155, 198, 283, 373; **Graduate Students,** 472, 477, 500, 518, 530, 534-535, 571-572, 707, 813. See also Southeastern states; Southern states; United States

G

Georgia: **Undergraduates,** 20, 123-125, 184, 198, 373; **Graduate Students,** 541, 548, 603, 813. See also Southeastern states; Southern states; United States

H

Hawaii: **Undergraduates,** 108, 205; **Graduate Students,** 531, 583, 609, 624. See also United States; Western states

I

Idaho: **Undergraduates,** 109, 130, 148-149, 327, 339; **Graduate Students,** 452, 532, 551, 758, 771. See also United States; Western states

Illinois: **Undergraduates,** 133, 151-153, 206, 288, 346; **Graduate Students,** 556, 568, 710, 759. See also Midwestern states; United States

Indiana: **Undergraduates,** 60, 138, 156-158, 187; **Graduate Students,** 471, 557, 573, 605. See also Midwestern states; United States

Iowa: **Undergraduates,** 1, 133, 162-164, 179; **Graduate Students,** 401, 556, 576-577. See also Midwestern states; United States

K

Kansas: **Undergraduates,** 79, 102, 129, 133, 174, 181-183, 247, 307, 328, 370; **Graduate Students,** 488, 527, 549, 556, 594, 599-600, 649, 671, 729, 754. See also Midwestern states; United States

Kentucky: **Undergraduates,** 94, 138, 187-188, 198; **Graduate Students,** 510, 557, 605-606, 759. See also Southern states; United States

L

Louisiana: **Undergraduates,** 198, 242; **Graduate Students,** 596. See also Southern states; United States

M

Maine: **Undergraduates,** 263; **Graduate Students,** 490, 621, 683, 691. See also New England states; Northeastern states; United States

Tenability Index

Some programs listed in this book can be used only in specific cities, counties, states, or regions. Others may be used anywhere in the United States (or even abroad). The Tenability Index will help you locate funding that is restricted to a specific area as well as funding that has no tenability restrictions (these are listed under the term "United States"). To use this index, look up the geographic areas where you'd like to go (always check the listings under "United States"), jot down the entry numbers listed after the applicant category that applies to you (Undergraduates or Graduate Students), and use those numbers to find the program descriptions in the directory. To help you in your search, we've provided some "see also" references in each index entry. Remember: the numbers cited here refer to program entry numbers, not to page numbers in the book.

A

Alabama: **Undergraduates,** 35, 97; **Graduate Students,** 415. *See also* Southern states; United States; names of specific cities and counties

Alameda County, California: **Graduate Students,** 770. *See also* California

Arizona: **Undergraduates,** 24-26; **Graduate Students,** 441. *See also* United States; Western states; names of specific cities and counties

Arkansas: **Undergraduates,** 242, 348; **Graduate Students,** 759. *See also* Southern states; United States; names of specific cities and counties

Austin County, Texas: **Undergraduates,** 322; **Graduate Students,** 744-745. *See also* Texas

B

Baltimore, Maryland: **Graduate Students,** 770. *See also* Maryland

Boston, Massachusetts: **Graduate Students,** 770. *See also* Massachusetts

Brazoria County, Texas: **Undergraduates,** 322; **Graduate Students,** 744-745. *See also* Texas

Bucks County, Pennsylvania: **Graduate Students,** 770. *See also* Pennsylvania

Burlington County, New Jersey: **Graduate Students,** 770. *See also* New Jersey

C

California: **Undergraduates,** 11, 54, 180, 334; **Graduate Students,** 418, 454-455. *See also* United States; Western states; names of specific cities and counties

Camden County, New Jersey: **Graduate Students,** 770. *See also* New Jersey

Chester County, Pennsylvania: **Graduate Students,** 770. *See also* Pennsylvania

Chestnut Hill, Massachusetts: **Graduate Students,** 511. *See also* Massachusetts

Chicago, Illinois: **Graduate Students,** 770. *See also* Illinois

Colorado: **Undergraduates,** 44, 71-73, 91, 115, 145, 321, 331, 382; **Graduate Students,** 459, 481-483, 502, 539, 564, 739, 746, 761, 821. *See also* United States; Western states; names of specific cities and counties

Colorado County, Texas: **Undergraduates,** 322; **Graduate Students,** 744-745. *See also* Texas

Connecticut: **Undergraduates,** 76; **Graduate Students,** 485-486, 509. *See also* New England states; Northeastern states; United States; names of specific cities and counties

Contra Costa County, California: **Graduate Students,** 770. *See also* California

D

Dallas, Texas: **Undergraduates,** 322; **Graduate Students,** 744-745. *See also* Texas

Delaware: **Graduate Students,** 515. *See also* Northeastern states; Southeastern states; Southern states; United States; names of specific cities and counties

Delaware County, Pennsylvania: **Graduate Students,** 770. *See also* Pennsylvania

DuPage County, Illinois: **Graduate Students,** 770. *See also* Illinois

Durant, Oklahoma: **Undergraduates,** 348. *See also* Oklahoma

F

Florida: **Undergraduates,** 4, 67, 89, 97, 107, 110-111, 128, 155, 191, 283; **Graduate Students,** 477, 500, 530, 533-535, 571-572, 707. *See also* Southeastern states; Southern states; United States; names of specific cities and counties

Florida, central: **Undergraduates,** 322; **Graduate Students,** 744-745. *See also* Florida

Florida, southern: **Undergraduates,** 62, 98, 322; **Graduate Students,** 472, 518, 744-745. *See also* Florida

Fort Bend County, Texas: **Undergraduates,** 322; **Graduate Students,** 744-745. *See also* Texas

Nursing Specialty Index

Use this index to access the more than two dozen different nursing specialties supported by the funding opportunities described in this directory. In addition to looking for terms representing the specialties that interest you, be sure to check the "General" entry; hundreds of programs are listed there that can be used to support study, research, or other degree-related activities in *any* nursing area (although the programs may be restricted in other ways). For your convenience, programs intended for either undergraduates or graduate students are clearly marked. Remember: the numbers cited in this index refer to program entry numbers, not to page numbers in the book.

A

Administration: **Undergraduates,** 69, 112, 129, 243, 247-248, 276, 280, 295, 397; **Graduate Students,** 455, 480, 535, 537, 549, 633, 638, 670-671, 673, 705, 713, 717, 767, 832-833

Anesthesiology: **Undergraduates,** 11, 31, 37, 94, 254, 280; **Graduate Students,** 408-409, 415, 418, 431, 440, 447, 451, 492, 494-496, 510, 515, 533, 538, 540-541, 546, 559, 567, 573, 588-589, 595-596, 604, 608, 621, 626, 632, 640, 648-651, 655-656, 666, 681, 683-685, 693, 699, 705, 724-726, 758, 762, 797, 807, 816-817, 828

C

Cardiology: **Graduate Students,** 736, 741

Critical care: **Undergraduates,** 15, 31, 158, 254; **Graduate Students,** 402-406, 425, 447, 524, 681, 736

D

Dermatology: **Undergraduates,** 87-88; **Graduate Students,** 499

E

Educator: **Undergraduates,** 181, 208, 254, 271, 389; **Graduate Students,** 483, 493, 522, 568, 599, 629, 633, 636, 665, 681, 697, 702-703, 719, 744, 746-747, 772, 789, 799, 824

Emergency: **Undergraduates,** 50, 61, 103, 245-246, 254, 273; **Graduate Students,** 521-523, 543, 570, 585, 601, 607, 613, 658, 681, 701, 727, 738, 752-753, 795

G

Gastroenterology: **Undergraduates,** 340-341; **Graduate Students,** 742, 773-774

General: **Undergraduates,** 1, 3-8, 10, 13-14, 16-17, 19-20, 24-31, 33-36, 40-41, 43-45, 48-49, 51-57, 59, 62-63, 65-66, 70-73, 75-78, 80-84, 86, 89, 91, 93, 96, 98-100, 102, 104-111, 113-120, 122, 124-127, 129, 131, 135-137, 141-146, 148-154, 157-161, 163-166, 168-172, 174-175, 177-185, 188-189, 191, 194-196, 198-201, 203-206, 209, 212-225, 229-242, 244, 247, 249-250, 253, 255-259, 264-270, 272, 274-275, 277-282, 284-292, 296-300, 303-306, 308-309, 311-314, 316-319, 321-323, 325, 327-328, 330-337, 342-344, 346-347, 349-350, 352, 354-363, 365-372, 375, 378-385, 388-390, 394-396, 400; **Graduate Students,** 401, 410, 412-414, 419-424, 426, 428, 430, 434-435, 441-443, 446-447, 449-450, 453-454, 456-459, 461, 464-467, 469-470, 472, 474-476, 478, 481-482, 484-487, 489, 491, 497-498, 500, 502, 504, 506-509, 511-513, 516, 518-520, 527-532, 534, 539, 542, 544-545, 548-550, 553, 560-561, 564, 569, 571, 574-575, 577, 582, 584, 586-587, 590-591, 593-594, 597-600, 602-603, 606, 609, 612, 614-616, 618-619, 624-625, 627-628, 630, 632-633, 635, 637, 639, 641-642, 644, 647, 652-654, 657, 659-664, 668-669, 671, 676, 680, 682, 686-687, 692, 694-696, 698, 702, 704-706, 708-710, 712, 714-716, 718, 720, 722, 730, 733-735, 739, 743, 745, 748-749, 754, 756-757, 759-761, 763-768, 770, 775-778, 780-785, 788-793, 798, 800-803, 805-806, 809-812, 815, 819-822, 824-825, 829-830, 835

Geriatrics: **Undergraduates,** 140, 211, 248, 254, 351, 384; **Graduate Students,** 468, 525, 583, 634, 673, 681, 794, 823

H

History: **Undergraduates,** 202; **Graduate Students,** 407, 417, 611, 620, 700

I

Informatics: **Undergraduates,** 64, 95, 254; **Graduate Students,** 473, 509, 514, 522, 681

L

Long-term care: **Undergraduates,** 107, 155-156, 158, 162, 183, 248, 276, 293-295, 324, 351, 373; **Graduate Students,** 530, 572, 576, 643, 673, 717, 794, 813

Lung and respiratory disease: **Graduate Students,** 517

M

Midwifery: **Undergraduates,** 46, 280, 353, 389, 391; **Graduate Students,** 427, 462, 632, 705, 796, 824, 826

N

Neonatal and perinatal: **Undergraduates,** 112, 260; **Graduate Students,** 536-537, 622, 688

Nephrology: **Undergraduates,** 9, 18, 167, 254, 261-262, 392; **Graduate Students,** 416, 433, 460, 581, 681, 689-690, 827

Calendar Index

Since most financial aid programs have specific deadline dates, some may have already closed by the time you begin to look for funding. You can use the Calendar Index to identify which undergraduate or graduate level funding programs are still open. To do that, go to the educational category that applies to you, think about when you'll be able to complete your application forms, go to the appropriate months, jot down the entry numbers listed there, and use those numbers to find the program descriptions in the directory. Keep in mind that the numbers cited here refer to program entry numbers, not to page numbers in the book.

Undergraduates:
January: 2, 10, 13, 34, 48, 52, 59, 83-84, 117, 126, 135, 161, 176, 192, 195, 198, 202, 208, 221, 253-254, 257, 267, 274, 285, 289, 293-295, 298, 301-302, 312, 320, 322-323, 325, 327, 329, 336-337, 354, 370, 374, 380, 388, 394

February: 1, 6, 26-28, 49, 57, 66, 77, 93, 99, 101, 105, 108, 127, 143, 164-165, 181, 189, 199, 203, 205, 232, 241, 251-252, 255, 259, 275, 281, 303, 309, 338, 343, 355, 358-359, 384, 390

March: 16, 29, 33, 36, 40, 46, 80, 86, 94, 100, 113, 137, 146, 154, 157, 169, 171-172, 179, 186, 204, 209, 220, 229, 233, 237-238, 240, 268, 276, 286, 310, 315, 333, 346, 366, 372, 376, 379, 391, 395

April: 3, 8, 14, 41, 43, 45, 54, 56, 64, 71, 76, 96, 112, 140-141, 150-151, 153, 159-160, 166, 177-178, 180, 183, 185, 194, 200, 211, 213, 222-223, 228, 231, 235, 269-270, 280, 290, 311, 317, 319, 324, 342, 344, 350, 352, 357, 385, 389, 398-399

May: 4, 19, 24-25, 42, 50, 61-63, 82, 89, 91, 98, 103-104, 106, 110, 116, 118-119, 124, 136, 147, 149, 156, 162-163, 168, 170, 175, 188, 196, 217-218, 225-226, 234, 245-246, 249, 260, 264-266, 273, 284, 291-292, 296, 304, 308, 316, 318, 330, 335, 347, 353, 362, 371, 375

June: 5, 7, 12, 17, 20, 22-23, 37, 53, 67, 69, 78-79, 102, 125, 129, 174, 182, 184, 215, 219, 239, 242-244, 247, 271-272, 282, 287-288, 299, 307, 326, 328, 334, 351, 360, 373, 400

July: 81, 230, 297, 332, 340-341, 377, 397

August: 55, 65, 210, 248, 300, 356, 378

September: 35, 70, 87-88, 122, 128, 216, 224, 236, 258, 305, 368, 381

October: 9, 18, 21, 32, 44, 51, 72-73, 95, 107, 111, 114-115, 145, 155, 167, 191, 250, 261-262, 306, 321, 331, 382, 392

November: 30, 38-39, 47, 58, 60, 68, 74, 85, 90, 92, 97, 121, 123, 130, 132-134, 138-139, 173, 187, 190, 193, 197, 207, 227, 263, 283, 339, 345, 348, 364, 386-387, 393

December: 11, 313-314, 349, 367, 369

Any time: 15, 31, 131

Graduate Students:
January: 411, 419, 432, 452, 457, 466, 468, 470, 497, 513, 542, 554, 574, 610, 617, 620, 622, 629, 647-648, 680-681, 709, 715, 717, 721, 723, 737, 745, 748, 750-751, 755, 768, 770, 785, 814

February: 401, 429, 441, 443, 476, 507, 520, 526, 528, 531, 561, 568, 577, 599, 609, 619, 624, 635, 678-679, 682, 686-687, 722, 769, 791, 799-800, 825

March: 407, 409, 415, 427, 431, 440, 446, 449-450, 453, 462, 475, 478, 492-494, 496, 510, 515, 533, 535, 538, 540-541, 559, 567, 569, 573, 583, 588-589, 591, 595-596, 602, 604, 608, 621, 626, 640, 649-650, 655-657, 663-666, 674, 683, 685, 693, 695, 699-700, 724, 726, 728, 731-732, 744, 756, 758, 762, 778-780, 783, 797, 806-807, 810, 812, 816-817, 826, 828

April: 408, 412, 424, 428, 435, 456, 461, 464, 473, 484-485, 490, 495, 506, 508, 512, 516, 519, 536-537, 550, 560, 563, 578, 584, 593, 598, 616, 625, 627-628, 630, 634, 643, 651, 654, 677, 705, 711-712, 716, 725, 741, 749, 764, 767, 772, 775-777, 790, 820, 822-824, 829, 834

May: 420, 434, 442, 472, 483, 491, 500, 502, 505, 517-518, 521-523, 529, 534, 543-544, 565-566, 570-571, 576, 582, 585-586, 590, 597, 601, 606-607, 612-613, 623, 632-633, 641-642, 644-645, 658, 661, 667-668, 676, 688, 692, 694, 696, 701-703, 708, 713-714, 727, 730, 733, 735, 738, 752-753, 757, 760, 763, 766, 781, 788, 795-796, 802, 811, 815

June: 414, 430, 437-439, 451, 458, 467, 477, 480, 486-488, 511, 525, 527, 546, 548-549, 587, 594, 600, 603, 639, 660, 670-671, 697-698, 706, 710, 720, 729, 754, 787, 794, 813, 835

July: 426, 638, 652-653, 719, 773-774, 789, 818, 832

August: 474, 489, 631, 673, 740, 801

September: 402-406, 499, 524, 718, 736, 792, 833

October: 410, 416, 421-423, 433, 436, 448, 454-455, 459, 465, 481-482, 498, 503, 509, 514, 530, 539, 552, 564, 572, 581, 659, 672, 675, 689-690, 739, 746-747, 761, 798, 809, 821, 827, 830

November: 460, 463, 471, 479, 501, 504, 547, 551, 555-558, 580, 592, 605, 636, 646, 662, 691, 707, 734, 759, 765, 771, 782, 784, 786, 804, 808, 819, 831

December: 417-418, 469, 562, 579, 611, 669, 742-743, 793

Any time: 425, 444-445, 447, 553, 575